MIND AND MADNESS IN ANCIENT GREECE

The Classical Roots of Modern Psychiatry

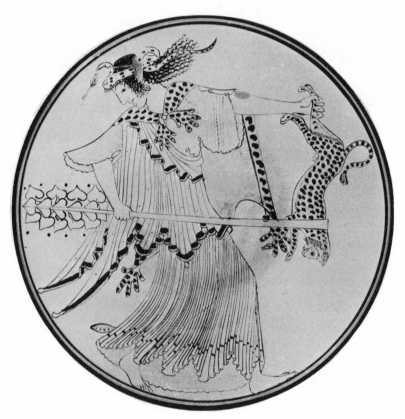

Maenad with leopard skin and headdress of hissing snake. She carries a thyrsus and a leopard cub.

Interior of Attic white-ground kylix by the Brygos Painter, fifth century B.C. Staatliche Antikensammlungen und Glyptothek, Munich.

Opposite: Agave carrying the head of Pentheus.   Ring stone intaglio. The Metropolitan Museum of Art, New York. Bequest of W. Gedney Beatty, 1941.

MIND AND MADNESS
IN ANCIENT GREECE

The Classical Roots
of Modern Psychiatry

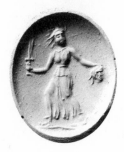

BENNETT SIMON, M.D.

Cornell University Press   ITHACA AND LONDON

Cornell University Press gratefully acknowledges a grant
from the Andrew W. Mellon Foundation that
aided in bringing this book to publication.

First published 1978 by Cornell University Press.
Published in the United Kingdom by Cornell University Press Ltd.,
2–4 Brook Street, London W1Y 1AA.

International Standard Book Number 0-8014-0859-8
Library of Congress Catalog Card Number 77-90911
Printed in the United States of America
*Librarians: Library of Congress cataloging information appears on the last
page of the book.*

For Nancy, in the asphodel meadows

Contents

Illustrations

Preface

> Ben-Zoma used to say: Who is wise? He who learns from every man. As it is said in the Scriptures, "From all of my teachers have I learned."
>
> —*Ethics of the Fathers, The Talmud*

This book is a product of the union of two passions, one for the Greek classics and the other for psychiatry and psychoanalysis. I first became aware of the possibility of such a union when I read E. R. Dodds's *The Greeks and the Irrational* as an undergraduate. Some ten years later, after I had completed medical and psychiatric training, the basic ideas of the book began to take shape. I learned at that time of other attempts at synthesizing modern concepts in psychiatry with classical studies, among them Werner Leibbrand and Anna-Marie Wettley's magisterial history of psychiatry, *Der Wahnsinn,* Philip Slater's *The Glory of Hera,* and the works of Pedro Laín Entralgo. Readers familiar with the writings of these authors will note many areas of convergence between their thought and my own.

The central problem in contemporary psychiatry is to understand and sort out the bewildering variety of ways in which we conceptualize the origins, nature, and treatment of mental illness. This book attempts to deal with that problem by exploring the thinking of Greek antiquity, a vital period in the history of psychiatry.

Even defining the scope of modern psychiatry is a formidable task. Yet without some sense of what psychiatry is, it is impossible to write anything about its history, let alone use the past to illuminate the psychiatry we know today. I shall explore this difficulty and sketch some previous attempts to define the connection between ancient and modern psychiatry before going on to discuss in detail the ancient precursors and analogues of contemporary models of mental illness. With an examination of Homer, the tragedians, Plato, and Hippocrates I explore the nature and origins of the two fundamental polarities in psychiatry today: the intrapsychic versus the social model of the origins and treatment of mental disturbance, and the medical versus the psychological model. The application of all of these models to the elucidation of one particular condition is presented in a case study of hysteria. I shall conclude with a consideration of the requirements for a synthesis of these divergent perspectives.

To those seeking an answer to the problem of which model is best and which models can be discarded, this work will be a disappointment. Rather, it is a contribution to the history, sociology, and basic value system of each of the modern models. The truth value of each model can be ascertained only if we are prepared to take full account of these dimensions.

It will become quickly apparent that I not only explore the precursors of psychoanalysis in ancient Greece but also use psychoanalysis as a tool in historical exploration. Despite the risk of methodological confusion, I have found psychoanalysis most helpful in clarifying the questions raised by thinkers in antiquity as well as their proposed solutions.

Perhaps, then, it would be fair to say that what began as a historical examination has become a statement of certain fundamental and inescapable problems that appear whenever people begin to think seriously about mind and its aberrations. I have, in effect, outlined some basic structures that, in various permutations and combinations, have become the building blocks of psychiatric theory and practice.

A work of this sort is ultimately a personal synthesis, and the choices of what to include and exclude are not governed solely by considerations of time and space. The reader who seeks a comprehensive picture of "psychiatry" in Greek antiquity will find that certain important topics are omitted or slighted, among them lyric poetry, rhetoric, history, and, most regrettably, the work of Aristotle. The Hellenistic and Greco-Roman periods require separate treatment. Similarly, important topics in folk psychiatry, such as the healing cult of Asclepius, various rituals, and the use of divination, oracles, and dreams, cannot be taken up in the detail they deserve. These topics might seem to widen the gulf between ancient and modern psychiatry, but if our definition of modern psychiatry were broadened to include such practices in modern times, the gulf would appear considerably narrower. If my choices prove useful to the reader, if they enable one to see familiar things in new ways, to that extent I shall have succeeded.

The list of individuals who have helped me is extensive, but perhaps a psychoanalyst may be permitted a measure of indulgence in tracing the sources of his work. My father, now deceased, and my mother, though they did not always understand my interests, encouraged a love of learning. My sister, Diana Maine, was my first teacher of Greek and Latin. At Erasmus Hall High School, Harry E. Wedeck showed me that the study of classical civilization is the study of *humanitas*. As an undergraduate at Harvard, exploring Greek and Hebrew along with premedical studies, I was exposed to the minds of brilliant scholars and gifted teachers. In particular, I owe much to Eric A. Havelock, and I have had the good fortune to continue a relationship with him over the years. My indebtedness to his work and to his encouragement is profound.

From several gifted clinical teachers at the College of Physicians and Surgeons I learned much about the virtues of the medical model. During my psychiatric residency at Albert Einstein College of Medicine I had the opportunity to work with Dr. José Barchilon and to profit from his seminars on psychoanalysis and literature. Dr. Milton Rosenbaum materially facilitated my pursuit of what must have seemed to him rather occult interests, and Dr. Morton Reiser gave support and invaluable criticism in the early stages of this work. Dr. Herbert Weiner, my mentor, encouraged me in collegial collaboration and with me coauthored "Models of Mind and Mental Illness in Ancient Greece," my first paper on the subject to be published. Over the years he has given unstintingly of his vast store of knowledge. Dr. William Grossman similarly gave me the opportunity to collaborate with him, and his continued interest in this work, as well as his careful reading of earlier versions of portions of it, have been invaluable. At the New York Psychoanalytic Institute, where I received excellent training in both the theory and the practice of psychoanalysis, Dr. David Beres helped me in very concrete ways to "know myself." Dr. Peter Laderman had previously been most helpful in that same endeavor.

Joseph Russo worked with me on problems in Homeric psychology. His critical reading of portions of this manuscript and his sustained interest are gratefully acknowledged. Terence Irwin often served as a critical audience and was most helpful in dealing with specific problems presented by Plato's dialogues. Dr. Charles Ducey, student, colleague, teacher, and comrade-in-arms, has been extraordinarily helpful in his careful reading of this work. Mary Lefkowitz read the sections on tragedy and hysteria. Dr. George Devereux of Paris has been most encouraging and has made numerous helpful suggestions. His published work has been of immense importance, though, unfortunately, his *Dreams in Greek Tragedy* appeared too late for me to use as extensively as I would have liked. Friedholf Kudlien of Kiel, from whose work on Greek medicine I have learned much, reviewed the chapters on the medical model.

Dr. Stanley Reiser encouraged me to undertake the book and assisted me in starting a Harvard undergraduate seminar on models of madness. Dr. John Mack, my chairman at the Cambridge Hospital, facilitated my writing and provided a model in his distinguished work on applied psychoanalysis. Drs. James Beck, William Binstock, Stanley Palombo, and George Vaillant read and commented on various portions of the text.

The Boston Psychoanalytic Society provided a climate of acceptance for interdisciplinary work. Its library and librarian, Ann Menashi, were immensely helpful. Moral support and opportunities to discuss portions of this work came from the Group for Applied Psychoanalysis and a study group on classics and psychoanalysis. The National Institute of Mental Health provided crucial material support.* A John Simon Guggenheim Memorial Fellowship allowed leisure for rethinking and reworking the sections on myth and tragedy.

Phil Patton, Paul Brasuel, Paul Scham, and Elizabeth Genovese helped as research assistants and translators of material in French and German. Barbara Behrendt and Kim O'Brion typed earlier drafts and Carol Kassabian skillfully prepared the final versions.

I owe a special debt to Maureen Fant, who did yeoman work in helping prepare the notes and in providing scholarly editorial advice. Her assistance in the revisions of the final manuscript was indispensable, as was her careful preparation of the manuscript for publication. She gave both criticism and encouragement at several crucial junctures.

The editors of Cornell University Press furnished substantial assistance in the form of two readers' reports. One anonymous reader helped me to achieve some economy of form and matter, and Diskin Clay saved me from numerous errors of fact and interpretation and gave me fair warning in instances where I chose to disagree with him.

It is with great sadness that I record my gratitude to my deceased wife, Nancy. She had read numerous drafts, commented enthusiastically and critically, helped with numerous details, and above all provided an environment in which it was possible to pursue this work. It was one of her regrets that she would not live to see the book appear.

My children, Jonathan and Amy, grew as the work progressed. At first mute observers, they later were interested and articulate participants in our dialogue.

For the help of all these and unnamed others, the only proper reward is a good book. Any shortcomings are my responsibility.

B. S.

Wayland, Massachusetts

---

*Grants no. 571-NH-6418, 1963–65, and no. IROI-MH-2459, 1973–75.

A Note on Transliteration

Since the method of transliteration used in this book may seem capricious, a word of explanation is in order. On the whole, I prefer to transliterate directly from the Greek, not through Latin, so that the word σωφροσύνη, for example, becomes *sōphrosunē*, not *sophrosyne*. Familiar proper names, however, are given in their most common form, invariably the Latin. Thus Achilles, Ajax, Circe, and Cyclops are used instead of Achilleus, Aias, Kirke, and Kyklops. Quoted translations retain the translator's orthography.

Citation of Classical References

The reader not familiar with classical sources can be quite perplexed by the variety of methods of citation. Classicists now tend to use as a standard format the one used in the *Greek-English Lexicon* of H. G. Liddell, R. Scott, and H. S. Jones, 9th edition (cited as LSJ). In this book, several forms of citation are used which represent a compromise between the forms familiar to classicists and those most usable by the nonspecialist.

Citations of the *Iliad* and the *Odyssey* of Homer are given in the form "*Iliad* 3.414–18," referring to Book 3, lines 414–18. Unfortunately, many of the commonly used translations do not use line numbers. Richmond Lattimore's *Iliad* does not, but his *Odyssey* does, as does Robert Fitzgerald's *Iliad*.

Citations of Plato's dialogues are given as, for example, "*Republic* 513A," referring to section 513, subsection A (subsections are A through E). This is the form of notation used in the standard Greek texts and in some English translations, notably the Loeb Classical Library editions. Benjamin Jowett's translation uses only section numbers, but this practice presents only a minor inconvenience. *The Republic* is also often cited by book (there are ten books). I prefer to cite passages by number and letter, however.

Similarly, in citing works of Aristotle I follow the numbering of the standard Greek texts, the form followed in many available translations. "*Poetics* 1453a27" refers to section 1453, subsection a (there are only two subsections, a and b), line 27. The reader can use the Loeb Classical Library editions or the volumes of *The Works of Aristotle Translated into English* (published by the Clarendon Press, Oxford). One work, the *Problemata*, is cited only by section, the commonest form of citation for this relatively obscure work, and the form used in the Loeb edition.

Fragments of the pre-Socratics are cited in the form used in the so-called Diels-Kranz edition of Greek text and German translation (H. Diels, ed., *Die Fragmente der Vorsokratiker*, with additions by W.

Kranz, 5th–7th eds. [Berlin, 1934–1954]). The form of citation is "Anaxagoras, B5," meaning the fifth fragment of Anaxagoras in the group of fragments designated B. In this book only B fragments are cited—that is, those that Diels and Kranz consider to be actual quotations. Fragments designated A are paraphrases. Unfortunately, no comparble English version exists. Kathleen Freeman's *Ancilla to the Pre-Socratic Philosophers* (Cambridge, Mass., 1948) is an almost complete translation of the B fragments, but the translations are often quite misleading. Geoffrey S. Kirk and J. E. Raven's *The Presocratic Philosophers* (Cambridge, 1957), though not complete, is far better. It contains Greek texts and translations of most of the more widely cited passages in the classical and philosophical literature as well as a useful commentary.

Citations to Hippocrate are difficult to present in any standard form. No complete edition of Hippocrates has been published in English, and the existing English versions do not consistently follow the format of the most widely used Greek text, E. Littré's ten-volume *Hippocrate: Oeuvres complètes* (Paris, 1849). Citations in this book appear in the form in which they can be located either in Littré (title of work, Littré volume number, and page) or in the Loeb Classical Library edition.

Other authors, including Galen, referred to only occasionally, are cited in a form in which they can be located in the Loeb Classical Library editions, or in the particular edition and translation that is specified in the note.

I

THEMES IN
THE STUDY
OF THE MIND

1

On the Babel of Tongues
in Contemporary Psychiatry

What is a psychiatrist? According to my definition, a psychiatrist is
surprisingly rare even within that group who have graduated from
psychiatric residency training and are spending their time treating
psychiatric patients. This rarity reflects a situation quite different
from that which obtains, for example, for graduates of violin training, of whom one might say that Jascha Heifetzes are rare. Most of
the people who claim to be fiddlers are at least playing the same
instrument, even if not so well as Heifetz. It seems to me that for
those who claim to be psychiatrists, not only are they not all playing the same instrument, but some are playing instruments the
others disapprove of or disbelieve, or even, in some cases, instruments whose very existence is unknown to others in the group.
                                        —F. Worden, "Questions about Man's
                                         Attempt to Understand Himself"[1]

Thus the state of psychiatry today: the musicians do not play the
same instrument, they could never form a symphony orchestra (who
could agree on the conductor?), but there is not complete cacophony.
From the noise a few themes emerge often enough to allow us to
distinguish variations on them. It is with a few of these themes that
this book will begin: as they are heard today and as they were played
in Greek antiquity.

The themes cluster around the difficult task of understanding
something of ourselves in the full range of our thoughts, feelings,
decisions, impulses, and actions, and around the way questions are
asked about human beings and their mental and behavioral life.

Since the very posing of the questions influences the answers, one
of the main issues in psychiatry today is where to begin. While it is
taken for granted that understanding the interactions between mind
and body is essential, it is far from clear whether the best initial
approach is with the interaction or with the mind alone.

A related issue is the question: What is a suitable explanation for
behavior? Shall we be content to understand people's motives? To
what extent can we assume that intelligible human motives are at

work shaping both the "psychopathology of everyday life" and the more severe forms of psychopathology? An explanation that states a physical cause or correlate of a piece of behavior is, for many people, more substantial than one that points to motive. While many, including myself, assume that both kinds of explanation are needed, the problem of where to focus one's energies and attention is very real.

We shall be considering how these issues apply to the understanding of mental functioning, particularly abnormal functioning. We shall talk about "mental illness," but we must always ask whether or not the term "illness" is accurate or useful for the phenomena we are trying to understand.

To illustrate some forms of these broad issues, let us first turn to Plato's portrait of Socrates as he sat discoursing in prison, awaiting execution, having chosen death over exile. His enemies wondered if he was mad for wanting to die; his friends were puzzled and deeply upset. Philosophy, or Socrates himself, seemed to have backed him into a corner. Is it madness to die in the name of a way of living, the "examined life"? Perhaps. Certainly there is more than a touch of perversity, stubbornness, and "Socratic irony" in his choice. How can we explain why Socrates calmly philosophized while he awaited the hemlock? He told his companions of his first encounter with the philosophy of Anaxagoras. He had hoped that, as advertised, it would deal with "mind," but was disappointed to find the philosopher "altogether forsaking mind or any other principle of order, but having recourse to air, and ether, and water, and other eccentricities" (*Phaedo*, 97B–98C). Such a philosopher, according to Socrates' caricature, would seek to explain Socrates' behavior in terms of the biology and physics of the muscles and bones that allow a man to sit. This kind of explanation is surely a "confusion of conditions and causes." Socrates sat in prison because he *chose* to place obedience to the laws of Athens ahead of personal survival. Moreover, he decided that to flee would be to betray his lifelong philosophical mission: to make men consider their ethical choices. Thus, for Socrates, the attempt to understand human behavior was first and foremost an inquiry into the motives and reasons people have for behaving as they do.

But surely these issues should pose a problem only for philosophers and other ethereal types, *Luftmenschen*, with no sense of the hard facts of reality. The problem, however, has also come to trouble practical people, those who treat the disturbed and who expect payment for their knowledge and their pains. The mind–body problem, the motive–cause problem, has become a territorial and professional issue as well as an academic one.

With that in mind, let us move from Socrates in prison in the Athens of 399 B.C. to a young neurologist vacationing in the countryside near Vienna in the summer of 1895. On the night of 23 July 1895 Sigmund Freud dreamed a dream, and the next day, puzzled and troubled, he wrote it down. That day he began to use a new method of understanding dreams, "free association," and more or less successfully decoded his own. If one looks for the turning point, this is certainly a suitable date and setting, for, with the work of Freud, the questions of whether to treat mind or body, who should treat the mind, and whether the mind should be "treated" or "understood" came to the fore.

Let us turn then to *The Interpretation of Dreams,* in which Freud presents an analysis of a specimen dream. The "Irma dream" came to be known as *the* dream specimen of psychoanalysis, for in its background, text, and interpretation it presents the core issues of psychoanalysis, which include most prominently the themes of mind and body, motives and causes.[2] Freud, then thirty-nine, was a fairly successful neurologist who had been devoting more and more of his time to patients with "nervous disorders," those many patients who seemed to live, indeed thrive, in the borderland between mind and body, between neurology and psychotherapy, a relatively recent term.[3] Prominent among these patients was a group bearing the time-honored title of "hysterics," and among them was a young widow called Irma. Freud had just completed his account of the treatment (which he had not yet begun to call psychoanalysis) and had mixed feelings about the outcome. "The patient was relieved of her hysterical anxiety but did not lose all her somatic symptoms," which is to say that some peace of mind had been achieved but she still suffered from the puzzling somatic complaints she had had at the outset. A friend and colleague, Otto (also a friend of Irma), had just reported to Freud that "she's better, but not quite well." Freud fancied some reproach in his colleague's words and tone. Furthermore, the patient, also a friend of Freud's wife, was expected to visit them a few days hence for his wife's birthday.

This was the preamble to Freud's dream, which, in part, ran as follows:

A large hall—numerous guests, whom we were receiving.—Among them was Irma. I at once took her on one side, as though to answer her letter and to reproach her for not having accepted my "solution" yet. I said to her, "If you still get pains, it's really only your fault." She replied, "If you only knew what pains I've got now in my throat and stomach and abdomen—it's choking me"—I was alarmed and looked at her. She looked pale and puffy. I thought to myself that after all I must be missing some organic trouble. . . . [There follow some scenes of medical examination.]

Not long before, when she was feeling unwell, my friend Otto had given her an injection of a preparation of propyl, propyls, . . . propionic acid, . . .

[and] trimethylamin (and I saw before me the formula for this printed in heavy type). . . . Injections of that sort ought not to be made so thoughtlessly. . . . And probably the syringe had not been clean.

Freud had already explained something of his method of dream interpretation—free association to the dream's elements—but even before that had argued that dreams could be "interpreted"; that is, "interpreting" a dream implies assigning a "meaning" to it—that is, replacing it by something which fits into the chain of our mental acts as a link having a validity and importance equal to the rest. As we have seen (in Chapter One), the scientific theories of dreams leave no room for any problem of interpreting them, since in their view a dream is not a mental act at all, but a somatic process signalizing its occurrence by indications registered in the mental act.

Thus Freud had reviewed and reflected on the respectable scientific opinion of his day, which asserted that dreams are epiphenomena; they register somatic events, but do not have a meaning or coherence of their own. He turned to the lay world and its belief that dreams do have meaning, but rejected the methods of popular dream interpretation that had flourished for many millennia. Dreams are not prophetic, they do not convey messages from another realm, yet they do say something about the individual. This was the gist of Freud's argument.

Along with his studies of dreams, or rather prior to them, Freud had studied hysteria and had reached conclusions that had been in the air from the middle of the nineteenth century onward. Such workers as Jean-Martin Charcot, Hippolyte Bernheim, and Pierre Janet, along with Freud, were coming to see hysterical symptoms as a kind of language that could be read or decoded.[4] Freud eventually became the most articulate and systematic exponent of the view that hysterical symptoms had meaning that could be read, and that motives, not physical causes, should be sought. A young woman waved good-bye to the lover who later left her, and her right arm became paralyzed. "If I forget thee, O Jerusalem, let my right hand forget its cunning" provided a more helpful clue to the mimetic language of the paralysis than did a search for lesions in the brain.

Of course, at this time Freud was becoming famous, indeed infamous, for his insistence on the importance of repressed and disguised sexual wishes that lay behind the symptoms of the hysterics (though he considerably broadened the definition of sexuality beyond the meaning of intercourse). In effect, Freud was beginning to affirm that the hysteric's so-called ignorance (the propensity to amnesias, for example) was a *motivated ignorance*. A sexual claim put forth by the body had to appear in disguise in order to accomplish its mission. Though we lack the details of Irma's treatment, we can surmise that

Freud construed her somatic symptoms to be a hysterical expression of the thwarted sexuality of the recently widowed young woman. (Greek doctors knew that virgins and widows were most susceptible to those diseases of the womb they called "hysterical.") Perhaps Freud's proposed solution was that she must either acknowledge her sexual wishes and then go ahead and have an affair with Herr S. or renounce all hope of winning him and look elsewhere.

How, then, did Freud interpret his dream? It revealed to him, after appropriate self-analysis, some mundane, unexotic, and unpleasant truths about himself. Essentially Freud concluded that his dream was a form of self-defense. Properly interpreted, the dream turned out to be a carefully contrived and disguised series of character assassinations aimed at patients and colleagues who had directly or indirectly reproached him for failure or negligence of any sort. Otto, who in real life had suggested that all was not well with the patient, in the dream is the kind of doctor who might use a dirty syringe. So much for the man who had hinted at reproach!

A scene (in the dream text) of Freud examining Irma's throat might or might not have had something to do with nocturnal movements or hidden disease in the dreamer's throat. It certainly did, however, have something to do with angry words stuck in his throat. These words and feelings were finally brought to light only by this curious kind of self-examination: dream analysis by means of free association.

Thus, in one stroke, Freud had radically altered the focus of his inquiry from medical to personal and interpersonal. He did not ignore doctors and physical illness, but looked instead at what doctors and patients, and doctors and their colleagues, may feel about each other. While his dream presents us with the formula of an organic chemical, the substances that cause trouble are the more subtle compounds of envy and self-righteousness which were undoubtedly injected into us early on in our lives with the dirty syringes that we still use long after they should have been discarded. "Know thyself" must apply to physician and patient alike. The "cure" is dependent on the physician's knowing that he himself suffers from the same diseases, as it were, that his patient does.

As if to complete the coup, Freud asserted that his method of looking at the mind, sick or well, was no longer necessarily in the province of doctors. Early in his career he spoke of doctors and patients, but by the end he was speaking of analysts and analysands. He had, in effect, brought to fruition the promise implied in the claim of the old Sophist Antiphon that he possessed a *technē alupias,* a craft for ridding the soul of distress.[5] He was a physician of the psyche.

This is the scope of the revolutionary change wrought by Freud. From our perspective, it might be more accurate to say that Freud actualized something that had been in the air in his own lifetime and inherent in the ways we have looked at the mind from Greek antiquity onward. The motives of an ethical act should be the proper focus of interest for a man, Socrates claimed. Certainly that was what was important for a student of the psyche. And so, for Freud, the proper concern for the student of the psyche in the twentieth century should be the study of the motives of behavior, especially as they appear in disguise.

The patients whom Freud treated were often deeply troubled, but by and large they functioned in their day-to-day lives and were not considered crazy or psychotic (a term introduced in the mid–nineteenth century).[6] Toward the end of the nineteenth century and the beginning of the twentieth, a few physicians who worked in mental hospitals, asylums for the severely disturbed, were making significant advances in clinical observation and were slowly beginning to define relatively discrete groups of patients who seemed to suffer from some common underlying disturbance.

Eugen Bleuler's classic *Dementia Praecox, or the Group of Schizophrenias* appeared in 1911.[7] Bleuler argued that a number of apparently discrete psychotic states could be grouped together on the basis of recurrent "primary symptoms," into a category he called "schizophrenia." This term embodied his theory that there were basically certain important "splits" in the personality functions of such patients, as a split between thought and affect (not multiple personality). Bleuler considered schizophrenia a disease, probably caused by some yet undiscovered toxin or metabolic defect. But he argued that, though ignorant of the physiological causes, we had to proceed and try to understand the psychological organization of the patients. He began to delineate the sequence of steps from the "primary symptoms" to the typical full-blown clinical picture so often seen in chronic psychiatric wards. Thus Bleuler posited a medical condition but did his research primarily on the description of the psychological state and its development. While he did not argue that there was no meaning to his patients' productions, he concentrated on description, collection, and classification. His colleague Carl Gustav Jung was arguing that the complexes Freud had discovered in his neurotic patients could be seen perhaps even more clearly in schizophrenics. In order to demonstrate degrees of typical schizophrenic thought disorder (that is, the failure to organize thinking around a goal) Bleuler gives specimens of patients' replies to questions. For example:

A hebephrenic patient, ill for fifteen years but still able to work and still full of ambitions, gave me the following oral answer to the question, "Who was

Epaminondas [the fourth-century Theban general]?":

Epaminondas was one of those who are especially powerful on land and on sea. He led mighty fleet maneuvers and open sea-battles against Pelopidas, but in the second Punic War he was defeated by the sinking of an armed frigate. With his ships he wandered from Athens to Hain Mamre, brought Caledonian grapes and pomegranates there, and conquered the Beduins. He besieged the Acropolis with gun-boats and had the Persian garrisons put to the stake as living torches. The succeeding Pope Gregory VII . . . eh . . . Nero, followed his example and because of him all the Athenians, all the Roman-Germanic-Celtic tribes who did not favor the priests, were burned by the Druids on Corpus Christi Day as a sacrifice to the Sun-God, Baal. That is the Stone Age. Spearheads made of bronze.

Bleuler analyzes the relative degree of connectedness of the thought sequences. The case illustrates a moderate degree of schizophrenic association disturbance. Purpose, the most important determinant of the associations, is lacking. The patient formally adheres to the question put to him, but in fact never speaks of Epaminondas; actually he covers a much larger group of ideas, but they are linked too loosely to provide a logically useful connection. There is no goal-directed concept that "can weld the links of the associative chain into logical thought."

We can point to certain issues that Bleuler does not address, though he has behaved as the good clinician, examining, diagnosing, and trying to construct a usable working framework within which a physician may operate. Physicians are accustomed to working with diseases whose etiology they do not understand.

Consider, however, the setting of the question (imaginary but not farfetched).[8] Professor Bleuler says to a severely disturbed patient, "Look here, my good fellow, I'm doing a book on mental illness, and I need some clinical material to illustrate my finding about intellectual processes in schizophrenia. Since you had a good education in a Zurich gymnasium, would you help me out by answering the question: 'Who was Epaminondas?' "

There are several frameworks and goals that the patient might use in his reply. First, he might feel like a student. He knows just a little about the subject, so, using the time-honored student device, he tells everything he knows that is even remotely connected to the question, hoping that *some* credit will be forthcoming. Second, his goal is not an examination answer, but a pathological one to help Bleuler's research. Third, the patient might use his reply to express his feelings toward the questioner or the question (he has been put on the spot). However confused the answer's facts and sequences, the images are clearly violent. He is masking his hostility toward Bleuler with the guarded and censored language used by those living in occupied countries. If we can see that the patient's goal is different from the professor's, we can see the reply as intelligible and goal-directed.

What this exercise illustrates, of course, is the kind of analysis that goes along with certain psychotherapeutic approaches to schizophrenia. These approaches, to some degree, bypass some of Bleuler's issues and focus more on the meaning of the schizophrenic production, which can be understood only by those who can understand the position and inner experience of the patient. Our alternate analysis of the case does raise the issue of different ways to approach the phenomena of schizophrenic thought. In brief, to treat schizophrenic thought as a symptom of an underlying disorder is to rely on a medical model of psychological disturbance. To treat the disturbance as a necessary and motivated deviation from the usual way of communicating is to use a psychoanalytic model of understanding.

We have moved from Socrates in prison to Freud interpreting his dream to Bleuler introducing the malignant disorder called schizophrenia. What must appear a capricious grouping—concerns with the grounds for ethical choices, the dreams of normal people and neurotics, and a major form of out-and-out madness—actually brings us back to the original problem: What are psychiatry and psychiatrists?

What is the psychiatrist's proper area of professional competence? A few years ago a sensitive study of draft resisters in prison appeared.[9] These young men had chosen imprisonment over exile. Written by a psychiatrist, not a philosopher, this study nevertheless dealt with some issues raised in the Platonic dialogues on the trial and death of Socrates, among them ethical issues and questions of choice. If psychiatry is the study of illness, then the author overstepped the bounds of his profession. If choosing to go to jail is itself a sign of illness, then he did not. The author might defend his work on the grounds that, as a psychoanalyst, he often dealt with people facing difficult choices. The hysteric, Freud suggested, chooses exotic suffering over life's ordinary disappointments. The schizophrenic, some therapists would say, in a sense prefers madness to the possible consequences of his feelings—homicide, suicide, or disintegration of the self. Or, one might argue, psychiatrists and psychoanalysts are accustomed to studying the lives of their patients to understand how they got where they are. Hence a study of how these men came to choose prison is proper for the psychiatrist.

Conversely, a psychiatrist committed to the view that schizophrenia is of organic etiology could argue that it is cruel to speak of the schizophrenic as having chosen to go mad. One might as well speak of a crippled patient as having chosen muscular dystrophy rather than face life. The hysteric, perhaps, could be seen as playacting at being ill, a first cousin to the malingerer, who marginally belongs to psychiatry. But a war resister or a philosopher—that is carrying things too far! Politics and the social order may concern us as private citizens but not as psychiatrists.

Thus we need a latter-day Socrates to ask us to examine our meaning when we say we are specialists. Specialists in what? Mental illness? Well, then, young man, what kind of illness is "mental" illness? As Socrates questioned poets, sophists, rhetoricians, and politicians, needling and cajoling them into defining their real proficiencies, so he would have to do with us.

A glance at both popular and professional literature on this topic reveals that at one time or another psychiatrists have claimed (sometimes by public demand) for their proper sphere people as diverse as hospitalized psychotics, criminal offenders, unhappy heterosexuals, happy and unhappy homosexuals, politicians, children who do not seem to want to learn, unhappy couples seeking divorce, unhappy couples not seeking divorce, the poor, the aged, the retarded infants, narcotics addicts, problem drinkers, and patients suffering from such illnesses as ulcers. Psychiatrists at times consider it their proper task to deal with people who are excessively selfish and self-centered (narcissistic character disorders), people who are excessively private (schizoid character disorders), and people who just seem never to make it in life ("inadequate personality"). Psychiatrists, of course, are far from unanimous about which of these (and more) pertain to their particular sphere.

To make matters even more confusing, psychiatrists are now only one group of professionals who deal with the "mentally ill." Psychiatry, as a profession, is relatively new.[10] Even newer, however, is the field of clinical psychology. Here are nonmedical professionals who treat the "mentally ill." Another professional category is composed of social workers, who work with "clients," not patients. The last decade or so has seen the rise of several kinds of nonprofessional who work, for example, with chronic schizophrenics. Various self-help organizations for the "mentally ill" have arisen, some of which insist on the blurring of what they consider artificial boundaries between normality and sickness. Thus what psychiatrists call psychosis, particularly schizophrenia, is seen by some as a form of pilgrimage, or transcendental voyage, where guides, not physicians, are required.[11]

Similarly impressive (or depressing) is any catalog of what are called therapies. A fairly representative list would include pharmacological therapies, electric shock therapy, psychosurgery, and, not too long ago, insulin coma therapy. Then there is psychoanalysis, with its extraordinary variety of approaches, as well as psychotherapy, group therapy, encounter group therapy, behavioral therapies, family therapy, psychodrama, and even poetry therapy, bibliotherapy, and heliotherapy. [12]

So many conditions, so many types of practioners, so many therapies! But somehow psychiatrists, psychologists, and all the others do manage. They do their work, they continue day to day in satisfying pursuit of their craft, and one begins to suspect that most practitioners also have a sense of how to cope with a multiplicity of therapists and therapies, as if there are ground rules for living though the ground rules are not clear. [13]

We have now seen something of the state of perplexity in the field of psychiatry and the study of mental illness at large. In the next chapter we shall consider in more detail some reasons why things are so complex in the study of mental illness, why these issues have not been neatly settled even by men and women of great goodwill and intelligence.

We have not had, and still do not have, our Socrates.

2

The Development of Models
of Mental Illness

> The science of mental disease, as it would develop in the asylum,
> would always be only of the order of observation and classification.
> It would not be a dialogue. It could not be that until psychoanalysis
> had exorcised this phenomenon of observation . . . and substituted
> for its silent magic the powers of language.
> —Michel Foucault, *Madness and Civilization*[1]

Why has the study of mind and mental illness been so difficult, and
why are we still uncertain about so many basic issues? By comparison with physical scientists, investigators and practitioners in the area
of mental illness must appear to progress as snails and to behave as
the blind men at the elephant.

But we are groping at a far more complex beast than the elephant,
the creature called man, and the study of man presents formidable
problems that have not beset the physical sciences. We shall consider
some of the principal difficulties in studying the more severe grades
of mental illness. The same considerations apply, however, to the
task of understanding and defining a wide range of mental disturbances, from the severe to the mild and transitory.

First, there are serious problems of definition and boundary. Every
culture, to my knowledge, has some category that can be called
"madness," but madness is not always easily distinguished from
other categories of thought and behavior. Further problems occur in
separating madness from states of disturbance that occur in connection with particular life events or stages of life: sickness, separation,
death, adolescence, old age, and so on. Generally speaking, each
culture has rough limits of expectable behavior in these situations,
but when does profound grief become pathological mourning?
Where does adolescent turmoil end and schizophrenia begin?

At what point do we draw the line between innovative and insane,
between visionary and psychotic? May not both labels be appropriate
at times? A person may be so innovative in his ideas about government that he is considered revolutionary. In our day we have heard

much about the use of mental hospitals for imprisonment of political deviants, particularly in the Soviet Union. This idea has ancient roots, for Plato proposed in his *Laws* that atheists whose lack of faith seemed to arise from ignorance rather than malice be placed for five years in a *sōphronistērion,* a "house of sanity."[2] While the practice is certainly a diabolical method of suppression, its feasibility rests in part on the unspoken assumption that anyone who opposes the system is mad, either because he does not believe the claims of his government or because everyone knows it is crazy to risk public defiance of the government. Thus if we speak of the statistics of mental illness, we must be certain who is included in those statistics.

Above and beyond the difficulties of defining the field of study, serious obstacles stand in the way of learning about people whom we would unequivocally consider mentally ill. For one thing, the phenomena to be studied are often fleeting or difficult for both observer and sufferer to describe. They may be difficult to replicate and validate, even with long-term observation and accurate record-keeping. In addition, some of the core experiences of the psychotic may be so idiosyncratic that they are difficult to put into the ordinary vocabulary of the culture.

Then there is the problem subsumed under the term "participant observer." Most of the characteristic phenomena of psychosis (withdrawal and delusions, for example) may vary considerably depending on the nature of the relationship between observer and sufferer. It is now well known that both the contents and the intensity of hallucinations may vary with the state of the relationship between therapist and patient.[3] The schizophrenic thought disorder might appear prominently when the patient takes a psychological test but less so when he is at work in his usual job. The phenomena, in short, are to a large but indeterminate degree dependent on the interpersonal circumstances of the moment. This notion, carried further, has led to oversimplified formulations whereby schizophrenic phenomena are claimed to be nothing but interpersonal phenomena. At the extreme, some argue that we, the sane, "create" insanity by what we do, say, and feel.[4]

We must also consider that the behavior and thinking of the psychotic person are upsetting to others, including those who might wish to observe, study, or help such people. When a schizophrenic begins a recitation of his uncensored sexual or murderous delusions, or demonstrates grossly inappropriate affect, even the most stalwart of therapists could wish he were elsewhere.

The effects of excessive fear or guilt on thinking are well known. These painful affects lead us to distortions in our own thinking, make us prey to inner fears and fantasies, and impel us to keep excessive distance from the patient. One result may be the search for a simple, easy theory of madness that provides some closure on fears and fantasies engendered in us. Such explanations may be couched in terms of possession or of sickness as punishment for guilt or oversimplified scientific-sounding hypotheses. Our anxieties may lead us to keep both psychological and physical distance to protect our own well-being and sanity. This distance in turn prevents us from getting close enough to the patient to learn more about him and from him. Thus the defensive and self-protective needs of the observer can interfere with empathy and detached inquiry.

Patients too may have self-protective needs and inner resistances to learning about their disturbances. They may take refuge in theories or fantasies affording some relief from anxiety, and the culture usually provides such ready-made explanations, be they magical and demonic theories of possession or scientific theories. There is undoubtedly an overlap between what the observers and the patients need to defend against, but we should not assume that these defensive needs are identical.

Psychotic phenomena vary widely over time and in relation to the observer. If a natural history of schizophrenia exists, independent of interventions, it is extremely difficult to ascertain what it is. One may develop false impressions about what it is that has helped or harmed the patient. The history of medicine amply documents the fact that only a few apparent successes in the treatment of difficult and puzzling conditions are necessary to enshrine the agent as therapeutically effective. (Great advances in medicine have been made by physicians who decided to *withhold* all available treatments and finally to establish their worthlessness.) Thus almost any theory of cause or cure of schizophrenia can easily find "proof." The converse is also true: the extreme variability of the condition may lead us to miss the fact that a particular agent or kind of intervention (such as psychotherapy) may in fact be effective. Furthermore, certain treatments may appear effective for reasons quite different from the rationale attending them.[5] Nonspecific relief may accrue from trust in the practitioner or the relief of putting oneself into professional hands. Likewise, the patient may understand the treatment in a completely different way from that intended by the practitioner. A paranoid schizophrenic may find transient relief in imprisonment for a minor crime because it gives him a real external persecutor, more comfortable to live with than his demonic inner persecutors.

Another problem is the task of ascertaining facts about mental illness and about mentally disturbed people. The patient must report his experience in socially intelligible terms; it must fit into culturally defined categories. There is a great deal of evidence, both cross-cultural and historical, that culturally defined categories shape both the patient's version of his inner experience and others' reports of his behavior.[6] Among the important categories into which the patient's experience must fit are the theories held by the practitioner to whom he comes. These theories are not unknown to the patient, since they form part of his cultural milieu. There is, then, the danger that the only facts that can be elicited or assimilated by the therapist are those consonant with his theory. Others will be ignored or reinterpreted. Of course, without theories, it would be difficult to know what to ask or how to elicit reasonably ordered data. There is thus a complex dialectical relationship among the reports of the patient's experience and symptoms, the cultural categories of mental disturbance, and the theories of the practitioner. New discoveries depend either on new theories and categories or on patients who insist on reporting experiences that fall outside the cultural expectations. At various times in the late Middle Ages and Renaissance, for example, a person who felt and acted in a decidedly peculiar manner might report that he had recently experienced an encounter with a demon or succubus. He would be taken for healing to a priest, who would confirm that such events did indeed happen and would apply appropriate diagnostic criteria to establish if this was such a case. He might be able to determine which particular demon was involved and to prescribe treatment. It was not until physicians began to claim rather energetically that many of these people were victims of illness, not demonic possession, that a rival theory was introduced. When certain judges, physicians, and patients began to accept the theory of illness, more people began to report their experiences in forms that fitted a medical-humoral theory.[7]

Further, we have good reason to believe that in many, perhaps all, human societies several theories of mental disturbance are available, though one of them may predominate at a particular time or place. Typically, a process of negotiation takes place between the patient (with or without his family) and the practitioner around the issue of whether or not this case falls within his theory and competence.[8] Certainly in our own day we see patients shopping for a therapist who will give them a diagnosis, rationale, and treatment that conforms to their expectations. These therapists may tend to find reconfirmation of their theories because they end up treating patients who agree with them about their problems. I believe that this process has a great deal to do with the difficulty of establishing objective facts in the area of mental illness and contributes much to the climate of polemic and competitive claims in contemporary psychiatry. Again, new discoveries are made and objective truths established only when practitioners (and patients!) can strike a balance between holding to their theories and being willing and able to assimilate new data.

Finally in our catalog of difficulties: What is the *goal* of the person eliciting information about a mental disturbance? The information that the psychotherapist is concerned with collecting is different from that which a judge or lawyer may require. The confusion that often ensues when a psychiatrist is called to court as an expert witness is evidence enough that lawyers and doctors are seldom interested in the same facts. Similarly, during the many centuries when the Church had contact with the mentally ill in Europe, theologians and clerics uncovered and recorded many facts about mental illness which might have been of interest to physicians and psychotherapists. They were recorded, however, in a context that made it most unlikely that they would be available or intelligible to anyone operating outside a theological framework. We shall see that the Greek poets and tragedians had insights about psychosis which were not incorporated into medical theory in their own day and not appreciated in psychiatric theory for over two millennia.

Given all these sources of difficulty, it is not surprising that there is a multiplicity of therapies and theories in psychiatry. There always has been. Religion and cult, whether pagan or Christian, have always offered remedies. Treatments for the rich have doubtless always differed from treatments for the poor. In one form or another, theology and philosophy have offered their consolations. Institutions that can be called hospitals for the mentally ill probably first arose in Islamic countries, and, for the fortunate, some hospitals have indeed been hospitable.[9] For the less fortunate there have been forms of incarceration and, for particularly dangerous patients, exile or death, by neglect or execution.[10]

To illustrate the variety of approaches, let us examine the state of psychiatry in a particular place and period, America from the mid-nineteenth century to the present. By the 1850s a number of large public hospitals had been established, the state hospitals, supervised by physicians but in fact offering no effective medical treatment. A few smaller institutions—hospitals, asylums, retreats—still practiced some variety of the "moral therapies" ("moral therapy" had been introduced from England in the early part of the nineteenth century).[11] Some neurologists practicing in general hospitals or sanitoria believed their patients had "nervous" diseases such as neurasthenia.[12] Later in the century Christian Science became a burgeoning form of treatment for both physical and mental distress.

During the first decades of the twentieth century the claims of physicians to be healers of the mentally ill had become rather firmly established and psychiatry was a respectable medical specialty. While effective medical treatments for psychosis were not much more readily available in 1920 than they had been before the turn of the century, some discoveries had enhanced the claims and credibility of the physicians. General paresis of the insane had been proven to be a late form of syphilis for which fever (malarial) therapy had provided some relief. Fever therapy was thus one of the first medical treatments aimed directly at eliminating the specific cause of a psychosis.[13] Still, the ascendancy of the physicians was based more on the hope that medicine could unravel the answers than on the experience that medicine could cure.

By the late 1920s the influence of psychoanalysis was making itself felt in American psychiatry. Freud and Jung had visited America in 1909 to receive honorary degrees at the centennial of Clark University, and their visit made a significant impact on professional and popular opinion. Psychoanalysis was welcomed by some psychiatrists and physicians, and a number of psychiatrists gradually acquired psychoanalytic training. Other psychiatrists were deeply suspicious of psychoanalysis and saw it as a dangerous kind of mysticism or faith healing (or, even worse, charlatanism). While psychoanalysis could and did claim therapeutic success in the treatment of the neuroses, its impact on the treatment of the hospitalized insane lay primarily in the hope engendered by its explanatory value rather than in any large-scale therapeutic triumphs. A few psychiatrists soon began to take psychoanalysis more seriously for the treatment of the schizophrenic, and in the 1920s Harry Stack Sullivan established a small ward for the psychoanalytically oriented treatment of young schizophrenic men.

In the 1930s, organic treatments of limited efficacy for schizophrenia appeared: electric shock and insulin shock.[14] These techniques quickly came into widespread use because they provided some treatment for severe conditions for which no other was available. It was not until the mid-1950s that the first drugs appeared (reserpine, followed by the phenothiazines) which seemed specifically, and often dramatically, effective in the treatment of schizophrenia. A few years later drugs for depression appeared and began to be widely used.

Another important development of the 1950s was the spread of open rather than locked hospital wards. This was the second unshackling of the insane, 150 years after Philippe Pinel literally removed the chains from the inmates of the Bicêtre in Paris. More active efforts at group participation and at increasing the responsibility given to patients were concomitants of this open–door policy.[15] Earlier discharges were encouraged to minimize the deleterious effects of long-term hospitalization.

Thus by the end of the 1950s the major mode of treatment for the most severely ill remained custodial hospitalization. Three main approaches, however, were now espoused and practiced by psychiatrists: psychoanalytically informed approaches, drug therapies, and the notions of the open-door policy and the therapeutic community. Overall, up to that point, though psychiatrists had their differences and disagreements, such a term as "the mentally ill" made sense to all; moreover, few disputed that the appropriate experts were psychiatrists, medical doctors with specialized training in psychiatry. Doctors were superintendents of the hospitals and professors of psychiatry in medical schools; even psychoanalysts opposed lay analysis.[16]

In the late 1950s and early 1960s several authors began to attack the assumption that "mental illness" is an illness, and so properly in the province of medical doctors. The most famous of these writers in the United States is Thomas Szasz, whose *Myth of Mental Illness* appeared in 1961. Szasz argued that "mental illness" is considered an illness not because its victims give evidence of medical or biological disorder but because of particular historical and social needs. He argued that the "sick role" for the "mentally ill" was convenient for doctors, patients, and the public because it begged and concealed certain moral issues. There is, in effect, a socially condoned deception in agreeing that so-called patients are ill and need doctors, a deception that, he argued, is ultimately destructive of human freedom and responsibility. Szasz sees that doctors who purport to be specialists in "mental illness" are authoritarian rather than authoritative in their relationships with their patients. Psychiatrists have no real expertise, *qua* medical doctors, in what are really "problems of living." Treatment is then only a method of social control, however carefully disguised.

In that book and others, Szasz tried to develop alternate models, involving, for instance, game theory or decision theory. It should be noted that his specimen illness was hysteria, a condition that particularly lends itself to analysis as a form of motivated miscommunication. He later argued that all so-called mental illness, including schizophrenia, was "manufactured" by society, which was making scapegoats of these individuals by casting them in the role of sick people, hence second-class citizens.[17] Turning his fire on forensic psychiatry, he also argued that psychiatrists should have nothing to do with legal proceedings.

To his credit, Szasz has raised a number of important and painful issues in such a way that they have become difficult to ignore. On the other hand, he has gone much too far in his assertions that deception and scapegoating are involved in the manufacture of mental illness. He has confused motivation with etiology, as if to argue that because lepers became outcasts, leprosy was caused by society's needs to have scapegoats. He has taken too literally the notion that labeling certain people as mentally ill shapes their behavior, and he has also sold short the importance of biological factors in the psychoses. He has helped to confuse the relationship between possible biological deficit and moral responsibility for one's behavior.[18]

In 1960 R. D. Laing published his first book, *The Divided Self,* which, from a different perspective, also attacked the notion of mental illness. In contrast to Szasz's early focus on hysteria, Laing concentrated on schizophrenia and schizoid states. His framework draws upon psychoanalysis and existential philosophy. For him, to speak of "mental illness" serves to avoid looking at schizophrenia as a human, all too human, response to serious pathogenic human situations, especially those that take place in the family of the so-called patient. He drew in part upon the body of clinical knowledge that was being accumulated by those who worked with the families of schizophrenic patients and in part upon his own clinical experiences. He emphasized the schizophrenic as victim of the conflicting needs of the parents, especially the need to disregard the future schizophrenic's right to a life of his own.

In later publications Laing reported on his own study of such families, and then began to expand the circle of what he considered the noxious influences impinging upon the persons who were "selected" by their families to become crazy. These patients were victims of the onslaughts not only of their families but of their families' families, and finally even of society as a whole. (He would certainly consider the house of Atreus and its psychotic offspring, Orestes, a case in point.) "Society" has remained somewhat loosely defined in his writings, sometimes meaning capitalist society, sometimes technological society, and sometimes unspecified. One sees in his work the suggestion that schizophrenics are the prophets and seers of our sick society, our Cassandras. They see that the emperor has no clothes and they suffer the opprobrium of all who proclaim such truths.

Laing has shown the courage of his convictions and has attempted to put into practice his ideas about how we should deal with schizophrenics. At the same time he has eschewed more serious scientific discussion of the possible role of biochemical and genetic defects, and has thereby discouraged a serious synthetic dialogue. Overall, he has, like Szasz, stated many important truths, but has left too much of importance in vague and ambiguous terms.[19]

The critique of the medical model offered by Szasz and Laing has been augmented by a line of thinking which has arisen among some sociologists. Such workers as Edwin Lemert and Thomas Scheff have developed what has come to be called social labeling theory and the corollary notion of secondary deviance.[20] In their simplest form, these theories argue that some behaviors may be disturbed or deviant ("primary deviance"), but it is only because of social interaction and social labeling that people become converted from peculiar or mildly asocial individuals, for example, into mental patients. Some sociologists have done empirical work on these alleged processes and have argued that there is such a thing as "the career of the mental patient," a pathway through society and its controlling institutions that continues to redefine the person as mentally ill. While these theorists have asserted that much of what we call the phenomena of mental illness would probably disappear or lessen were our labeling processes to change, they concede that social labeling alone cannot account for all of what we call mental illness.

Another development that should be mentioned in this sketchy survey of the recent history of psychiatry is what has come to be known as the sociology of mental illness, which aroused great interest in the 1950s and 1960s. This term covers a heterogeneous body of research that attempts to correlate form and frequency of mental illness with important demographic, economic, and social-class variables. An indirect result of this research, along with the older stream of anthropological inquiries into culture and mental illness, has been the calling into question of the validity of the narrow definition of certain forms of aberrant or unusual behavior as "illness," hence as belonging in the purview of medical practitioners.

A major work in the sociology of mental illness was A. B. Hollingshead and F. C. Redlich's *Social Class and Mental Illness.* [21] Based on a survey of New Haven, it purported to show that serious mental illness was much more prevalent in the lower socioeconomic groups than in the upper ones. While some of their data and interpretations have been controverted, one finding has not been disputed. They documented what a great many people already knew, that the poor tended to be treated with such organic therapies as electric shock, insulin shock, and drugs, the upper classes with verbal psychotherapy. One effect of the critiques of and attacks on the medical model has been systematical examination of the premises underlying various ways of looking at mental illness. Beginning in the early 1960s, Humphrey Osmond and later Miriam Siegler used the terms "models of mental illness" and "models of madness" as a way of organizing the various theories and working models in psychiatry. Their efforts clearly defended the medical model against both psychoanalysis and various social psychiatric theories. The medical model is *the* standard by which they define the dimensions of their study of other models, and by which they judge them. In a 1966 paper, "Models of Madness," Siegler and Osmond discussed schizophrenia and delineated six major models: medical, moral, psychoanalytic, family interaction, conspiratorial, and social. [22] They also compared the models along these twelve dimensions: definition or diagnosis, etiology, behavior (how it is to be interpreted), treatment, prognosis, suicide, function of the hospital, termination of hospitalization, personnel, rights and duties of the patient, rights and duties of the family, rights and duties of society. (They have since added two more models, impaired and psychedelic, and have somewhat modified their list of dimensions, principally by adding goals of model.)

In their recent *Models of Madness, Models of Medicine,* Osmond and Siegler have presented the most extended and detailed discussion to date of the concept of models of mental illness.[23] Nevertheless, their bias in favor of the medical model is still apparent. They argue that the medical model is, in fact, several: a clinical, a research, and a public health model. The framework of models they have so carefully constructed is getting so cluttered that we can scarcely see the outlines. It should be noted that their main focus is schizophrenia; they devote little attention to neurosis or character disorder.

A less comprehensive but more careful and illuminating attempt to classify the diversity of models has emerged from a series of studies by Leston Havens, *Approaches to the Mind* (1973). Rather than "models," Havens speaks of four major "approaches": descriptive-organic, psychoanalytic, interpersonal, and existential. He does not claim that these four approaches adequately describe the entire psychiatric scene at the time he began (the 1960s), but that they cover much of what was thought important. He notes that each model takes off from a specific kind of patient and, in a sense, is strongest with that kind of patient. He stresses the complexity of the relationships among the theoretical assumptions, the working method, and the observations that are made. The role and activity of the therapist-observer, rightly emphasized, are different in each of the four approaches, and each approach generates a different body of "facts" about the patient. The facts of the descriptive-organic approach are the signs and symptoms exhibited by the typical or ideal patient and the points in the course of his illness at which they appear. The existential approach, by contrast, generates information about what it feels like to live in a state of despair, and about the despair the therapist can feel when in close contact with a person in this state.

Havens's analysis permits a greater appreciation of the complexity of each model than Osmond and Siegler's diagrammatic approach. An important message in his book is that there is no need to despair over the seeming confusion in psychiatry today, that, though we are not yet ready for the grand synthesis of all approaches, a proper understanding of the major ones reveals that we have made great progress in our understanding of mental illness.

Perhaps we are getting closer to minimizing polemic and maximizing honest debate. Some impressive bodies of data on schizophrenia have been accumulated. Medical and biological research has become much more sophisticated even in the last ten years, and the earlier claim that "behind every twisted thought lies a twisted molecule" has yielded to more precise thinking about the ways in which biological defects may be implicated in behavior and thinking.[24] Careful research has established a genetic factor in schizophrenia. Family-interaction studies have also demonstrated that the schizophrenic's symptom picture seems to make sense within the family context.[25] Many so-called symptoms seem to be imitations of family style, rebellions against it, or mockery of it.

Even psychoanalysis, notorious for difficulties of collecting and systematizing data, has reached a stage in its approaches to schizophrenia at which it can provide useful data for later integration with other hypotheses. Thus, even though there has been much disagreement on details of formulation of etiology and of psychotherapeutic approach, there has been a surprising amount of agreement on certain essentials. For example, the schizophrenic is terrified of both closeness and excessive distance.[26] He walks the narrowest of tightropes in human relationships—too much to one side and he may kill or be destroyed by persons he needs and loves, too far to the other and he may die lonely and abandoned. It will be possible in time, I believe, to get even greater agreement and specificity in the formulation and description of the psychodynamic functioning of the schizophrenic.[27] In any case, diversity of opinion and approach, if properly channeled, can lead to progress.

I have gone into this much detail about the state of the art of understanding psychosis and the notion of models of mental illness for several reasons, among them to illustrate my understanding of the core issues in the field of psychiatry today. The questions addressed by the notion of models of mental illness represent the starting point of and the justification for the inquiry about mind and mental illness in Greek antiquity. In a 1966 publication Dr. Herbert Weiner and I attempted to use the notion of models of mental illness to gain a long term perspective on certain perennial issues in psychiatry.[28] We assumed that such contemporary difficulties as those I have outlined are reflections of perennial unresolved issues in the field. It seemed then that ancient Greece might well be a suitable place to begin an investigation of the nature and history of these issues. Specifically, we suggested that it was crucial to examine the division among medical, intrapsychic, and interpersonal (field-theory) approaches to mental illness. This cleavage was already present in the ancient Greek material. At the same time, it seemed that it could be useful to students of classical antiquity to reconsider some familiar material from the perspectives of human behavior. With a few notable exceptions, the study of abnormal mental life as represented in the literature of antiquity had been treated in a fragmented and concrete way. Earlier workers tended mainly to describe and catalog cases of overt madness in Greek and Roman literature and ignored elementary insights and constructs made available by modern psychiatry.[29] Further, mind and its disturbance tended to be considered separately both by classicists and by historians of psychiatry and psychology. The broader social context of the representation of mind and of mental disturbance had not been taken into account.

Accordingly, we proposed to study ancient Greece from Homer to Plato and to divide the available material into three main models of mind and mental illness: the poetic (mainly Homeric), the philosophical (mainly Platonic), and the medical (mainly Hippocratic). We did not then (nor do we now) claim that these models are the linear ancestors of the contemporary, but rather that one might usefully examine them as exemplars of important issues that have persisted in modern psychiatry. The medical model is unique, as a relatively direct line runs from ancient to modern medical views about mental illness. The poetic model provides a suitable vehicle for examining issues raised by social-causation or field theories of mental illness. The modern models I have in mind are embedded to some degree in the works of the interpersonal school of psychiatry and even more in the theory that society causes mental illness and in the notion of social labeling. The Platonic material is the vehicle for examining notions of disease or disorder as a result of imbalance among the component portions of the mind. The idea of a structure called "mind" which has parts finds a modern counterpart in classical psychoanalytic theory, with its emphasis on the existence of a psychic structure divided into parts according to function.

In effect, we shall be using antiquity and the present to mirror one another and thereby to reveal new aspects of each and new relationships of each to the other. The inquiry is not strictly historical or cross-cultural. It is best considered a structural approach, which aims to isolate and define certain building blocks that have gone into the construction and generation of theories of mind and mental illness. Nor do we claim that these structures are to be considered as necessarily *the* basic elements of thinking about mind and madness, but rather as intermediate constructs that can help us organize and classify our theories and practices.

An important premise of Greek science is exemplified in the aphorism *Opsis tōn adēlōn ta phainomena,* "The phenomena are only the visible aspects of what is hidden beneath." The belief in an underlying order of things and the conviction that ordered inquiry can reveal what is hidden are values that we acquired from the Greeks and continue to share with them. In that spirit, let us begin to look.

3

The Greeks and
the Irrational

The fanatacism with which all Greek reflection throws itself upon
rationality betrays a desperate situation; there was danger, there
was but one choice: either to perish or—to be *absurdly rational*.
—Nietzsche, *Twilight of the Idols*[1]

Over the past centuries, classical scholarship and the study of the
human psyche have intersected at many points. One of the most
famous examples of this meeting is Robert Burton's *Anatomy of Melancholy* (1621), which treats nearly every variety of human passion
and urge. Though not a physician, Burton was thoroughly familiar
with both classical and contemporary medical literature. An intro-
verted, celibate Oxford don and cleric, he dubbed himself Democritus Junior, after a famous melancholic of the late classical tradition.
The work is a tribute to the enduring influence of classical antiquity
on the educated people of his day. We can surmise from the little we
know of Burton's life that the book must have served an important
therapeutic function, a testimony to the power of scholarship to
ward off melancholy.

Burton, though not the first, was certainly the most thorough and
the most famous writer to appeal to the popular interest in madness
and melancholy through the wealth of material from classical antiquity. His work on the "English malady" apparently aroused a sympathetic response in his melancholic compatriots, but English madness still had to be viewed through classical lenses.

Burton's easy allusions to Greek physicians also point to the long-
standing and intimate connection between clinical medicine and the
Greek medical traditions. Through the eighteenth and even the early
nineteenth centuries, Galen, Hippocrates, Aretaeus, Caelius Aurelianus, and other Greek and Roman physicians were quoted as authorities on medical matters in general and mental illness in particular,
almost as colleagues. Ancient cases can be juxtaposed with the cases
and opinions of living colleagues, by way of either agreement or
disagreement. Benjamin Rush (1745–1813), a signer of the Declara-

tion of Independence and the so-called father of American psychiatry, can thus cite Galen and Aretaeus when he argues for his theory that madness originates in the blood vessels and is always accompanied by fever.[2] For many centuries, then, there was an easy intimacy among doctors, though they might be separated by a millennium or two.

Pinel, writing at the beginning of the nineteenth century, still quotes the ancient doctors and medical encyclopedists, but with a difference. Pinel appeals more to what he considers the investigative spirit and observational acumen of Hippocrates, for example, than he does to the contents and conclusions of ancient medical thought. And as the century proceeds, a new spirit of careful observation, inquiry, and assembling of data takes hold, and we find only passing mention of the ancients. James Prichard in England, Jean-Etienne-Dominique Esquirol in France, and Isaac Ray in America cite the old Greeks and Romans as only little more than curiosities, no longer as the sources of important opinions or facts.

Thus nineteenth-century medicine and psychiatry broke new ground and were no longer bound by the teachings of antiquity. But in another area a new link slowly developed between classical studies and the vicissitudes of the human psyche. In part this link was a function of developments in psychiatry that were to lead to dynamic psychiatry and psychoanalysis. In a larger sense, a *Zeitgeist* manifested itself in the novels of Dostoevsky, in the early psychoanalytic investigations of Freud, and in the interests of a few classical scholars in Germany.

In a later chapter I shall say something of the great German-Jewish classical scholar Jacob Bernays, who was known for his interpretation of Aristotle's notion of catharsis (1851). As important as his view of catharsis (which emphasized a medical rather than a moral interpretation) is his profound interest in the relationships among reason, passion, and ecstasy. The spirit, if not the content, of Bernays's work seems to have influenced a young and promising classical scholar named Friedrich Nietzsche.[3] His first book, *The Birth of Tragedy* (1871), greatly disappointed many of his classical colleagues, but eventually his line of thinking was to prove influential even among classicists. His arguments centered around the idea that tragedy arose from the synthesis between the serene Apollonian and the ecstatic orgiastic Dionysian elements in Greek culture, that the conflict and tension between the two was an integral part of Greek culture:

These two distinct tendencies [the Apollonian and the Dionysian] run parallel to each other, for the most part openly at variance; and they continually incite each other to new and more powerful births, which perpetuate an antagonism only superficially reconciled by the common term "Art"; till at last, by a metaphysical miracle of the Hellenic will, they appear coupled with each other, and through this coupling eventually generate the art-product, equally Dionysian and Apollonian, of Attic tragedy.[4]

Elsewhere he wrote that the Greeks spoke so much of moderation because they knew how immoderate they could be. With Nietzsche's work new questions had to be addressed, among both classical scholars and other intellectuals, which might have been subsumed under the epigram "The Greeks and the Irrational." E. R. Dodds, in his magisterial work of that title (1951), paid homage to another great classical scholar, Erwin Rohde, an associate and supporter of Nietzsche. Rohde's *magnum opus* on Greek religion and civilization was entitled *Psyche: The Cult of Souls and Belief in Immortality among the Greeks.* It is certainly of more than passing interest that Rohde chose that title at a time when such terms as psychiatry, psychotherapy, and psychoanalysis had only recently been (or were soon to be) introduced.

At the end of the nineteenth century and the beginning of the twentieth, classical scholars at Cambridge were bringing contemporary anthropological concepts to bear on Greek studies. Sir James Frazer's *Golden Bough* begins with an examination of the nature of a strange priesthood in Roman antiquity and frequently returns to the Greeks and Romans. Jane Harrison, F. M. Cornford, Gilbert Murray, and others contributed to the recognition of the primitive in Greek religion and culture. Although there has been much scholarly reaction to their primitivizing excesses, they too raise issues that may well prove more enduring than some of the answers they gave.

About the same time, Freud and the early psychoanalysts testified to the enduring pull of classical antiquity by their readiness to turn to Greek mythology. These early analysts had, by our standards, a good classical education, and some were serious amateur classical scholars. But something more than his gymnasium training in Latin and Greek allowed Freud to choose the term "Oedipus complex," to speak of narcissism, and to invoke the notion of Eros as found in the "divine Plato" to support his own concept of libido.[5] It seems that Freud sensed that the Greek myths, especially as presented in tragedy, were already profound analytic statements about human psychology. He saw Sophocles' *Oedipus Rex* not merely as a convenient illustration of his newly discovered "complex," but as an almost close-to-conscious attempt at analysis of the inner workings of the mind.[6] In effect, the Greek myths, especially as expressed in poetry, had already done some of the work of identifying and dissecting the crucial elements in human motivation.

While Freud had at most a cursory acquaintance with the classical scholarship of his day, he and his circle were interested in and influenced by the works of Sir James Frazer, including *The Golden*

Bough. Freud was interested not only in the contents but in the spirit of such works, namely, the assumption of the persistence of the primitive within the civilized. Beginning with his earliest psychoanalytic writings, he equated the primitive stage of humanity with the childhood of each human being, and then equated both of those with the unconscious. Thus there is an important congruence between Freud's interest in the influence of the unconscious on the conscious and the interest of the Cambridge group in the primitive and ritual underpinnings of sophisticated and rational Greek cultures.

But Greek culture affords us much more than a case study in the interrelationship between the primitive and the civilized, the irrational and the rational. The Greeks themselves, or at least a few, were explicitly interested in such issues and began to articulate important questions and interesting answers. The relationships between sane and mad, rational and irrational, mythological and scientific were topics of dialogue for the Greeks. As far as we know, they were the first to take up and consider these issues in extended and explicit form.

The Greek Models[7]

In a very important sense the three models into which I have divided Greek literature—the poetic, the philosophical, and the medical—correspond to lines of cleavage in Greek culture. I do not have in mind an image of sharp and clear divisions, but rather something more like the lines along which a crystal breaks. For some of the Greeks, such as Plato, the lines were more sharply drawn. For him philosophy and poetry were at war; he banned the poets from his republic. In many respects philosophy and medicine shared important areas of interchange, though philosophy drew more upon medicine than medicine upon philosophy. Overall, Plato viewed medicine as one of the crafts—a particularly important one, but not a serious rival to his own method or interests.

Medical writers were more concerned than philosophers about distinguishing the two disciplines. A few medical writings argue emphatically that medicine is based on clinical experience and practical knowledge, while philosophy is based on *a priori* frameworks. In the fifth and fourth centuries we do not hear much about rivalry between medicine and philosophy in the treatment of the human "soul," but by later Hellenistic antiquity, and certainly by Christian times, the sense of competition was keen. "Doctors of the soul" and "doctors of the body" were in some measure rivals, though the Greeks, it seems, were eager to try to heal such breaches. Greek culture, as agonistic as it was, was also marked by a pragmatic and synthesizing spirit.

Each of the three models will be examined from four viewpoints: (1) the representation of mind and of ordinary mental activity, (2) the representation of disturbance of mind, (3) the treatment of disturbance of mind, and (4) the relations between the craft of the practitioner (poet, philosopher, or doctor) and the theories of mind and mental disturbance.

At this point we must be content with such general terms as "disturbance of mind" and "therapy," recognizing that they apply more literally to medicine than to poetry. In the course of my treatment of the individual models the specific senses in which these terms are relevant will become clearer. Homer was not a therapist, yet in some significant way the Greeks saw poetry as a form of therapy. Plato spoke of "healing of the psyche" largely as a metaphor borrowed from medicine. At the same time, he defined what were for him the really important disturbances of the psyche and proclaimed his philosophy and his method as the appropriate means of healing.

This leads to another consideration in my choice of the term "model" rather than "theory." Greek medicine definitely had a theory about what caused mental disturbance, a theory that justified the kinds of treatments used. Homer clearly did not have a theory of mind or mental illness, though he had much to say that involved mental life, and he had attitudes and assumptions that underlay what he said. Plato had theories, but they were not explicitly about the disturbances with which the doctors were concerned. The term "model" is used to designate the manner in which a particular thinker or creative writer described mental activity, the kinds of explicit and implicit assumptions he made, and any statements that may suitably be considered actual theories. I do not use "model" here to mean analogy, though I shall discuss some important analogies to mind. Today we speak of computer models of the mind, or the mind as transistor and transducer of experience. "Models," in the sense of analogies, are a part of what I call "models of mind," for these analogies often shed light on some important underlying assumptions in the minds of the thinkers I am considering. Hence "model," as I use it, is a compromise between the need to find a term broader than a formal theory yet narrow enough to differentiate one set of viewpoints and assumptions from another.

Several threads run throughout the material, uniting the ancient and modern. These threads represent important issues in contemporary psychiatry and have in large measure determined my choice of both the ancient and the modern models I discuss. The first centers around the notion of a structure of mind. Is there indeed such a structure? The notion of mind as something fixed and internalized was not firmly established in earlier antiquity (it is absent from the Homeric poems) and many contemporary theories have tended to redefine, if not discard, the notion of a structured entity called mind. As we shall see, both Plato and Freudian psychoanalysts posit an internalized mental structure that has an organization and whose parts have particular functions.

If we accept the notion of a structure, what is its nature and what are its component parts? Is the substance of mind unique, or is mind composed of elements common to the outside world, either biological or chemical? Is the structure of mind analogous to other structures, such as that of society? And finally, do defects in the structure or in its parts or in the relations among the parts lead to abnormal mental functioning? The medical models, both in antiquity and in the present, posit a material structure or at least a material substrate to mind, and view disturbances in the functioning of that material as more or less directly leading to disturbances of mental life and of behavior. Other models do not deny the existence or importance of such a material but regard its functioning or malfunctioning as incidental to their main concerns.

A second issue has to do with the relative importance for mental life of forces arising from within the person and forces arising from outside. How can these forces be characterized? Is the person able to control them or must he merely endure and react passively? Are external and internal forces in conflict, or are both necessary for the functioning of the mind? How does the mind mediate between or integrate external and internal forces? Is human mental life the product of nature or of nurture, or, if of both, how do they interact? What are the forces, internal, external, or in combination, that lead to disturbance of the mind? The ancient medical theories speak of the influence of climate, geography, air, and water on the internal qualities and humors of the body; food too is important in shaping the balance among the internal substances. Mental disturbances come from humoral imbalance, and the humors in turn are influenced by these external factors. The corollary of this view, of course, is that changing the external factors, including modifications of site and ways of living, can favorably influence the internal balance and restore proper mental functioning. Drugs are but one method of achieving such modifications. All of this is subsumed under the ancient medical notion that "regimen" is crucial to health and disease. For Plato, in contrast, among the factors vital for health within the soul are goodness and badness within the society and within the soul itself. Finally, in general, modern theories of mental disturbance are more sophisticated than the ancient ones in their attempts to understand the integration of these various factors as well as the pathways by which a particular factor influences mental functioning. Though the "nature–nurture" problem has not been solved, modern theories are better suited to a consideration of the complexities of interaction of many forces.

The third issue that runs throughout these discussions is the relationship between theory and practice. Are they always consonant? What happens when data do too much violence to theory? If theory and practice are in fact intimately and organically related, what brings about and maintains that connection? Is there a subtle way in which the mind that is described in the theory is in fact a reflection of the mind of the theorist? Finally, is it possible that the way the theory accounts for disturbances of mind is also a reflection of the kinds of thing that disturb the mind of the practitioner in the course of his therapeutic activity? These questions have not been sufficiently explored in the works on the history of psychiatry or on contemporary psychiatric theories.

II

THE POETIC MODEL

4

Mental Life in
the Homeric Epics

You know, doubtless, that the sage Homer has written about practically everything pertaining to man.
—Xenophon, *Symposium*

The Homeric epics are the earliest works of Greek literature to survive.[1] Undoubtedly masterpieces of a long tradition of Greek heroic poetry, they tell stories that must have been sung long before Homer. Insofar as they embody historical actuality, it is the thirteenth-century world of the Mycenaeans, whose traditions and memories were told, retold, and elaborated through the lays of countless bards.[2] Homer put together his monumental works sometime in the eighth century B.C. To a significant degree they were composed as oral epics and written down soon after their composition, which coincided with the introduction of alphabetic writing (the Phoenician alphabet) into Greece. Some scholars have argued that because they were created when a predominantly oral-traditional culture was acquiring the art of writing, these poems possess a unique vitality and a marvelous balance of the intricate and the spontaneous.

The poems are heroic epic. They tell of the deeds of heroic warriors, their struggles with their enemies, their encounters with their gods, and, often most tragically, their enmity for each other.[3] They are a compilation of myths from many sources built around believably human heroes.

Heroic poetry is the repository of the culture's ideals and a consolation to those living in less heroic times. By its implicit standards, we are all living in less heroic times than those of the tales. Heroic poetry commonly appears at a time when heroes are gone and their absence is mourned. Thus the tales recounted in the *Iliad* and *Odyssey* were probably first told not long after a war (the Trojan?) waged by Mycenaean chieftains. We know from archaeological findings that by the twelfth century the kind of warrior aristocracy and social organization implied in the poems were in decline.

Heroic poetry consoles us by holding up a vision of our deepest ideals and aspirations, of what it is to strive beyond measure and to risk going beyond proper human bounds. The heroes are just close enough to us and human enough to serve as models, but sufficiently remote and superhuman that we need not require ourselves to reach their level. Such poems tell us what it was like in the old days, when men who were close to the gods, or even children of the gods, walked the earth. The old days are comfortably set in the long ago, either ancient times or the timelessness of childhood dreams.

Heroic poetry at its best records far more than the glorious deeds of noble fighting men. In its affective shadings, in its multiple allusions to every aspect of human life, a great epic shows us men in turmoil and conflict. Myth portrays action, tells a tale, and suggests a moral. The rendering of myth in epic, however, introduces a new dimension, best termed tragedy. Out of the clashes of arms and will that mark these poems, a certain reflectiveness on the human condition emerges. Reflections on loneliness, old age, death, the lot of the human race occur throughout the poems.

The epic hero is rewarded for his labors by victory and consoled for his losses by the immortality that comes from having his story told over and over through the generations. *Kleos,* glory and fame, the knowledge of an undying memory, is the greatest reward. The afterlife of the Homeric hero is a miserable world of flitting shades who drift aimlessly and endlessly in the underworld. But undying fame, particularly that which comes from having progeny to continue the heroic line, can somehow sustain one in that empty and bloodless existence. Achilles, in both the *Iliad* and the *Odyssey,* comes closest to damning war and denouncing the entire heroic ethos as just not worth the grief they bring. When Odysseus sees his shade in Hades, Achilles proclaims that he "would rather follow the plow as thrall to another man, one with no land allotted him and not much to live on, than be a king over all the perished dead" (*Odyssey,* 11.488–91). Odysseus is able to console Achilles by telling him that his son, Neoptolemos, has been a mighty warrior.

It is no wonder that Aristotle could see but a short step from the Homeric epics to the great tragedies of the fifth century. For Aristotle, as for us, there is a continuity and timelessness in the tragic portrayal of the human condition, the relations between man and gods, between man and fate. In this sense, the psycholgoy of Homeric man is not so different from that of the fourth- or fifth-century Athenian, or from our own.

Yet in another sense (not really recognized by Aristotle) the two ages differ greatly in the ways in which that psychology is conveyed and in the language with which it is described. Important and far-reaching changes in language, especially that portraying mental life, had taken place in the centuries between Homer and Aristotle.⁴ But let us look at Homer's language and his sense of the way people think, feel, and behave.

Psyche

Apart from the intrinsic interest and importance of the term *psuchē* in Homer, it is worth examining for the profound metamorphosis it underwent in fifth-century philosophy and then in Plato.⁵ The Platonic usage is familiar and intelligible to us, the Homeric stranger and more remote.

The opening lines of the *Iliad* introduce us to the term, saying that when a man is slain, his psyche goes to Hades while his corpse (he himself) remains and, if unburied, is spoil for the animals of the field and the birds of the sky. A part of the man seems to continue its existence in Hades.

The *Odyssey* (Book 11) provides us with a more extended description of what this psyche and its existence in Hades are like.⁶ The dialogue between Odysseus and the psyche of Achilles in Hades conveys a dreary and joyless existence after death. In the *Odyssey* the psyches cannot speak; they flit about like shadows, have no intelligence, and can speak only after drinking the blood of slain animals. Only the seer Tiresias has the power of speech and the use of his wits, by dispensation of the goddess Persephone. The shades are compared to shadows; their substance is that of figures in dreams. Hades is a faraway place (not clearly an "underworld" in Homer), difficult of access, situated near "the village of dreams" (24.12).

In Hades, Odysseus meets the shade of his mother, who has died of longing for him sometime during his twenty-year absence from Ithaca. When he tries to embrace her but cannot, he asks if she is merely an "image" (*eidolon*) sent by Persephone to increase his grief (11.210–14). This question is subtle and implies that Odysseus wonders if she is a deceptive image, not really his mother or her shade. Obviously, a real mother would rush to embrace her child.

She explains that she is not an image, but that after death "the sinews no longer hold the flesh and bones together, but all [the parts] are subdued by the strength of the flaming pyre, and when the spirit [*thumos*] first leaves the white bones, the soul flutters out like a dream and flies away" (11.219–22).⁷ This, then, is the limited immortality that people may achieve: their psyches are released and continue on after death.

While in Homer the psyche usually first appears after death, it may also, curiously, leave a person when he loses consciousness and, presumably, return as he awakens. Psyche is sufficiently concrete to leave the body through a spear wound and also carries a connotation of "breath," though this usage is only remotely discernible in Homer.[8] Other uses of the term in Homer indicate that the psyche is sacred. One can swear by one's psyche, as by the head or knees. It is ascribed only to human beings, not to animals.

Clearly psyche defies easy definition or classification in our own psychological terms. It somehow is a part of oneself, and yet is more a replica of the self than a part. It is important to note that Homer has no term for "self" or "oneself," so that Homeric language cannot pose such a question as "What is the relation of the psyche to the self?" Psyche is abstract, yet seems to have (as do most mental terms in Homer) a concrete physical sense.[9]

We can gain some further appreciation of the Homeric notion by considering what psyche is *not*. It is never portrayed as a thinking, feeling, reflecting, and deciding part of the living person. Thus it is not a psychic agency in our sense of the term. It seems to carry on some of these functions after death, but as a continuation of the whole person, not as an agency of faculty.

Erwin Rohde, in his *Psyche,* was the first to suggest that the psyche is a double, or alter ego.[10] He wished to place the Homeric psyche in the context of the widespread human belief in the existence of another self. This double is variously represented as something surviving after death, or as a shadow. While this approach has some value, it raises more problems than it answers, particularly since the significance or function of belief in doubles in the various primitive groups mentioned by Rohde is not at all clear.

Psychoanalytic formulations about doubles originate with Otto Rank's famous work *The Double.* [11] Rank agreed with earlier writers that the double is a defense against fear of death and total oblivion and argued that the belief in a double reflects a persisting early stage in the individual's development of his sense of self. It is a "reflection," another that is at once a self, by means of which the person comes to a new kind of integration of the self.[12] Further, Rank argued that for the individual (most of his examples are taken from modern literature) the double represents some disavowed or unacceptable part of the self. Some of this is seen in this clinical example:

An elderly man, obviously suffering from mental and physical deterioration, was convinced that another man lived behind the mirror in his room. The other looked exactly like him and had the same trade—he was a toolmaker. This other man had stolen his toolmaking equipment and pawned it, thus depriving him of his last chance to make a living, and had seduced and run off with the patient's wife (who in fact had left him a few years before). Thus the old man, feeling helpless and vulnerable in the face of internal forces (disability and despair) and the external forces that beset lonely aged people, devised another self. The double helps account for his otherwise unbearable feeling and his pitiful lot. He does not have to acknowledge that *he* may have driven his wife away (or that she preferred another man), since he feels that all this was done to him. In addition, the double functions to relieve an otherwise unbearable loneliness.[13] I believe that Rank's formulations afford some useful perspectives on the Homeric portrayal of the psyche. The psyches we encounter in Hades are an unhappy lot. When they have the opportunity to speak, they are always grieving, nursing injuries, complaining of injustices, and bemoaning losses. The split-off or undesirable aspect of the self that may be represented in the psyche in Hades is the aspect that must endure passively. It is not unacceptable for a hero to be injured or aggrieved; but to be impotent or passive cannot long be endured. In a sense, the shades in Hades may express feelings not just about being dead but about being worse than dead—alive and unable to act, the epic hero's nightmare.[14] And death has another terrible aspect—the possibility of being forgotten. Epic deeds make one immortal, provided there are progeny or poets to carry on the memory. From this perspective, the living Odysseus' descent to and return from Hades has a poetic logic. For the story of the *Odyssey* is the story of a man who in life has had to endure and has been able to do so. Furthermore, he has been symbolically reduced to oblivion, the self-declared "no man."

If we shift for a moment to a Platonic perspective on the nature of psyche, we can form a clearer picture of the Homeric notion. Psyche, for Plato, is capable of functioning as one's ethical and cognitive core, and as such is frequently equated with the self. For Plato, psyche makes decisions and can make responsible choices; it certainly can be held responsible for its choices. Thus Plato's myth of the journey to the abode of the psyches, the myth of Er at the end of the *Republic,* emphasizes responsible choice. There the psyches draw lots to decide the order in which they may *choose* among the available lives in their next incarnation. "The blame belongs to him who chooses. God is blameless" (617E). In this myth, in fact, Odysseus is the one who makes the most of his choice, though he has in fact drawn the last place. Thus what Plato emphasizes as the essential and desirable features of the psyche are in Homer represented by the activity of the living man. Psyche in Homer, if we view it as a kind of double, is the passive, enduring, and nonautonomous aspect of the self, a fading memory of the person; in Plato it is immortal and vital.

We shall now consider how the Homeric man is activated, because, though psyche is alive, it is not an animating and activating force for the living individual. We shall look at the representation of dreams in the epics, for there we may begin to see the essential outlines of the Homeric portrayal of the living man and his mental life: he is activated by an external agent.

Dreams[15]

At the beginning of Book 2 of the *Iliad,* Zeus, pondering how best to destroy the Greeks and avenge Achilles' honor, decides to send a dream to Agamemnon which will lead him to make a foolish move. Zeus instructs "evil Dream" to go to Agamemnon with a message. Dream, disguised as Nestor, stands beside the sleeping Agamemnon and repeats Zeus's instructions to Agamemnon to gather his armies in the expectation of capturing Troy that day. This incident is typical of the Homeric representation of dreams and contains a number of striking features.

First, the dream is a person, or a personified agent. Second, the dream is an external agent descending upon Agamemnon, not originating from within him. The dream is not, as for Plato, a result of an activity of one or another part of the psyche (such as the appetitive part, which can express all kinds of wild desires while the rational part sleeps). It is not a result of somatic perturbations, as the Hippocratic doctors and Aristotle will assert.

There is also a stereotype about the dream in Homer: Dream finds Agamemnon asleep and positions himself at his head—Homer appears to be intuitively aware of the source of dreaming—but here too, consistent with the dream as external agent, the space where it is located, as it were, is outside the dreamer.

Next the figure of Nestor, a real person, is fused with that of Dream. But for the dreamer (and for poet and audience) this fusion is quite natural. The content of the dream, too, is hardly strange or exotic; it is quite close to the wishes and waking thought of the dreamer. Dreams in Homer generally do not require symbolic interpretation.[16]

Overall, the portrayal of dreams and dreaming embodies and typifies, albeit in somewhat more explicit form, the characteristic Homeric attitudes toward mental life.

Characteristics of Mental Life

The terms for the inner agencies of mental life are not clearly and systematically distinguished. In the dream discussed above, Zeus ponders "in his heart." The Greek is *phrena,* a term associated with intellectual activity, but not purely intellective either. Homer also uses several variants of the root that has come to signify "heart" in English (*kardia* and *kēr*) which are used in similar, though not necessarily identical, contexts. The most intellective term in Homer for an organ or agency of mental activity is *noos,* but even this cannot always be equated with "mind."[17] Despite several decades of scholarly activity aimed at delineating the precise boundaries and meanings of the various mental terms, it is difficult to render these terms consistently, let alone in a manner that consistently corresponds to English usage, poetic, popular, or scientific.

This state of affairs may also be contrasted with Plato's use of mental vocabulary. Though not always successful, Plato aims for clear and consistent definitions of his terms.

Homer makes no clear or consistent differentiation between organs of thinking and organs of feeling or emotion. To a large degree, all of the terms of mental functioning are amalgams of mind and heart or of thinking and emotionality. The agencies of mental life are rather concrete and overlap with physical organs. Thus *phrenes* (mind or wits) also signifies the leaves of the diaphragm, or perhaps even the lungs. I have mentioned psyche, which, while it does not correspond to an organ of the body, has overtones of something quite physical. *Thumos,* another common Homeric term, is an entity or organ that swells within the person yet can leave with death or fainting. It can carry on a dialogue with the person, who frequently addresses it; on occasion his *thumos,* or "another [*heteros*] *thumos,*" may speak up. The heart (*kradie*) that Odysseus addresses when he says, "Bear up, O my heart; you have suffered worse than this" is also the physical heart that can be penetrated by a spear.

Of all the terms for mental activity, *noos* is probably freest of any specific physical connotations. *Psuchē* partakes of the physical, but seems to be less concretely physical than most of the other terms.

Of course, every modern language has terms that are both mental and physical. We readily speak of a "broken heart" and talk of courage as "guts." (Courage derives from the same root as *cardia* via the French *coeur.*) When one speaks in such terms, one does not make exquisite distinctions between body and mind or between thought and feeling. Since Plato, however, we have had available another level of discourse about mental life, and at this level we do aspire to make clear distinctions among agencies of mental life, between mind and body, and between thought and emotion. But in Homer there is no articulated concept of a psychic structure or function. Thus when Homer speaks of organs or agencies of mental activity, he makes no attempt to indicate any organization or interrelationship among them. It is not as if they were parts of some whole. Needless to say, any term that could be rendered as "structure" is absent from Homer's lexicon, and the phrase "structure of mind" could not be rendered into Homeric Greek. Nor do we find in Homer any assumption of a hierarchy, of a layered organization of these parts, an assumption that becomes central in the Platonic psychology.

Similarly, no term for "function" exists in Homeric Greek. Later Plato can speak of the tasks of the rational part of the psyche, and this way of speaking comes much closer to describing and ascribing functions. Homeric Greek does not organize mental life into such categories as perception, sensation, cognition, memory. It is rich in part functions, particular concrete aspects of mental functioning (recognizing, reminiscing, exhorting). There is no attempt to relate these part functions to each other and no way to articulate such propositions as "Memory is a part of the process of learning."

Further examination reveals lack of clear distinction between structure and function. The same term may designate both the organ and the end result of the organ's function. Thus *noos* is the agency or the part that seems to see ahead and plan, but the same word can designate the plan itself. *Thumos* can designate both the locus of an impulse and the impulse itself.

Another aspect of what might be called concreteness in mental terminology appears in the words for visual activity. Homer has terms that denote "to stare," "to glare at," "to notice," but no one word that can be translated as "to see."[18]

It would be misleading, however, simply to group all of these observations under the rubric "concrete versus abstract thinking." By comparison with Plato, Homer lacks terms of abstract discourse about mental life. A certain measure of physiological concreteness is probably characteristic of the vocabulary of mental life in all languages, especially in regard to stages of feeling. Students of comparative Indo-European philology have argued that certain terms were probably more abstract in the root Indo-European language than they have become in its descendants.[19] There is some reason to suspect that "psyche" is one such term, that the concrete meaning of "breath" was a later acquisition. Thus, over time, terms might move from concrete to abstract and vice versa. It would be more accurate to say that Homeric language has its own categories, or even its own kinds, of abstraction.[20] It is better to characterize Homeric language as relatively deficient in terms useful for making analytic propositions than as deficient in abstract terms per se.

Two other areas of interest appear to lack abstract or general terms in Homer. One is the body. Bruno Snell has pointed out that Homer's lexicon contains no term easily translated as "body" or "the body" (let alone the physical element in such a phrase as "the mind-body distinction").[21] *Sōma* typically means a corpse, *demas* physical shape or form (as in "lovely in shape"). The Homeric somatic vocabulary emphasizes limbs, muscles, points of articulation of limbs, bones, and so on. Clearly this is a functional vocabulary—the vocabulary of warriors, athletes, men who observe traumatic wounds.

It does not necessarily bespeak a lack of a concept of body or capacity for such a concept. If one were to consider the vocabulary of such a sport as hockey, one might find a situation not too unlike the Homeric. "Body" is used in such a phrase as "a body check." We are interested in speed in some instances, in agility in others, and in bulk in some. As for mental vocabulary, we are not interested in hockey players' IQs but in their "wits" or "know-how" or "guts." Abstractions depend less on the capacity to make them than on the need to produce them.

Similarly Homer has no term for "person" or "oneself." He does not even have a generic term for man or woman, male or female. He has words for young man, old man, maiden, married woman, and so on. Here too one must consider the relation between the need for a category and the existence of a term for it. Philosophy and census taking may require a term for person, but Homer has other aims. A particular end appears to be served by the concreteness of Homeric language, which makes public and observable the ongoing stream of inner mental life. Thus, by using such particular vision words as *derkesthai,* to glance, and *paptainein,* to peer, the poet emphasizes aspects of the activity of looking that are observable to others.[22]

In like manner, the familiar Homeric simile, as applied to the description of mental processes, serves the same end—making public and observable that which is internal and idiosyncratic. Thus Penelope lies awake worrying about the safety of her son Telemachus, "pondering whether her blameless son would escape death, or whether he would be overcome by the arrogant suitors. Such things as a lion thinks when he is afraid, in a press of men, when they form a circle to entrap him "[23] (*Odyssey,* 4.789–92). The image of the lion carries the burden of making vivid and easily apparent to the audience the rather complex state of Penelope's feelings: apprehension, restlessness, the encroaching sense of helplessness in the face of a growing threat, and also a certain defensive hostility. This method of portraying the inner working of the mind is quite characteristic of Homer. Homer stresses the universal and the general in mental life and tends to suppress the highly personal and the idiosyncratic. Consider the extreme contrast between Homer in the *Odyssey* and James Joyce in *Ulysses.* Molly Bloom (Joyce's Penelope) is lying awake just after Leopold has slipped into bed after a night's wanderings with Stephan Daedalus. Curious about where he has been, she muses about his behavior:

only for I hate having long wrangle in bed or else if its not that its some little bitch or other he got in with somewhere or picked up on the sly if they only knew him as well as I do yes because the day before yesterday he was scribbling something a letter when I came into front room for the matches to show him Dignams death in paper as if something told me and he covered it up with the blotting paper pretending to be thinking about business so very probably that was it to somebody who thinks she has a softy in him because all men get a bit like that at his age especially getting on to forty he is now so as to wheedle any money she can out of him no fool like an old fool and then the usual kissing of my bottom was to hide it not that I care two straws who he does it with or knew before that way though I'd like to find out . . . one woman is not enough for them.[24]

Content, style, syntax, lack of punctuation, all combine to emphasize the most personal and inward aspects of Molly Bloom's mental life. Joyce obviously attempts to make the hidden visible and intelligible, but he is at least as much interested in what differentiates the mental content of the individual from that of another as he is in the universal similarities. Homer is clearly far more interested in the commonalities.

Homer has a marked tendency to ascribe the origins of mental states to forces or agencies outside the person. In Book 1 of the *Iliad*, when Achilles is about to slay Agamemnon, who has just announced his intention to take away Achilles' concubine, Achilles forbears because Athena comes down, pulls him by his hair, and says, "Cease" (1.210).[25] If a man can sing, it is because a god has given him "song and lyre." The outside agencies are often divine but may be other people, drugs, or even strong emotions.

Energy, strength, courage frequently appear as if infusions from a god. A man's strength is frequently called sacred (*hieros*). In Book 13 of the *Iliad*, Poseidon comes down to try to encourage the disheartened Achaeans to fight off the Trojan onslaught against the ships. Poseidon comes upon two heroes, Ajax the son of Oileus and Ajax the son of Telamon, disguises himself as the seer Kalchas, and

> striking
> both of them with his staff filled them with powerful valour
> and he made their limbs light, and their feet, and their hands above
>   them,
> and burst into winged flight himself, like a hawk.
>
> [*Iliad*, 13.60–62][26]

Thus what might have been portrayed as each man's firm resolve to fight hard is in fact portrayed as the work of an outside agent. In the dialogue between the heroes and the disguised god, the god/seer encourages them. This passage illustrates an important point in the Homeric presentation of motivation, what has been called Homer's "two-tiered" presentation of motive. Here he presents a divine source and intelligible human sources. Poseidon is the divine source, but the heroes are themselves men of great courage and strength who ordinarily are the sorts of men to encourage themselves and each other. It can be argued that the divine intervention is not really redundant, for Poseidon, or the belief in him, represents a shared ideal, or ideal part of the self, for each of the heroes. From the perspective of individual psychology, we might consider Poseidon as a "projection of a self-representation," that is, a part of the self that is externalized and related to as if it were another person.[27] From the perspective of group psychology, the god is also a representation of something shared, something that unites the group, a common ego ideal of the sort that is extremely important in group process.[28]

This passage also shows Homer's tendency to describe inner life as a kind of personified interchange or interaction between a man and his parts. "The spirit [*thumos*] inside my breast drives me," or "my legs and arms are willing." While Homer can and occasionally does use "I want," "I am eager," and the like, he overwhelmingly prefers to talk of one part of the person doing something to the whole. And so thoughts and feelings are described as initiated by a source other than the person—a god, another human, or a part of the person.

Thus we see two related ways of rendering mental life in Homer: the use of an external person or personified agent to initiate mental activity, and the presentation of the inner mental activity as a series of interchanges. A particularly vivid example is seen when Achilles is driving his chariot to battle to avenge Patroklos. We would expect him, in this situation, to press on to battle and at the same time to be apprehensive about whether or not he will survive the day, knowing he is fated to die young. But observe how Homer portrays his mental state.

Achilles first addresses his steeds, Xanthos and Balios, urging them to bring him back alive and not to leave him dead on the battlefield, as they did Patroklos. Xanthos, enabled to speak by Hera, tells Achilles that he will be spared, but not for long; that they cannot save him, for it is the will of the deity that he die. Achilles replies that he knows his fate but will not "cease before the Trojans have enough of battle" (*Iliad*, 19.4). This portrayal of inner states by means of dialogue is powerful poetry. At the same time it indicates a kind of spilling over of the boundaries of the self, and this aspect has attracted the interest of several classical scholars. Hermann Fränkel in particular has formulated a characterization of Homeric man that captures the essence of this phenomenon.[29] He views Homeric man not as an "I," an ego, a closed and private entity, but rather as an "open force field," having no structural bounds that would help separate it and insulate it from the effects of forces all around it. Lacking structure as it does, it cannot be represented by any coherent, articulated concept of the self; instead we have a collection of parts, *thumos, kradie, phrenes, noos,* as well as limbs, strength (*menos*), courage, and the like, which seem to infuse the various parts. Their sum represents the ego or whole mind, including the man "himself" and his character.

Fränkel argues that the tendency for frequent and sometimes petty interventions of the gods into human affairs is most easily explained in terms of his picture of the Homeric man and is consonant with the Homeric conception of mind as open and unstructured.

Yet, as Fränkel has also pointed out, and as is obvious to any reader of Homer, the characters of the poems are neither puppets nor fragmented men. Though a man has many parts that may move his whole, and though he is subject to external and divine influences, he acts as a whole. The parts are rarely shown in conflict with one another.

This de facto integration and integrity of the character at once differentiates the Homeric view of mental life from the view we find expressed in various kinds of psychopathology, especially extreme forms of psychosis. A schizophrenic may talk of influences from the outside, mysterious forces putting ideas into his mind, people reading his mind, and one part of him telling the rest what to do. Distinctions between inside and outside typically are blurred in the severe psychotic state. But apart from important descriptive and phenomenological differences between the Homeric account and the psychotic account, the most striking difference is the sense of integration and wholeness that attends the Homeric character. The schizophrenic is struggling mightily to keep his integrity and to prevent even further fragmentation and disintegration of the self. While there is much to be learned from a consideration of the similarities among the Homeric (which is in many ways typical of what we have come to call the thinking of "primitives"), the thinking of psychotics, and the thinking of children about mental processes, it is also important to note the differences.[30] The Homeric mode of describing mental life is considered *normal* by the characters in the poem and is presented as such by the poet. In the next section I shall discuss what the Homeric man considers unusual or abnormal in his own terms.

In discussing the issue of the wholeness of the Homeric man, we must remember that he is a man in a group and of a group. No man is alone in Homer. When physically isolated, heroes discourse with human-like agencies—deities, dream figures, or parts of the self. Other people or representations are always intensely present.

In this respect, significant differences may be noted between Homer's two epics. The *Odyssey,* of course, concentrates on one hero, the *Iliad* on several. But even more important, the *Odyssey* is the story of a man who is threatened with extinction and with the danger of being stripped of all that defines the Homeric hero as an individual. Odysseus is the hero who proclaims himself "no man." He is repeatedly either disguised or bearing a false identity or withholding his true one.[31] Washed up on the shore of Phaeacia, he is naked and starving, threatened with death, close to oblivion. The *Odyssey* is in many ways a poem of inwardness, as we can see in the descriptions of certain mental processes. Decision making in the *Odyssey* is typically a debate within the hero, or between parts of himself, rather than the intervention of a god who makes the decision for him. To be sure, we find examples of both kinds of decision making in both poems, but the emphasis differs.[32] All in all, the *Odyssey* focuses far more than the *Iliad* on what it is to be in danger of isolation from one's group, whether the group consist of comrades, family, or the human race. Odysseus is not only alone, he is a loner. In fact, Odysseus is portrayed as though he were an only child.[33] In a sense, the portrait of Odysseus is consonant with the sense of inwardness that appears in Greek lyric poetry and later in tragedy.

It is important to remind ourselves that in attempting to analyze the inner lives of Homer's heroes we cannot go beyond a description of his words and the manner in which he presents their experience. We simply cannot know the inner experience of mental life for the heroes who lived in Mycenaean times or for the audience that listened to the Homeric tales.

Disturbances of Mental Life and Behavior

At the opening of Book 23 of the *Odyssey,* the faithful old nurse Eurykleia runs to tell her mistress, Penelope, that Odysseus has returned and has killed the suitors. Penelope, who has been asleep, is incredulous at first and answers (ll. 11–16):

> Dear nurse, the gods have driven you crazy [*margēn*]. They are both
>   able
> to change a very sensible person into a senseless
> one, and to set the light-wit on the way of discretion [*saophrosunēs*].
> They have set you awry; before now your thoughts were orderly.
> Why do you insult me when my heart is heavy with sorrows,
> by talking in this wild way [*parex ereousa*]. . . ?

Thus the description of disturbed mental activity follows along the same lines as the description of more ordinary mental states. "The gods have driven you crazy." This is quite typical of the language used to describe someone who is acting, according to the speaker, a bit "touched in the head." It is typical too that the poet does not describe a floridly psychotic state, but rather uses language not unlike "You must be crazy to think that . . ." In contrast to characters in the tragedies, no one in the poems is considered out-and-out mad.

The incidental vocabulary here, however, certainly suggests the obvious—that the poet and the audience know about mad people and madness.

Overall, there is no notion that mental disturbances arise from a disorder or derangement within a mental structure, since there is no notion of a structure. Nor can one detect evidence of a concept that an alteration in the relationships of different parts of the mind is a cause of mental disturbance or tension. Homer certainly describes situations of internal conflict, generally between one impulse and another, with both oriented toward an action. A conflict characteristic of the *Odyssey* concerns the timing of action: now or later? Such a conflict occurs at the beginning of Book 20, where Odysseus is torn between the impulse to kill the suitors now, while they are sleeping with the servant girls, and the sober thought of waiting to form a more systematic plan.

Though no frank madness erupts in the poems, we find important situations of tension, conflict, and behavior that seem to go against the best interests of the heroes. In the *Iliad* the "wrath of Achilles," which is destructive to the Greeks, the Trojans, and Achilles himself, is traced to the "plan of Zeus" and the interactions of the heroes and the gods. In the *Odyssey* Penelope's suitors are blinded by Athena to their coming destruction by Odysseus, but they have plenty of motivated folly of their own.

Another disturbance prominent in the *Odyssey* is excessive forgetting.[34] Throughout the poem Odysseus is in danger of being made to forget his homeland, his wife and son, his very identity. The Lotus Eaters, Calypso, Circe, and the Sirens threaten oblivion. Here too, as in the description of ordinary mental activity, agents (including deities) act on the person, and the person passively receives these influences.

Dodds, in the first chapter of *The Greeks and the Irrational*, elaborates on the notion of *atē*, infatuation, in the Homeric poems. In Book 1 of the *Iliad*, the quarrel between Agamemnon and Achilles is dramatized. A plague has struck the Greeks, and the prophet declares that the Greeks are suffering because Agamemnon has taken captive the daughter of a priest of Apollo. Agamemnon reluctantly agrees to return her, thereby averting the wrath of Apollo (who has sent the plague). He demands, however, that he be given in recompense Achilles' girl captive, Briseis. Achilles is furious, and in the public assembly he begins to draw his sword to kill Agamemnon, but he is restrained by Athena, who promises that he will be rewarded three times for the loss. All of this means a terrible loss of face and of *timē*, honor, for Achilles (while Agamemnon fears the loss of his *timē* if he yields to Achilles). Achilles decides to withdraw from the battle and the Greeks suffer tremendous losses. He refuses offers of recompense and reconciliation until his friend Patroklos, wearing Achilles' armor, has been slain in battle. Finally (Book 19) Agamemnon offers Achilles a formal apology and munificent gifts; Achilles relents. The gist of the scene in Book 19 is that Agamemnon, in his zeal to save his own status and *timē*, has brought tremendous loss of life to his own army. He explains now that the responsibility lies not with him but with Zeus, Destiny, and Erinys. "What could I do? It is the god who accomplishes all things" (19.90). He then tells how Zeus was deluded (*asato*, a verb form of *atē*) by Hera when she arranged for Heracles to be born after Eurystheus, who later forced him to undergo his famous labors.[35] Zeus was enraged when he found out Hera's tricks and

> swore a strong oath that never
> after this might Delusion, who deludes all, come back
> to Olympos and the starry sky. So speaking, he whirled her
> about in his hand and slung her out of the starry
> heaven, and presently she came to men's establishments.
>
> [*Iliad*, 19.127–31]

Thus a bevy of deities—Zeus, Fate and the avenging Fury, and the goddess Atē—were involved in deluding Agamemnon. Even the gods were once able to be deluded, but Zeus threw Atē out of Olympus and now she hovers over the heads of men to bring them troubles.

Dodds has placed this kind of apology and exoneration in the framework of the adaptive needs of a culture where shame and public loss of face are important. The role of Delusion (Atē) is to serve as a socially acceptable explanation of how a great chief (even a great god) can do something stupid and destructive. We shall return to Dodds's explanation and argue that, while essentially correct, it does not go far enough.[36] The ubiquity of divine intervention, including the use of Atē in nonexotic situations, requires something more than the notion of a face-saving device in a shame culture.

In later Greek literature, *atē* does have the sense of a snare and a delusion, but also more generally of the fate and downfall appropriate to someone who has done a serious wrong. The Erinyes, whom Agamemnon accuses, become a major carrier of actual insanity, particularly in the tragedies built around the story of Orestes, who murdered his mother.

It is worth asking why clinical insanity does not occur in Homer when it is frequent in the tragedies. Madness was undoubtedly known to the poet and his audience, but it is likely that the literary and narrative purposes of the poet did not require the portrayal of mad heroes. We do not know, however, if the versions of the myths in which a hero goes mad were available to Homer; if they were, he chose not to use them. It is also possible that Homer suppressed such tales as unseemly. Scholars have pointed out numerous instances where Homer either ignored or suppressed mention of various magic rituals, superstitions, and the like which must have been known in his day.

It is difficult to decide this issue, but one can see a certain continuity between Homer and tragedy in the language of madness. *Mania* and *lussa* and their cognates denote in Homer primarily the raving frenzy of battle and of warriors. In tragedy they are the principal terms for madness. *Lussa* and *mania* personified are portrayed in vase paintings.[37] *Lussa,* incidentally, is probably related to *luk,* wolf, and so in Homer it might connote the ferocity of a wild animal.[38]

Apart from this continuity of vocabulary, an episode in Book 6 of the Iliad involves three figures who in later traditions were considered victims of madness but who in Homer were afflicted with blindness, loneliness, and foolishness, which might be considered the equivalents of madness. The passage as a whole is worth considering both because of its relation to later cases of madness and because it illustrates the tensions to which Homeric heroes are subject.

The scene is fierce battle; the Greeks are winning, though the Trojans are rallying. Diomedes, among the mightiest of the Greeks, is raging in battle. He encounters Glaukos, a Trojan; each admires and fears the prowess of the other. Diomedes asks Glaukos who he is and what his origins are, since he fears he may be an immortal in disguise. Having once fought unsuccessfully against a goddess, Diomedes feels that to risk such an encounter again would be the height of folly.[39] He tells the story of Lykourgos, who attacked the god Dionysus and was blinded, to illustrate the danger. By the fifth century, Lykourgos's punishment had become madness, a version represented in several (lost) tragedies and in vase paintings.[40] Thus Lykourgos blind seems equivalent to Lykourgos mad.

Glaukos replies that it is useless to inquire about his generation:

> As is the generation of leaves, so is that of humanity.
> The wind scatters the leaves on the ground, but the live timber
> burgeons with leaves again in the season of the spring returning.
> So one generation of men will grow while another dies.
> [*Iliad,* 6.146–49]

He continues with his genealogy. He is the grandson of Bellerophon, who slew the Chimaera. Bellerophon, falsely accused of trying to seduce a king's wife, was sent on missions from which he was not expected to return. Finally winning the king's favor, he marries his daughter and seems, for a while, to be favored by the gods.

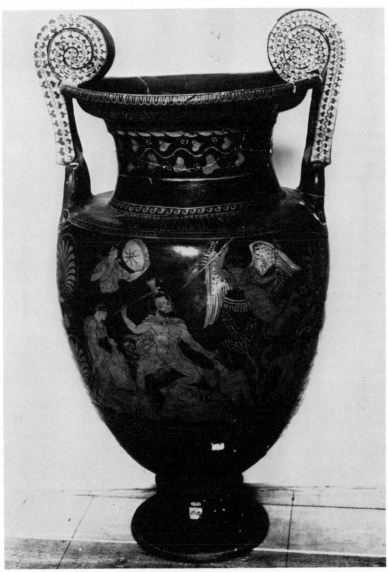

The madness of Lykourgos. Lykourgos, driven mad because he opposed the worship of Dionysus, has already killed his son, Dryas (left), and is about to slay his wife. Lyssa, the winged goddess with goad, is creating the delusion that his wife and child are vines that he is to cut down. At upper left is a Maenad with tambourine, an allusion to the role of Dionysus in the story.

Lucanian volute krater, c. 360–350 B.C. Museo Nazionale, Naples. Photograph of the Office of Antiquity of the Province of Naples and Caserta.

But he too became hateful to all the gods,
And alone wandered over the Alean plain [the plain of wandering],
Consuming his own heart, shunning the pathways of men.

[*Iliad*,6.200–202]

Now in later tradition, Bellerophon is listed as a melancholic (see Chapter 12). How or why this transformation was made is not clear, since Homer calls him neither blind (like Lykourgos) nor mad. Probably the figure of a man wandering in isolated places, all alone, suggests a madman. For the Greeks (as epitomized in Homer), a man without a group is not a man.[41]

These myths, inserted in the speeches of the two warriors when they encounter each other, warn that either opposition to the gods or merely their caprice can destory the mightiest of men. It is with some relief that the two antagonists discover that they are related by ancient ties of guest-host friendship: an ancestor of Diomedes had entertained Bellerophon, Glaukos's grandfather. They agree not to fight each other, but to exchange gifts and seek opportunities to fight with other antagonists. Glaukos, however, exchanges gold armor for bronze, because Zeus "stole away his wits." Matchless in war, he is fooled in gift giving. His father sent him off to war with the injunction

always to excel [to be *aristos*] and to be superior to all
others, and not to bring shame to the race of your fathers,
who were by far the noblest in Ephyre and in wide Lykia.

[*Iliad*, 6.208–210][42]

Thus we have a sequence that unfolds the tensions and dilemmas of the Homeric hero. He must excel at all times, be the best in battle, lest he disgrace his ancestors. At the same time he must not exceed himself, for it is dangerous to overreach and enter into combat with a god. Thus the hero must constantly check his own prowess. Latent in this set of injunctions is the dual admonition not to disgrace the father by poor performance and not to risk the dangers of surpassing him. Next, though the heroes must fight, they also must recognize and maintain the nexus of guest-host relationships that provide a check on their readiness for continuous warfare. Yet even in this relationship, which relaxes hostilities, they must take care to exchange gifts shrewdly. Glaukos fails in part, and it can only be because the gods took away his wits. Presumably Glaukos's foolishness is venial and does not signify that he has seriously violated the thrust of his father's injunction. But the passage suggests the narrow line that a hero of an aristocratic warrior culture must tread. Later Sophocles will give us in Ajax an example of how failure to live up to social (and parental) requirements and to avoid *hubris* leads to the kind of shame that generates murder, madness, and suicide.

Perhaps the answer to why Homer at most only hints at madness can be found in the epic form, which has certain capabilities that the tragic does not. Epic allows for an unending story, and so greater potential for action. As long as a hero can act (which means fight) he does not have to go mad. Glaukos can fight elsewhere. Tragedy requires situations in which action either is blocked or has shattering consequences that cannot be undone. Epic time is never ending; tragic time is short and intense, and allows no return.

There is a curious corollary of the fact that irrationality, as it appears in the poems, is basically caused by the gods, namely, the assumption of a rationality in the gods or in the universe. The gods may choose sides, have passions and strong feelings, but they also have their plans and schemes. Thus if a man acts irrationally, it is because a god is carrying out a carefully calculated plan to help one hero and hurt another. There is a method to human madness and human folly, but the method belongs to the mind of the god. As we shall see in a later chapter, madness in tragedy is still linked to explicit divine intervention. The link between human madness and divine rationality remains, but tragedy carries the link a step further. Tragedy presents a more sharply focused picture of the gods as integral parts of the hero's character.

Several centuries after Homer, Plato constructed a model of the mind in which it is seen as a battlefield with several warring parties. Madness is the victory of one party, the wild impulsive part of the mind. Thus the assumption remains that madness is a result of intentionality, though here the intentionality belongs to one party within the person rather than to a god. It is important to bear in mind that the assumption that intentionality underlies madness is central to all later psychodynamic theories of mental disturbance. All these theories posit personified agents within the person intent on pursuing their own interests. Madness and folly are caused by the fifth columns and Trojan horses within each of us, powerful forces that will attempt to subvert or destroy in order to carry out their mission. The nature of these forces and the details of their composition, origin, and location are seen as variable. There must be reasons why one age or culture emphasizes an external location while another locates them within the individual.

Let us turn now to the way Homer presents relief for the hero's distress and redress for his folly and irrationality. The Homeric hero, as I have suggested, is beset not only by external perils but by the ever present danger that he will not live up to the stringent demands of the heroic code. What, short of total victory, can relieve or console him, for no one in the poems is always and everywhere a victor? The answer is words, words that give meaning to the hero's distress.

These words emphasize that there is a rationality behind seeming irrationality or caprice, and this rationality provides consolation.

Relief for Distress

Just as the sources of mental distress, including apparently irrational behavior, are presented as external to the individual, so are relief and cure seen as originating from outside. The gods, who can relieve distress as readily as they can cause it, are the most obvious source of relief. Drugs, wine, food, sex, and friendship can also help. But, to the extent that there is a professional who administers relief, it is the poet.

As we have seen, no one in Homer thinks by himself, but rather engages in an interaction or dialogue, be it with another person, with a god, or with a part of himself. Relief, too, comes in an interactional setting.

The ideal relief for the hero is action, usually revenge. But revenge is seldom immediately feasible, and the hero must wait. Thus when Achilles threatens Agamemnon, Athena tells him to wait. Then she comforts him with the promise of threefold restitution for his loss. When Agamemnon does take Achilles' woman, he becomes not only angry but sorrowful (*Iliad,* 1.349–430). He goes alone and weeping to the shore but is soon joined by his mother, Thetis, a sea nymph, to whom he has prayed. He complains that his short life deserves an extra portion of honor, not Agamemnon's abuse. (Achilles is the "child" in the *Iliad;* he has with him his mother and his childhood tutor, Phoenix.) Thetis comforts him as he tells the story of the insult. He extracts from her the promise, which she will fulfill, that she will use her influence with Zeus to punish Agamemnon and avenge his dishonor by causing the death of many Achaeans. Agamemnon is forced by the Greek setback to plead with Achilles to return to the fray.

As I have emphasized, the Homeric epics contain no frank madness. The main problems are those embedded in the story line itself. The wrath of Achilles, for instance, is not only the theme of the *Iliad,* it is the principal disturbance from which Achilles suffers. Achilles' wrath is not called a disease, but it is a disruption in the order of things, a powerful source of disequilibrium in the social order. The poem opens with his wrath and proceeds to show its dire consequences for Achilles, for the Greeks, for Patroklos, and finally for the Trojans. His wrath against Agamemnon is finally assuaged in the course of the events following Patroklos's death, but toward the Trojans Achilles remains implacable.

As the last book of the *Iliad* opens, we see Achilles still distraught, even after Patroklos has been buried and funeral games have been held, after he has obtained restitution from Agamemnon and many Trojans have been slaughtered. Achilles' grief and sleeplessness force him once more to drag Hector's body around Patroklos's tomb. This book is a dramatic tour de force and a powerful resolution of the tensions of the poem as a whole. But we can also see in it a working through and resolution of Achilles' wrath and grief. Side by side with this sequence of change in Achilles, we see his poignant interchange with Priam, which finally allows Priam too some resolution of his mourning for Hector. Thus Achilles and Priam, each in his own way and then in a moving scene of mutual admiration, are relieved of their burdens. In this scene of two people working through enormous emotional pain, we can speak of therapy and can examine in some detail how it takes place.

Achilles has carried things too far—this is the message with which Book 24 opens. The gods and goddesses debate his refusal to give up the body of Hector for proper burial and bemoan his maniacal drive (*phresi mainomenis*) to abuse the body. Achilles has destroyed pity and has no sense of shame or reverence. At the same time, it is clear that Achilles imagines that Patroklos will not allow him to rest. He cannot eat, sleep, or take pleasure in a woman.

The gods are explicit in their diagnosis—Achilles does not know how to grieve and to relinquish grief.

> For a man must some day lose one who was even closer
> than this [Patroklos], a brother from the same womb,
>   or a son.
>   And yet
>   he weeps for him, and sorrows for him, and then it
>   is over.   [*Iliad,* 24.46–48]

In technical psychiatric terms, this is a state of pathological grief, a state of mourning that cannot run its course.[43] "Mourning" is, of course, a feeble term, scarcely adequate for the immensity of agony and suffering that Achilles inflicts on others and endures himself.

Priam, for his part, has been nearly destroyed by Hector's death. Unable to eat, drink, or sleep, he lies in the courtyard and covers himself with dust and dung. Clearly he will die of grief and can be saved only by the return of Hector's corpse for funeral rites and mourning. (Remember that Achilles, when he heard of Patroklos's death, rolled in the dust, and his companions feared that he could commit suicide [*Iliad,* 18.22–34].)

As is typical in Homer, the problem is worked out on two levels, divine and human. Parallel to Achilles' unrelenting rage is Hera's unrelenting bitterness and quest for revenge against the Trojans. She cannot forgive Paris and the Trojans for judging her less beautiful than Aphrodite. Zeus stills her wrath and forbids her further interference. He points out that it is unseemly to be angry forever; all the other gods are able to pity Hector. Hera yields to Zeus's plan to summon Thetis and urge her to instruct her son to return Hector's corpse for ransom. Thetis is herself in mourning for her son, who is destined to die soon. The gods and goddesses welcome her to Olympus and offer her solace. In effect, she must be relieved of enough of her own grief to be able to allow Achilles to ransom the body, and finally to relinquish his grief.

The gods agree on Zeus's plan.[44] Iris, the divine messenger, will instruct Priam to go to Achilles' tent, with Hermes as guide; Thetis will convey to her son the divine injunction that he return the body.[45] Thus, at a divine level, there must be some relinquishment of bitterness, acceptance of the limits of rage, and a firm reestablishment of pity. How does this take place at the human level?

Iris has commanded Priam to go to Achilles' tent. Hecuba, distraught at the prospect, accuses him of being mad or a fool or possessed (*daimonie*). She herself is unrelentingly bitter and announces that, were she to have the opportunity to capture Achilles, she would eat his liver raw. Priam must ignore her rage. He assembles the ransom and arrives at Achilles' camp.

Here some of the most moving interchanges of the entire poem are to be found, centering around two kinds of frank recognition. The first is that of the enmity between the two men, and the second, more compelling because of the first, is their common humanity. Hermes has urged Priam to entreat Achilles in the name of his father, mother, and child. Priam enters and supplicates the man who has slain Hector and so many of his other sons. Achilles and his companions stare at him in amazement, as they might stare at a fugitive who sought asylum after killing a man in his own country. This amazement is the beginning of a rapprochement between Achilles and Priam which will end with their gazing rapturously in amazement at one another (24.629–32). Priam asks Achilles to think of his own aged father, Peleus, yearing to see his only son, and in doing so to pity the father of Hector. This appeal moves Achilles, stirring in him "a passion of grieving for his own father."

> He took the old man's hand and pushed him
> gently away, and the two remembered, as Priam sat huddled
> at the feet of Achilleus and wept close for manslaughtering Hektor
> and Achilleus wept now for his own father, now again
> for Patroklos. [*Iliad*, 24.508–512]

Achilles is moved to pity (a term used frequently in Book 24) and explains how suffering comes from the gods and is the common lot of mankind, Greek and Trojan alike. But endless grief will not bring back the dead. Achilles arranged to have Hector's corpse properly washed and anointed and laid out. After he had lifted the corpse onto a litter,

> he groaned then, and called by name on his beloved companion:
> "Be not angry with me, Patroklos, if you discover,
> though you be in the house of Hades, that I gave back great Hector
> to his loved father, for the ransom he gave me was not unworthy.
> I will give you your share of the spoils, as much as is fitting."
>
> [*Iliad*, 24.591–95]

In these lines we see Achilles working through his grief and need for revenge. Out of a realization of the humanity he shares with Priam (and Hector with Patroklos), he puts aside the guilt, shame, and sense of outrage he has been nurturing.

He can now turn to the needs of Priam. He urges him to eat, knowing full well what it must mean for the old man to accept food from his son's killer. In order to have him eat and relinquish his grief, he proceeds, in typical Homeric fashion, to tell a story, the tale of Niobe. Her children had been slain by divine wrath when she claimed that they were more beautiful than Apollo and Artemis, "but she remembered to eat when she was worn out with weeping" (24.613). This tale within a tale, an epyllion within an epic, is an important device of consolation and restitution for the characters in the poem.

The use of a myth accomplishes several ends. In its manifest content it demonstrates how even the most grief-stricken parent allowed herself the comfort of eating. It contains the implicit injunction to follow the example of the gods and demigods of long ago. It is an invitation to the consolation of seeing oneself as part of a larger scheme.

A subtler aspect of this story comes closer to the core of the process of psychotherapy. Achilles offers Priam more than support and comfort and reinstatement in the order of things. As is often the case in Homer, comparisons are multifaceted and have several meanings. For instance, if Homer likens Priam to Niobe, suggesting that he has a maternal side, Achilles is likened to Apollo. Achilles, however, is also a grieving parent, in that he has lost someone dear to him. Priam is thus both a destroyer (via his son) and the distraught parent. As Achilles nurtures Priam in both a paternal and maternal way, Priam is allowed a transient regression to a childlike position. One could demonstrate still other overtones, but the important point is that the tale allows for several simultaneous identifications for both Priam and Achilles: male and female, destroyer and destroyed, parent and child, active and passive, bereaver and bereaved. Thus the experience (transient and largely unconscious) of a number of identifications allows one a more thorough working through of profound sorrow and distress. These multiple identifications not only allow a new integration but constitute a certain enlargement of the humanity of the characters. Something more than persuasion is involved, something that reverberates in deeper layers of the soul. This use of the story as a part of therapy within the poem is also a paradigm for the poem's therapeutic effect on the listener.

We see evidence that the story has been effective therapy for both Achilles and Priam: they eat. They then join in admiration of each other. Finally Priam requests that Achilles set up a place for him to sleep, for he has not slept since he learned of Hector's death. Achilles, anxious that Priam's "heart might have no fear," provides a resting place and assures him of a truce to allow twelve days for the mourning, cremation, and funeral rites for Hector. Priam sleeps, and then Achilles goes to sleep, lying at the side of his beloved Briseis.

Thus we see how Homer has elaborated a complex picture of what is needed to resolve the turmoil and sorrow of the human heart. Action alone does not suffice; discharge of emotions is not enough. The acceptance of a common humanity and a common mortality begins to achieve some therapeutic effect. At first it only allows Priam and Achilles to mourn at the same time, separately, each for his own sorrows. But the realization that each can empathize with the other brings them closer and allows for something more than pity to surface. Finally, both the disease called the "wrath of Achilles" and the implacable grief of Priam are brought to some resolution by a profound realization not only that each can be in the other's place but that each has within him parts of all others: man and woman, mother and father, parent and child, sister and brother, friend and foe, beast and human.

The essential features of the kind of therapy we see emerging within the poems can be summarized: (1) It is initiated from outside the person. (2) It involves or is initiated by a divine agency. (3) It involves an emphasis on the place of the individual within his group, defined as those now alive, his forebears, and his posterity. (4) The disease represents the hero's falling out with the social order. He also disrupts the social equilibrium of others. (5) Frequently, by means of a tale within a tale, the disorder is defined in terms of the larger social order as a recognizable disorder. (6) The cure is provided by a socially available model and precedent for ways to handle distress or despair. (7) The help is made effective not only by the support and intervention of other people or gods but by the process of "working through," whereby the afflicted person can get in touch with inner identifications and parts of himself which had previously not been available or allowed.[46]

It can be readily seen that some of these points can apply equally to the experience of the audience that hears (or reads) these poems, that individuals in that audience, or the audience as a group, can find relief from their own tensions and distress with the aid of the story. But before we can elaborate further on this issue, we must turn to an investigation of the relationship among poem, poet, and audience.

5

Epic as Therapy

... for though a man have sorrow and grief in his newly-troubled soul, and live in dread because his heart is distressed, yet when a singer, the servant of the Muses, chants the glorious deeds of men of old and the blessed gods who inhabit Olympus, at once he forgets his heaviness and remembers not his sorrows at all.
—Hesiod, *Theogony* [1]

Sleep, baby, sleep,
Thy father watches the sheep,
Thy mother shakes the dreamland tree,
And down falls a little dream on thee. . . .
—Traditional Lullaby

The singing of lullabies and the telling of stories are surely among the oldest and most universal of uniquely human activites. Perhaps we shall never know how they arose or the precise biological function they served. But who among us has not understood from earliest childhood the soothing power of song and tale? If we were to seek the precursor of all art and therapy, we might plausibly look to these early enchantments between mother and child. Certainly the very form of the poetic performance affords a tangible, bodily pleasure, especially in cultures where song and poetic performance are institutionalized and ritualized parts of daily living. [2] The rhythm, the music, the familiar structure of the poem must evoke memories and feelings referable to the early childhood experience of being held by, sung to, and comforted by the mother. The very familiarity of the story must carry a measure of comfort and reassurance. Its contents awaken, intensify, and clarify certain feelings within the listener. In ways we do not fully understand, the experience of the tale also permits a release of painful emotions. If this release is to take place, the story must be about people sufficiently like ourselves that we may identify with them and their plights. But the characters must not be so like us that, unable to distance ourselves, we identify with them too literally. The good storyteller regulates both the degree to which his listeners participate in the tale and the degree to which they observe the action.

Undoubtedly participation with an audience, even an imagined one (as when we read a story), can be a source of consolation. We are not alone in our sorrows; others have felt as we do and may even share our private grief. The shared experience of listening to a tale that expresses the group's fundamental values, beliefs, and aspirations serves to restore us to and reintegrate us with that group.

The poets have always known about their ability to heal sorrow. We should not be surprised to find Hesiod, in the seventh century B.C., singing of the power of epic song to comfort and bring blessed forgetfulness of pain.

Where does the healing power of the story lie—particularly a story embedded in such an elaborate work as an epic poem? It cannot lie only in the story's lulling and narcotic effects, important as they are.

The poetic performance invites the individual to rejoin the larger community and to use the communal, socially valued pathways for definition and release of tensions. The poem allows each person to redefine and restore his relationship to his family, his clan, his ancestors and gods, and ultimately all human beings.

I have also alluded to another aspect of the story as therapy in my discussion of the tale within a tale: the possibility of multiple identifications with the positions and plights of various characters, which enlarges our potential for self-expression and self-realization. Especially in such a genre as the epic, the characters are heroes, and insofar as we can identify with them, we may momentarily share their heroism and again get in touch with our heroic ideals.

All of these considerations apply to some extent to all storytelling, in every age and culture. Here, however, we must consider some features of the Homeric poems more relevant to their healing power, and so increase our understanding of the way in which mind and mental distress are portrayed in the poems; that is to say, the Homeric model of mind and mental illness. I believe that Homeric psychology, the Homeric view of mental life, is embedded in the form, composition, and presentation of the poetry—an argument that has not been developed in classical scholarship.[3]

The argument rests on two important features of the Homeric epics: that they are traditional and that, in some sense, they are orally composed. The view that these two features are, in effect, synonymous—that is, that traditional is necessarily oral—is known among Homeric scholars as the Parry-Lord hypothesis.

Let us begin with some general features of heroic epic poetry. First, it is traditional in form. Certain phrases, a special elevated diction, certain episodes (for instance, kinds of battles), and a certain meter characterize such poetry. The effect of the traditional language and format of the tale is to present even quite recent events as though they were part of the heroic past. Creating a past of its own, heroic poetry does not reproduce, it idealizes.

This poetry defines and presents in pristine form the ideals of the culture, especially its aristocratic and heroic ideals. Thus, though the story is set in a particular time, its ideals are timeless. Heroic epic at once derives from a traditional heritage and transmits it to the next generation.

Next, I would argue that orally composed poetry makes use of and gives expression to archaic modes of thought, often called primitive thinking. Its archaism lies in the fact that it is characteristic of earlier epochs of the human race and of each individual (childhood), and of the processes of unconscious thinking in adults.

In general terms, it appears that the Homeric model of mind I have outlined would be highly adaptive and well suited to the communal need to preserve certain time-honored values and archaic ways of thinking. This model of mind emphasizes the communal and collective rather than the individual, the public rather than the private and idiosyncratic, the intensive and constant interpenetration of the life of each person with the lives of the other members of the group. It also emphasizes the influence that people (and divine agents) exert on each other and plays down the autonomy of each individual. Such a public and traditional model of mind serves to buttress a sense of continuity from generation to generation; it is less useful for a society that wishes to perpetuate the ideal of change from one generation to the next. It is important for a conservative culture that "mind" be accessible to traditional influences.[4] In this context one sees the importance of the gods as causes and initiators of mental activity, for the gods embody what is considered oldest and most valued.

Heroic poetry arises when heroic values and the aristocratic structure of the culture are under threat and undergoing change.[5] It is an attempt to reverse the flow of time and to assert the importance of values less viable than they once had been. It is likely, then, that heroic epic is not so ancient in any culture as it purports to be. Since the cultures that have produced heroic epic tend (with exceptions) not to have written history, however, this idea cannot be proved.

Let us turn to the work of Parry and Lord.[6] Milman Parry was an American classical scholar whose work is a landmark of twentieth-century Homeric studies. In 1928, after several years' study in France, Parry published the first of his works on Homer, *L'epithète traditionelle dans Homère*. He began with an examination of a feature of the poetry that is at once apparent even to the most casual reader—the prolific use of fixed epithets. He argued that these epithets, or formulae, are not embellishments or ornamental archaisms, but rather are a central feature of the poems' construction. In that thesis he laid down the beginnings of several ideas that would become more explicit in his later works, principally his idea that the Homeric poems are constructed by heavy, if not exclusive, reliance on a variety of stable and traditional formulae. He eventually argued that almost every phrase in the poem represented, in some form, a formula; these formulas may be precise phrases (as the epithets are) or syntactic or metrical-syntactic sequences.[7] Certain phrases, or their metrical and syntactic equivalents, for instance, can occur only at certain points in the line. Thus, he argued, the Homeric poems, far more than anyone had previously imagined, are constructed of certain standard linguistic and metrical building blocks. Formulas, in this sense, are familiar to us from fairy tales, folktales, and the Bible. Every fairy tale begins with "Once upon a time" or "Long, long ago," and the child who insists that a story begun some other way is not a proper story is well within his rights. Parry also assumed that since these elements are traditional, they are subject to stringent rules against change and modification. The third step in his argument (not fully explicit in his first work) is that poetry composed so extensively of formulae is not only traditional but orally composed. Written poetry, let alone prose, he argued, betrays its origins by virtue of its being less formulaic than oral poetry. He attempted to show that even the Alexandrian Greek epic known as the *Argonautica,* a conscious imitation of Homer, showed slight but consistent differences from the Homeric poems in its use of formulae and in formulaic use of meter.

Parry's arguments were at first based almost entirely on the internal evidence of the Homeric poems, but later he began to study oral poetry as composed and performed in rural Yugoslavia, where he found storytellers in nonliterate sections of the society. Comparison between them and the Homeric bards was, he felt, valid. This work, conducted with and later extended by Albert Lord, led to the notion that in true oral compositon, traditional thematic motifs are skillfully woven to make a plot. Lord's ideas extended the concept of the formula to include traditional storytelling motifs, the building blocks of the extended tale. This concept implies that oral poets do not have to memorize poems, but rather have to master the *units* and learn to assemble them.

Although some controversy has surrounded this hypothesis, I agree with those scholars who assert that Parry and Lord have demonstrated an oral, formulaic, and traditional character for the Homeric poems, though not necessarily that the received *Iliad* and *Odyssey* were composed under the conditions of oral composition and performance which they studied in Yugoslavia.[8]

What degree of originality and poetic creativity can we allow

Homer? Parry and, to some extent, Lord do not answer this question, but rather emphasize how much of Homer is best understood as following from the requirements of tradition. They tend to see the choice of epithet as traditional and as metrically required. Other scholars emphasize, and I believe rightly, that the epithets are skillfully used and carefully chosen for their dramatic relevance. At the least, the traditional epithets are skillfully exploited by the poet.[9] The Homeric poet was probably highly innovative and creative within his own tradition and perhaps even was considered innovative or, more likely, great because he was so quintessentially traditional.

In Homer and later Greek tradition (and in the creations of other cultures that twentieth-century students of oral literature have examined),[10] one can see that the poet does not memorize a poem that he has composed in private, nor does he recite from memory a poem he has learned from someone else. He composes more or less on the spot, in front of his audience. He is able to do so because he has a large repertoire of traditional themes, language, and meter. The implication is that there is no "received text" of the poem. If several poets are asked to sing the tale of the homecoming of Odysseus, their songs are likely to vary considerably. Further (and here the evidence from Yugoslavia is convincing), no poet sings the tale in the same way at each performance.[11]

An analogy close to our own experience is the fundamentalist or revivalist sermon, especially one directed to an audience of limited literacy. The preacher takes a familiar biblical passage and draws not only upon the familiar tales and themes but upon language traditional to sermons. The audience influences the composition of each sermon. In every sermon the preacher must strike a balance between tradition and innovation.

The audience plays an important role in oral composition. An author of written works may always have some audience in mind, but he does not have before him one he must satisfy then and there. The poet, as it were, negotiates with his audience. He must tell a tale that will please his listeners in a manner that will interest them. Some of this is of course conscious. An extreme example comes from Lord's Yugoslavian studies: a bard who sings a battle story in both Christian and Moslem districts will make either the Crusaders or the Turks victorious, depending on the religion of his audience.[12] At a more automatic and unconscious level, the mood and the mind of the audience and of the performer become closely interwoven. Havelock has offered the example of a jazz performance where a minimally fixed score is used. The music played has much to do with the "vibes" that pass between musician and audience. If the performance is to be successful, rapport and mutual sensitivity must develop between audience and performer. Here too innovation and tradition play their parts. The performer must satisfy both his and the audience's needs for a blend of the familiar and the different. The bard must know how to read his audiences' wishes.

If the poetic performance goes well, the audience becomes immersed in the story and identifies with the characters. Similarly, the poet must lose himself in the telling and blur the boundaries between himself and his characters. Here too a delicate balance is necessary—both poet and audience must be more deeply immersed in the tale at some times than at others. Devices are available to help regulate this movement in and out of the poem. One device that brings the audience close is the poem within a poem—a scene in which a bard performs before an audience.[13] Another is a reminder by one character that what all of them are now doing "will be a song for men in time to come."[14] This device too brings the audience close and sets up an infinite regress.

E. A. Havelock has provided us with a vivid reconstruction of the audience's experience.[15] He stresses the strong element of sensuous pleasure for both poet and audience in the physical act of poetic recitation. The poet commits his lungs, larynx, and tongue, his arms, and a whole set of bodily reflexes to the act of rhythmic production. The listener finds the experience perhaps even more emotionally absorbing and gratifying than does the performer; he is involved through his ears and eyes and responds with his mind and entire nervous system. It is the extreme pleasurableness of the physical participation in a recital that makes it such an effective learning process. This level of gratification enhances the possibilities for bard and audience to become absorbed into the poem. In a sense, the experience of audience and poet can be considered an artistically controlled blurring of boundaries of the self or as a series of transient experiences of merging with the poem and with its characters. To reap the benefits of the poem, we must "lose ourselves."[16]

The Greek tradition gives us some explicit statements about the way the bard conceptualizes his activity, though we cannot deduce his inner experience from these statements alone. He is the servant of the Muse, who breathes into him and teaches him. Both *Iliad* and *Odyssey* begin with invocations to the Muse. The bard is an instrument upon which the Muse plays to produce a song. The poet sees himself not as an autonomous creator of original poetry but as one who has received a gift from or has been inspired by external sources.[17] These sources may be divine (the Muse) or human (his teachers). It is not only his "inspiration" that comes from without but his very craft and skill. The Heliconian Muses both "breathed into" Hesiod (*Theogony*, l. 31) and "taught him" (l. 22). Hesiod's belief in the extrinsic source and quality of his song is paralleled by the attitudes of the Yugoslav bards interviewed by Lord. The bards may state that they are singing the same song exactly as they learned it, although an observer can detect many differences in detail from performance to performance. Little allowance is made for or importance attached to the mental gifts or idiosyncrasies of the bard as prime factors in the creation of the poetry.[18] There is no place even for the notion of composition. From the bard's viewpoint, he does not compose and then perform his composition; he simply reproduces the song as it is. Thus we see again, in the attitude the bard takes to his own role, the irresistible tendency to favor external over internal determinants of mental activity. In this formulation of bard-audience interaction, the form of the poem is defined as the poem-as-performed. The "gift of song," the song, and the performance are not clearly distinguished conceptually or operationally.

Some three centuries after Hesiod, Plato wrote an account of the experience of the poetic performance. In the *Ion,* Socrates addresses a rhapsode, a professional reciter of Homer. The rhapsode is not the oral epic bard I have been discussing but rather a man who recites a written text from memory. Nevertheless, Socrates' words to him are relevant to the situation of bard and audience. He says (533D–533E):

This gift . . . you have is not an art, but . . . an inspiration. . . . The Muse . . . first gives to men inspiration herself; and from these inspired persons a chain of other persons is suspended who take inspiration from them. . . . Do you know that the spectator is the last of the rings which as I am saying derive their power from the original magnet?   [*Ion,* 535E][19]

Plato's version of the flow of feeling in the poetic performance captures something of what the oral-epic composer at work in front of an audience must have thought of his inspiration. He is subject to influences outside him and, at the same time, is a focus of influence radiating out to others.

In essence, then, the image of the bard's mental processes, as recorded in Homer and Hesiod and elaborated by Plato, is consonant with the general tenor of the Homeric portrayal of mental life. The mental event is initiated by outside influences, and interaction is felt to occur between the initiator and the person who experiences the event.

The process by which the bard acquires his craft is important in this regard. Becoming a bard obviously requires training and takes hard work. Like much of learning in preliterate societies, his seems to take place in a master-apprentice relationship. He learns by imitating and identifying with his master, who has learned by a similar process. Such a close personal relationship is the sine qua non of learning in a culture that has no books and no schools. The education of a bard probably draws heavily upon the kinds of intense identification and transient blurring of ego boundaries that are involved in the relationship among poet, poem, and audience.[20] Thus the objective correlate of the bard's subjective experience of being taught by the Muse is an intense relationship with his teacher.

We are now in a position to clarify several points. In addition to seeing that the accounts of the mental processes of the bard in Homer, Hesiod, and Plato are consonant with the tenor of the Homeric portrayal of mental life in general, we can now see that the portrayal of mental life in Homer is consonant with the conditions of oral-epic composition and performance in the following ways:

Oral Epic Poetry	*Homeric Model of Mind*
1. The bard receives and transmits the poem; he does not (subjectively speaking) compose it. He gets the poem from the Muses; objectively, he gets the poem from his teacher, and from the "tradition."	1. Mental activity is initiated externally by a god, another person, or a part of the person.
2. The poem is created in the setting of an interchange among poet, audience, and traditional poetic materials.	2. Mental activity is portrayed as a personified interchange rather than a purely internal activity.
3. The poem consists of traditional, common material rendered in traditional ways.	3. Mental activity is preferably portrayed as if visible, public, and common rather than private and idiosyncratic.
4. No distinction is made between the "gift of song" and the song itself. Composition and performance are one.	4. No clear distinction is made among the organs of mental activity, the activity itself, and the products of the activity (no structure-function distinction).
5. The blurring of boundaries among poet, audience, and characters in the poem is integral to the performance.	5. The self or person is defined in a field of forces in a series of interchanges with others.

We can enlarge on this comparison in several directions. For one thing, we can now see a context for the apparent inconsistency with which the Homeric man is presented: as a collection of parts that nevertheless functions as an integrated whole. The poem's composition reveals that it is constructed of a number of building blocks—thematic, metrical, lexical, and so on. Yet the process of poetic integration yields a poem not easily reducible to its component parts. The character of each of the main heroes was undoubtedly a given of the tradition, as were their interactions, yet there is also room for a subtlety and uniqueness of character that goes beyond any traditional or stereotyped model available to the poet.

I have argued that an important aspect of the poems' healing effect (as suggested by Hesiod) resides in their ability to foster identifications of audience with characters. We can now see that the conditions of composition and performance encourage blurring of boundaries and thereby facilitate the identification of audience with character (or merging of audience with the poem). This blurring is more characteristic of childhood thinking and dreams than of adult and waking thinking. In this sense, oral epic poetry exploits an aspect of normal childhood thinking that is still available to the adult and the Homeric model of mind fits the poetic requirements of the bard. Thus, in brief, the poems' form and content cooperate to induce transient modes of thinking and feeling that promise to restore us to a lost childhood state, a state of greater closeness with caring and protecting objects. (Poetry can also evoke some of the frightening aspects of childhood, but probably provides means of mastering them.)

The poems are replete with the language of enlargement and expansion of the self. A hero who is filled with tremendous courage and strength by a god is a recurrent feature of the *Iliad*. The descriptions of the power of the gods must evoke childhood feelings about the grandiose and powerful self.[21] Simultaneously, the power of the gods acts as a check on the grandeur of even the most powerful heroes. Thus another aspect of the poems as therapy is its ability to enlarge the stature and enhance the self-esteem of the listeners while placing some limits on the grandiose self.

One more aspect of the relationship between the poetry and the portrayal of mental life is worth considering. I refer to psychic intervention by a god in the form of *atē*, delusion, to account for a hero's doing something foolish or shameful. Dodds has shrewdly seen that in the warrior aristocracy of the *Iliad,* shame, face, and honor assume particular importance in the relationship among the heroes. Therefore, when Agamemnon finally acknowledges that he was wrong to take Achilles' woman, he invokes the notion of *atē,* a divine agency that made him do it. Dodds argues that this is a way to save face in a society that places a premium on the dangers of shame. He suggests that the ease with which Homeric heroes can invoke an external agent as explanation for their behavior serves as a psychological, or social-psychological, defense mechanism. The need to project unacceptable impulses or actions onto a source outside the self is especially intense in a shame culture.[22] I would qualify Dodds's point of view on two grounds. First, the data now available do not indicate that shame as a social stricture is any more consistently associated with the extensive use of projection than is guilt. But more important for this discussion is the observation, made by Dodds himself and other scholars, that *virtually every kind of mental activity, including the most trivial and ordinary, can be ascribed to an outside source.* Thus we need a broader construct than that implied in psychic intervention as a defense mechanism. Recasting psychic intervention as a subdivision of personified interchange allows us to see this phenomenon in the context of oral epic poetry. The demands of the poetic performance, with its special rapport between audience and poet, encourage a psychological world view that finds it most natural to portray private mental activity publicly as a process of continuous interchange between persons.[23] I would extend this argument to say that the entire range of devices for portraying mental life must be understood in terms of the interaction between audience and poet.

In summary, I have argued that the answer to the question of why such a model of mind and mental disturbance is found in the Homeric epics must be approached by asking, "Why and how do Homeric epics exist?" Such an approach, I believe, usefully locates a mode of thinking within a particular literary and social context. This notion will also prove useful in examining the portrayal of mental life and mental illness in Greek tragedy, where we find a significant alteration in the relationship among the poet, his work, and his audience. Greek tragedies are clearly composed in writing yet are in many ways still embedded in habits of the oral tradition. As we shall see, there is a corresponding shift in the relationship between the individual and the group within the tragedies—tragic heroes, especially in Sophocles, stand out as far more alone and autonomous than the heroes in epic poetry. Similarly, the Platonic dialogues, which represent an even greater break with the habits of an oral culture, are associated with a sharper definition of the individual and present a clear notion of the mind as private and internal.

This discussion of the Homeric model of mind has several implications for contemporary models of mental illness. For one thing, if we view the bard as analogous to a healer or therapist, we can point to an interesting congruence between the craft or activity of the healer and the model of mind and mental disturbance with which he works. Thus, if the Homeric model of mind is one of the bard at work, we might attempt to extend this notion to activities that are more explicitly designed as therapy. There is much to be gained by considering that the model of mind and mental illness held by a particular therapeutic school must go hand in glove with the theories in the mind of the practitioner about what he does and how he does it in his work with his patient. We may then devise a formula for the "theory" of the bard *qua* therapist: the bard is a participant with his patient in a process of healing that exploits a rhythm of dedifferentiation and reintegration of the individual. It is a controlled process, with the bard having the greatest, but not the sole, responsibility for regulating pace and rhythm. This formulation is a useful way of looking at modern theories of mental illness that emphasize transactional and interpersonal aspects of illness and of therapy.[24] Therapists of this orientation have tended to view themselves as participant observers. I suggest that it would be useful to consider them also as participant regulators in a process of dedifferentiation and reintegration of the self. We could also speak of controlled regression, and the bard as a participant regressor. Like the bard, such therapists are also subject to a process of blurring and reestablishment of ego boundaries, just as their patients are. This notion is quite consonant with these therapists' views of therapy and accounts of their experience as therapists.

One other implication of this view of the context of the Homeric model of mind is the relationship of the individual to the group, or the definition of the individual vis-à-vis the group. It is my contention that theories of mind and mental illness which emphasize the mind (or the person) as a concentration and condensation of forces within a larger field of forces are embedded in contexts where individuals interact closely with each other as integral parts of the social whole. Theories that view each individual mind as a discrete entity walled off from all others make different assumptions about the relationship between the group and the individual. Medical models of mind have their own assumptions about the individual and the group, but I believe these assumptions are disguised in the anatomical and physiological language characteristic of those models.[25]

In sum, models of mind and mental illness contain certain presuppositions about the individual and the collective, and these presuppositions are operative in the "group" that consists of the healer and the patient.

6

Mental Life in
Greek Tragedy

Savage and unexampled enormities, horrifying to heaven and earth
alike, my mind within me is churning up, wounds and murder and
death that slithers along the limbs. Too trivial are the deeds I
recall—those things I did as a girl. 'Tis time for deeper passion;
now I am a mother, more impressive crimes are expected.
—Seneca, *Medea* [1]

Greek tragedy is rich indeed in its descriptions of the inner lives of its
heroes and heroines. This richness is the starting point of our inquiry. The interior of the person is illuminated with far greater intensity in tragedy than it is in epic poetry, and what is revealed tells
us much about conflict and pain and the attempts to defend against
them. Tragedy reveals a great interest in madness, which it shows as
arising from a matrix of deep ambivalence and unbearable conflict.
The focus is on the individual hero, but the interplay of powerful
social forces with internal conflict is never neglected. Tragedy, moreover, depicts attempts to treat madness and its consequence, and we
find an extraordinary subtlety in the portrayal of the play of internal
and external forces. The very richness and intricacy with which madness is presented invite us to consider the mind of the playwright
who can write of such powerful conflict while exerting artistic control over his material. For this reason we shall examine ancient and
modern views of the relationship between madness and creativity.
Tragedy's importance in the civic and religious life of Athens com-
pels us to consider how audiences may have used these performances
to deal with their own internal burdens, and to deal with a broader
question: Is theater therapy?

When we speak of Greek tragedy, we have before us only a frac-
tion of the plays performed at Athens during the fifth century B.C.,
some thirty out of nearly a thousand. Only the plays of Aeschylus
(525–456), Sophocles (496–406), and Euripides (485–406) have survived, but the testimony of antiquity is that these three were the
greatest of the tragedians. Their very popularity must have been a
factor in the preservation of some of their plays, despite the ravages

of time, the burning of libraries, and the caprice of schoolmasters, pagan and Christian.

Playwrights submitted sets of dramas consisting of three tragedies and a satyr play to judges, who selected the three best sets for the public competition at the Great Dionysia, the spring festival of Dionysus. One day was devoted to the work of each playwright, and at the end of the festival first, second, and third places were awarded by audience acclamation. The winner, crowned with an ivy wreath, held a place of honor similar to that of an Olympic victor.

Religious and solemn as these performances were, they were also occasions of emotional release. The satyr play provided an element of hilarity, appropriate to a celebration of Dionysus. But Dionysus Eleutherios, Dionysus Lusios, the god of liberation and release, also allowed the unspeakable and the unthinkable to be performed before the entire city. For three days a year the public could witness murder, madness, and incest.[2]

We know little of the origins of these extraordinary performances. The word *tragodia,* literally goat song, suggests that tragedy had its origin in ritual.[3] The Cambridge School of classicists revolutionized classical thought at the turn of this century with its emphasis on the ritual character of tragedy as the drama of the dying god or the corn spirit.[4] My own view follows more recent scholarly thought, which holds that the ritual origin of tragedy can never be proved and that Athenian tragedy as an art form evolved from something far removed from ritual. For the Greeks the power of tragedy derived from its artistic rendering of issues and emotions that earlier ritual may have expressed, not from its literal repetition of a particular ritual or associated myth. It is the artistic element, I believe, that allowed the playwrights' awesome spectacles to touch on deep-seated fantasies and fears in such a way that audiences could draw enrichment and pleasure from the performances.

The plays succeed because of the skill with which the tragedians show the interplay of conflicts at various levels. Conflicts between man and gods, between man and man, between one ideal of honor and another, between one part of the hero and another, between projections of one part of the self and another—all must be congruent and integrated. In the macrocosm are the themes of conflict between civilization and barbarism, between harsh tyranny and the recognition of basic human affections and affiliations. The heroes of tragedy who go mad (they are always *driven* mad) do so when their world is collapsing around them. Their madness is part of a frantic attempt to hold on to what they know and think right. Their world involves issues of the state, the gods, the family, and the microcosm of their own conflicted ideals and passions.

Aristotle suggested that tragedy should deal with stories of horrible events within the family, and pointed out that the great tragedies dealt with a few famous houses.[5] Because these are royal families, they can be used to bring together many levels of meaning and to touch many issues, including politics, social conditions, the relations between men and women and between humans and gods, and the world of timeless, universal unconscious fantasy and dreams, where kings, queens, princes, and princesses can represent for us all the most immediate familial objects of our childhood fears and passions.

Consider Aeschylus' *Oresteia,* the story of Agamemnon's return from Troy, his murder by Clytemnestra and Aegisthus, Clytemnestra's murder by her son Orestes, his subsequent madness, and its resolution in an Athenian court. What does the trilogy "mean"? The trilogy can plausibly be interpreted as:

1. A tragedy of war and its aftermath.
2. A theological drama—the conflicts between the Olympian and chthonic deities.
3. A representation of the conflict between patriarchal and matriarchal societies or values.
4. A representation of the growth of civil law in Athens.
5. A tragedy of a family curse.
6. A domestic tragedy about enmities among husband, wife, and children.
7. The tragedy of Orestes torn between love for his mother and a hatred of her bred of his loyalty to his father.
8. The tragedy of Orestes torn by an "unnatural" love—a conflict over unconscious incestuous wishes that are symbolically represented and warded off by matricide.[6]

This list suggests the multiple levels of conflict that enter into the experience of the characters in the drama and the multiple levels that are integrated by both the artist and his audience. Examples of extreme forms of conflict, such as Medea's over the killing of her children, are not merely isolated specimens of clinical psychiatric material, accurate though they are as clinical descriptions; rather they are one part of an intricate and harmonious design.

Harmony and balance are key terms in any discussion of Greek tragedy. The characters themselves, especially the chorus, plead the necessity of harmony and balance, neither too much nor too little— not too much reverence for one god at the expense of another. Imbalance is typical of the tragic protagonists. The chorus in Euripides' *Hippolytus* sings of "unfortunate harmony" (ll. 161–64), a part of women's nature. In the *Agamemnon* the chorus sings of the grim "balance of payment" in war, because Ares exchanges young men for funeral ashes (ll. 437–44).

Or consider madness and harmony. There is a fine detail involving balance in Euripides' description of Heracles' imaginary journey, part of the delusional rage that culminates in his murder of his wife and children. He hallucinates that he is attacking the citadel of Mycenae, tearing down with crowbars the Cyclopean walls, walls carefully fitted and measured with the plumb line (*Heracles,* ll. 943–46). Madness and geometry are played contrapuntally. A typical antonym for madness, in both Plato and the tragedians, is *sōphrosunē,* moderation or temperance. The task of the playwright, then, is to provide a temperate portrait of the most unharmonious and immoderate features of human mental life, a task epitomized by the ancient critic Longinus, who said, "Even in the Bacchanalia, one must be sober."[7] The portrayal of mind at its most conflicted and most disturbed occupies a unique place in tragic art because it is also a reflection of the task with which the playwright must struggle. In brief, he must have sufficient access to the most powerful irrational forces within himself so that he can portray them yet retain enough control to present a play that can be enjoyed by the audience. He must let down his own censorship in just the right measure so that the audience in turn can lower its own defenses. Madness is theater gone berserk.

The Greek tragedies are representations of people in action, contemplating action, and justifying action to themselves and to other characters. By means of dialogue, monologue, and chorus, each play depicts both the inner life and the characteristic modes of interaction of the principal characters. Aristotle defined tragedy as an "imitation of action" (*praxeos mimēsis*) based on the portrayal of the habitual character (*ēthos*) and the thinking (*dianoia*) of the protagonists.[8] The plays are replete with terms for mental life, terms that are part of the portrayal of a wide range of intellectual activities and a great variety of feeling states.

This concentration of mental terms is quite apparent in the opening scenes of such a play as *Medea.* Sophocles' *Antigone* is rich in words meaning stupid, senseless, mad. *Oedipus Rex,* of course, is explicitly about knowing, seeing, and understanding, and their interplay with ignorance, blindness, and misunderstanding.[9] We find a more detailed vocabulary of emotional response in tragedy than in epic poetry. Likewise tragedy is more explicit than Homeric epic in distinguishing between intellect and emotion while exploring their vital interrelationship.

While it is true that tragedy contains examples of Homeric personified interchange (for example, "he spoke unto his heart," *Antigone,* l. 227), they are rare; the more typical tragic mode would be "he thought" or "he knew." Some sense of the external origins of thought and feeling remains in tragic discourse. Medea is "stricken in heart with love of Jason" (l. 8), but even this kind of language is less habitual in tragedy than in Homeric epic. Homer would tend to insert a divine agency in the chain of mental causation; tragedy does not. In fact, Euripides has Hecuba assert that it was not Aphrodite who made Helen and Paris do what they did but Helen's own lust and love of luxury (*Trojan Women,* ll. 981–84).

In tragedy the gods generally do not initiate thoughts and feelings, however active they may be. The conspicuous exception to the pattern is the instance of madness: in all the cases we know in tragedies extant and lost, a divine agency drives the protagonist mad.[10]

In Homer, decision making often involves a god's intervention to tilt the balance as the hero ponders whether to do one thing or another. Moreover, the Homeric language of coming to a decision is periphrastic: "My *thumos* urged me to do this, but another *thumos* prevented me."

An example of hesitation before a decision is finally reached is seen in the speech of the guard to Creon in the *Antigone* (ll. 223–36). He is afraid to tell Creon that someone has covered the corpse of Polynices and that the guards have failed in their duty to prevent the burial of the "traitor."

> My mind [*psuchē*] kept saying many things to me:
> "Why go where you will surely pay the price?"
> "Fool are you halting? And if Creon learns
> from someone else, how shall you not be hurt?"
> Turning this over [*helisson*], on I dilly-dallied.
> And so a short trip turns itself to long.   [ll. 227–32][11]

Compare this passage with the opening of Book 20 of the *Odyssey,* where Odysseus does not make his decision until Athena appears and assures him of her help. The word *helisson,* turning about, is used in both passages, and the contrast is instructive. In the *Antigone* it is a metaphor describing a mental process; in the *Odyssey* it is part of the description of Odysseus himself, tossing and turning in sleeplessness. In the *Odyssey* passage, the mental processes are made manifest and explicated by similes, by a little tale that Odysseus tells himself, and by personified interchange. The personified interchange takes place between Odysseus and parts of himself (including his *thumos*) and between Athena and Odysseus. The analogous personified interchange in the *Antigone* is an inner debate that does not strike us as unusual.

The most famous inner debate in tragedy is surely Medea's speech in which she decides to kill her children for revenge, changes her mind several times, and finally decides she must kill them, knowing it is wrong to do so.[12] As the speech opens, she seems to debate whether or not to take her children with her into exile or to leave them in Corinth, but as it proceeds the debate shifts to whether or not she should take leave of her children by killing them. At first only the chorus is present, but later her children join her:

> Oh Children, O my children, you have a city,
> You have a home, and you can leave me behind you,
> And without your mother you may live there forever.
> But I am going in exile to another land
> Before I have seen you happy and taken pleasure in you   [ll. 1021–
>   25]
> For, once I am left without you,

. . .

> Sad will be the life I'll lead and sorrowful for me.
> And you will never see your mother again with
> Your dear eyes, gone to another mode of living.
> Why, children, do you look upon me with your eyes?
> Why do you smile so sweetly that last smile of all?
> Oh, oh, what can I do? My courage has gone from me,[13]
> Friends, when I see that bright look in the children's eyes,
> I cannot bear to do it. I renounce my plans I had before, I'll take my children away from
> This land. Why should I hurt their father with the pain
> They feel, and suffer twice as much pain myself?
> No, no, I will not do it. I renounce my plans.
> Ah, what is wrong with me? Do I want to let go
> My enemies unhurt and be laughed at for it?
> I must face this thing. Oh, but what a weak woman
> Even to admit to my mind these soft arguments.   [ll. 1036–52]

. . .

> Oh! Oh!
> Do not, O my heart [*thume*], you must not do these things!
> Poor heart, let them go, have pity upon the children.
> If they live with you in Athens they will cheer you.
> No! By Hell's avenging furies it shall not be—
> This shall never be, that I should suffer my children
> To be the prey of my enemies' insolence.   [ll. 1056–61][14]

Though this speech is in some respects unique even in the tragic corpus, it is representative of the inner debate and changes of resolution that are typical of tragedy. Inner debate is, in fact, incorporated into tragic diction. Certain compounds (usually with the prefix *meta-*) denote a change of mind or a wish to take back what one regrets having said.[15]

What about the "organs" of mental life in tragedy, and how does tragic usage compare with Homer's? Terms familiar from Homer—*thumos, psuchē, kardia, phrēn*—can be found in the two passages cited. The fluidity of their use in tragedy appears, in general, to be quite comparable to the Homeric style. They are not technical psychological terms with specific applications.

These terms have become more metaphorical than they were in Homer. *Thumos* and *psuchē* in Homer, it will be recalled, can leave the body, and overlap with "breath" and "breath of life" as well as denote functions that we would designate "psychological." Such terms as *thumos* and *psuchē* in tragedy are way stations, as it were, toward more technical philosophical usages.[16] They come to resemble our own use of somatic terms for feelings ("he has no guts") and seem less literal in their relation to the body than in Homer. In a sense, they are more abstract, which is another way of saying that their use reflects a greater degree of mind-body differentiation than is expressed in Homer.[17]

In tragedy we become acutely aware of the two levels of mental functioning, the emotional and the intellectual. If nothing else, the distinction between the choruses and the speeches tends to force this awareness on us.

Let us consider, to begin with, the contrast between two sections early in the *Medea*. Jason has jilted Medea to marry the daughter of Creon, king of Corinth, and Medea is beside herself. Her entrance begins a series of lyrical interchanges among Medea, the nurse, and the chorus of Corinthian women.[18]

Medea: Ah, wretch! Ah, lost in my sufferings.
　　　　I wish, I wish I might die.
Nurse: What did I say, dear children? Your mother
　　　　Frets her heart and frets it to anger.
　　　　Run away quickly into the house,
　　　　And keep well out of her sight [stay far from her eye].　[ll. 96–101]

　　　　　　　　　．　　　．　　　．

Medea: Ah, I have suffered
　　　　What should be wept for bitterly. I hate you,
　　　　Children of a hateful mother. I curse you
　　　　And your father. Let the whole house crash.　[ll. 111–14]

　　　　　　　　　．　　　．　　　．

　　　　Oh, I wish
　　　　That lightning from heaven would split my head open.
　　　　Oh, what use have I now for life?
　　　　I would find my release in death
　　　　And leave hateful existence behind me.　[ll. 144–47]

Note the bodily terms in these lines: at line 99 she "frets her heart" and "frets it to anger" (*cholos*, akin to *cholē*, bile); at line 101: "stay far from her eye."

Contrast this section with Medea's speech at lines 214–66. Though taut with emotion, it is primarily an argument, an explanation, a kind of legal pleading. Its intellectual tone is set in the opening lines, where Medea tries to assuage any anger or reproach felt by the women:

> Women of Corinth, I have come outside to you,
> Lest you should reproach me; for I know
> That many people are overproud, some when alone,
> And others when in company. And those who live
> Quietly, as I do, get a bad reputation.   [ll. 214–18]
>
> But on me this thing has fallen so unexpectedly,
> It has broken my heart. . . .   [ll. 225–26]

The theme of personal justification for being so distraught is now amplified into a discourse on the plight of women in general, on how difficult marriage is, even at its best. The woman must submit—to the will of her husband, to the mores of the husband's family, to the dangers of childbirth. In effect, she asks the chorus to consider her arguments and to understand her quest for vengeance.

The contrast, then, between the lyrical sections (ll. 96–212) and the iambic, more prosaic speech (ll. 214–66) is partly the contrast between emotion and reason. But it is also a matter of one cause pleaded on two grounds: feeling and reason.[19]

In this context, it is well to review some recurrent features of the choruses in Greek tragedy. Since they are set to music and accompanied by dance, they mobilize bodily response in the audience far more than do the speeches and they contain more fancy and wish-fulfilling fantasy. Themes of escape are common—"would that I were a bird," "would that I were elsewhere." Extended similes and metaphors—somewhat in the Homeric manner—are common. They tell little tales that comment on, add to, and show other emotional aspects of the action at hand. For example, when Antigone is being led to the cave where she will be buried alive, the chorus recalls the story of Lykourgos, who went mad and was imprisoned in a rock vault because he disobeyed the will of Dionysus   (*Antigone,* ll. 955–62):

> Remember the angry king,
> son of Dryas, who raged at the god and paid,
> pent in a rock-walled prison. His bursting wrath
> slowly went down. As the terror of madness went
> he learned of his frenzied attack on the god.
> Fool, he had tried to stop
> the dancing women possessed of god,
> the fire of Dionysus, the songs and flutes.

As I argued in Chapter 4, the tale serves, as if by means of free association, to show a number of facets of the situation, some of them contradictory. Here the chorus sympathizes with Antigone and raises some hopes of her release. At the same time, she is compared to Lykourgos, who was mad, and the chorus hopes her madness too will subside. Often the content of the choral odes deals specifically with more primary-process states, such as sleep and dreams, reverie and imagination. Note the explicit praise for the gratifications of dreams and imagination in Euripides' *Iphigenia in Tauris* (ll. 452–455):

Even in my dreamt imaginings I would like to be in my own home and city, because there is pleasure in the dreams pleasant sleep brings, and one is grateful for this source of richness which is open to everyone.[20]

Prominent among the emotions experienced and articulated by the chorus are pity, fear, and terror. The chorus in Euripides' *Orestes* sings (ll. 831–33):

What sickness or what cause of tears, what is more pitiable in any land than to shed with one's hand the blood of one's own mother?[21]

The singers in the *Ajax* chorus repeatedly express their fear for Ajax and for themselves as they see him mad (ll. 139, 227, 253). And the choruses both in Sophocles' *Electra* (l. 1408) and in the *Trachiniae* (l. 1044) shudder with fear (*phrittein*).[22] Terror and pity, of course, are prominent among the emotional states Aristotle lists as characteristic of the events of the tragedy and of the effects produced on the spectators.[23] It is important that the chorus experiences them.

Even more than the emotions themselves, the choruses feel for the sufferings and plight of the heroes; they *identify* with the protagonists in many respects. *Mimēsis*, imitation, though not mentioned in the tragedies, describes a mental function of the choruses. (I understand *mimēsis* in the sense implied in Plato's *Republic*, a combination of imitation and identification.) Words compounded with *sun-* (together) are prominent in the tragedies.[24] *Sunalgein*, to suffer together with someone, is an important example. In the *Ajax* (ll. 283–84) the chorus appeals to the hero's wife, Tecmessa, to tell the tale of Ajax's madness:

How at the start did this catastrophe
Swoop down? Tell us: we share the pain of it.

Part of the movement and development within the play occurs when a character comes to *feel for* another character with whom he has previously been at odds. Thus, by the end of the *Ajax*, Odysseus has come to argue that Ajax should be given a proper burial, not treated with contempt. In Odysseus we see what Aristotle calls *philanthropia*—a sympathy for one's fellow man based on a common human identification—overcoming the ethos of hating one's enemy. It is of a piece with Priam's plea to Achilles to ransom the body of Hector, an appeal based on the common humanity of Achilles' father, Peleus, and of Priam himself.

The chorus clearly serves an important function in bridging the gap between audience and hero. The sympathetic identification of chorus with protagonist is an invitation for the audience likewise to feel for and with the hero. The more dreamlike features of the choral odes stir up the fantasies of the audience. The choral music and dance movements convey the hero's and the chorus's internal states, and by a kind of contagion induce in the audience the feeling states portrayed on the stage.[25]

Thus the chorus emphasizes the nonverbal and the affective "reasons" for coming to sympathize with the hero. The hero's argued pleas provide a more intellectual basis for such an identification. The choruses, then, constitute a kind of detailed portrayal and exploration of the emotional side of human behavior. The iambic speeches of the main characters and their interchanges constitute an analogous exploration of the more reasoned and calculating parts of the human psyche.

I have elaborated on one sense of the term "identification," namely, coming to a sympathetic appreciation of the plight of another person. The term also has a more literal sense, the act of identifying particular people. Identification or misidentification of important persons in one's life is a prominent motif in Greek tragedy: *anagnorisis,* recognition, is crucial in many of the plays. I shall attempt to show that this kind of identification also entails a complex mixture of emotion and intellect, and I shall use some psychoanalytic modes of interpretation to illustrate the connection between the two senses of identification. Identifying with another's plight is a necessary part of knowing oneself and one's relatives correctly. Forces that interfere with empathy and sympathy for others also interfere with full recognition of all the parts of oneself.

Readers of the *Poetics* will recall that recognition is a central feature of Aristotle's conception of the most desirable and best sort of tragedy (for example, 1452a22–68). Gerald Else, in his excellent commentary on Aristotle's *Poetics,* argues that, while such scenes do not occur in the majority of tragedies, Aristotle has good reason for according recognition such importance.[26] Recognition scenes are an integral part of the formal structure, an intellectual element, as it were, that allows for the optimal stirring up and handling of the intense emotions of tragedy. In his *Interpretation of Dreams,* Freud compared the process of Oedipus' recognitions to the unfolding of a psychoanalysis.[27] Both Aristotle and Freud offer explanations of the impact of a successful tragedy. These explanations are, in fact, complementary rather than mutually exclusive.[28] Aristotle emphasizes the formal features of the play that create the optimal degree of audience response; Freud emphasizes the role of unconscious fantasy and defense against fantasy.

When we examine the theme of recognition in Euripides' *Iphigenia in Tauris* we see the complementary nature of these two modes of explanation, as well as the complex mixture of intellect and emotion that is entailed in identification and misidentification. Conflict and ambivalence, not mere ignorance, interfere with recognition of one's own kin. The plot is based on a version of the myth in which Iphigenia does not die, sacrificed by her father at Aulis, but at the last moment is carried by Artemis to the land of the Taurians. There shipwrecked Greek sailors are sacrificed as offerings to Artemis, and Iphigenia officiates. Iphigenia's brother, Orestes, whom she last saw when he was a young child, is now shipwrecked on this strange Black Sea shore. The story is set in motion with Iphigenia's dream and her interpretation, or misinterpretation, of it (ll. 42–58):

> These new night visions which the night comes bearing,
> I shall relate to the bright sky, if perhaps that might be a remedy.
> I seemed in my sleep to be dwelling in Argos, that I had escaped from
>   this land.
> I was sleeping in the midst of the maiden's quarters,
> And the surface of the earth was shaken with a quake.
> And I fled outside and standing there saw the coping of the palace
>   falling down,
> And the whole roof hurtled down from its topmost parts to the
>   ground.
> And only one column, so it seemed to me,
> Of my father's palace remained, and from its top parts
> Fair hair flowed loose and it took on the voice of a man.
> And I wept as I sprinkled water on it (him), as if it (he) were slated
>   for death,
> Carrying out this office I hold in the ritual slaughter of strangers.
> Thus I interpret this dream: Orestes is dead, and it was he for whom I
>   performed this rite.
> For the columns of the house are the male children,
> And those on whom I cast my ritual waters die.
> And I have no other loved one to whom this dream can pertain.[29]

In terms of formal construction of the plot, it is important that Iphigenia misinterpret this dream; she must believe Orestes dead if the subsequent failure of recognition is to be effective. If we take a psychoanalytic approach to this material and posit that the manifest content of the dream portrays the fulfillment of an unconscious wish, then Iphigenia *wishes* that the males, including Orestes, were dead. She also wishes that she were the one to sacrifice and slaughter Orestes. I suggest that Iphigenia is torn by unconscious conflict in her feelings toward her brother. The unconscious rage is in part displaced rage at her father, who was willing to sacrifice her for his own material glory; in part it reflects outrage and jealousy that Orestes was preferred—he was not offered for sacrifice. The males of the house are, in this sense, the cause of her misery. The other object of her rage is the relationship between Helen and Paris—the illicit lust that caused her own father to agree to sacrifice her. Although spared by the (virgin) goddess Artemis, she herself never achieves sexual gratification and remains unwed. The recognition of the Greek stranger as Orestes ultimately depends upon Iphigenia's discovery that Orestes shares her rage at Helen. Thus the realization that Orestes is indeed a friend allows her to work through some of her unconscious rage and jealousy, to relinquish enough of her ambivalence to be able to recognize that he is her brother, a *philos*. One could carry this construction further by examining the imagery and the symbolism of the dream. In symbolic terms, the dream also expresses the wish to destroy and castrate the males in her life (Agamemnon, Paris, and even her beloved brother, Orestes) rather than passively suffer outrage because of the sexual desire of those around her. It can be argued, then, that unconscious ambivalence is at the heart of Iphigenia's failure to recognize her brother. *Iphigenia in Tauris* has generally not struck its audiences and its readers as the greatest or the most tragic of the Greek tragedies; yet it and *Oedipus Rex* are the only two extant plays that conform to Aristotle's prescription for a really great tragedy, namely, a precisely timed sequence of recognition and reversal. This sequence is the formal structural counterpart of the process of coming to grips with unconscious ambivalence.

Recognitions and misidentifications are the basic stuff of which the great myths of all nations are made, particularly the myths of the birth of the hero.[30] Euripides' *Ion,* dealing explicitly with an abandoned child who comes to recognize his true parents, and *Iphigenia in Tauris* seem to represent the limits of this theme in tragedy and to mark the boundary between tragedy and comedy. Ultimatley, the recognition of the other is a crucial aspect of the recognition of the self.

Recognition is also very much related to the theme of tragic knowledge, as embodied in the Aeschylean formula of *to pathei mathos,* knowledge through suffering (*Agamemnon,* l. 177). "Knowledge through suffering" and "recognition" are the counterparts in imaginative literature of the Socratic call to "know thyself." At the same time, they deepen and extend the Socratic notion to include the most fundamental knowledge of man in relation to the earliest objects of childhood knowledge and desire—his family.

Orestes in Aeschylus and Euripides

Murder, suicide, and madness: these are the most prominent of the catastrophes portrayed in tragedy. Madness in metaphorical terms—

"You are mad if you think you can do this"—is extremely common in the plays of the three great tragedians, and virtually any kind of extreme passion can be matter-of-factly labeled mad. But frank clinical madness, complete with hallucinations and delusions, induced by a god or goddess, is also rather common. In Aeschylus, most famous is the madness of Orestes, brought on by the Furies as they seek vengeance for his slaying of his mother. The onslaught of the Furies begins at the end of the *Choephoroi* and is the main theme in the *Eumenides*. The first play of the trilogy, *Agamemnon*, depicts the prophetic madness of Cassandra (though there it is not explicitly labeled as madness). In *Prometheus Bound*, Io appears, driven mad by the gadfly sent by Zeus and Hera.[31]

Sophocles' most vivid mad play is his *Ajax*, and several lost plays probably also depicted madness (*Athamas, Alcmaeon*) and even feigned madness (*Odysseus Mainomenos*).

Three extant plays of Euripides have madness and its resolution as the central theme: *Heracles, Orestes,* and the magnificent *Bacchae,* his last play. *Iphigenia in Tauris* contains a scene depicting Orestes in a sudden fit of madness, and the *Trojan Women* presents Cassandra as mad. In fact, Longinus wrote that Euripides devoted special care to love and madness.[32]

The playwrights present clinically accurate and believable pictures of men gone mad.[33] Psychoanalytically informed critics have also argued that several of the plays are quite accurate from a psychodynamic viewpoint in the manner in which they present the onset, exacerbation, and relief of madness.[34]

If the causes of madness could be epitomized in a single sentence, it would be this: Madness comes from conflict. Along with conflict, ambivalence plays an important part. Intense ambivalence is not necessarily located within the individual, but rather is embedded in the very fabric of the play. Walter Burkert points out that the tragedies contain many overt references to sacrifice, including a number that deal with human sacrifice as part of the plot (for example, the Iphigenia plays; Euripides' *Hecuba, Heracleidae, Phoenissiae;* Sophocles' lost *Polyxena*). Murder in the tragedies is typically framed in the language and imagery of a sacrifice; the most outstanding examples are in Aeschylus' *Oresteia* and in Euripides' *Heracles* and *Bacchae*.[35] What is conveyed by the repeated reference to sacrificial ritual, in a word, is ambivalence. Deeply embedded in the ritual is a mixture of love and aggression toward the victim, be it animal or human. The animal to be ruthlessly slain is lovingly adorned. Human sacrifice certainly connotes a deep ambivalence toward the son or daughter who is offered as a gift or placation demanded by the gods. Freud, in *Totem and Taboo*, suggested that the origins of Greek tragedy have to do with the slaying of the primal father by the band of brothers.[36] However dubious the historical truth of Freud's construct, his arguments about totemism and sacrifice as expressions of guilt and ambivalence are valid. The extant plays dealing with madness are in fact deeply colored with language, imagery, and plot involving ritual and ritual sacrifice. Even the apparent exception, the *Ajax,* is connected with sacrifice by virtue of the form of Ajax's madness—the slaying of animals in place of humans.[37]

It is also important to recognize that in Greek tragedy sacrifice and madness have in common their ordination or provocation by the gods. Agamemnon slays his daughter because Artemis demands that he do so, not because he wishes to do so. The notion that the gods cause madness covers up the deep conflicts and guilt that must be at work somewhere in the life of the culture. How petty and oversensitive are these divine agencies who, for a slight to their honor, will wreak havoc, cause madness, and bring down mighty houses and cities!

Thus madness in Greek tragedy is inseparable from religion and from feelings about the gods. That feeling, a mixture of reverence, dread, occasional affection, and dutiful obligation, bespeaks an attempt to cope with emotions and wishes that must also exist between parents and children and between the sexes.[38] In the very play where Hera drives Heracles to madness and murder of his kin, Heracles proclaims that the gods cannot operate by the petty rules and ruthless habits of mankind. How could one believe that one's parents were so malevolent? Thus out of a matrix of conflict, ambivalence, guilt, and sacrifice grow the dreadful madnesses of the Greek stage.

The *Oresteia of Aeschylus*

Orestes first appears at the opening of the *Choephoroi,* the second play in the trilogy of the *Oresteia.* Toward the end of the play (l. 930) he murders his mother, Clytemnestra, and in the closing scene (ll. 1021–25) experiences the onslaught of the Furies and the madness they induce. His madness and its resolution in an Athenian trial are the themes of the last play, the *Eumenides.* It is fitting that overt madness should finally burst forth in the trilogy, for from the opening chorus of the *Agamemnon* there is an atmosphere of dread and anguish, of unnameable fears and terrors. Seething resentment, black rage, and bitter, unresolved grief frame the action of the play. The many references to dreams and night terrors, combined with the raving prophecy of Cassandra, create an atmosphere of minds tottering at the brink of madness. There is scarcely a respite as the second play in the trilogy picks up the motifs of unassuaged grief, rage, and bitterness and the terrors of the darkness of dreams (*Choephoroi,* ll. 32–36):

Terror, the dream diviner of
this house, belled clear, shuddered the skin, blew wrath
from sleep, a cry in night's obscure watches,
a voice of fear deep in the house,
dropping deadweight in women's inner chambers.

The chorus further speaks of "bitter hatred" (*pikron stugos,* l. 80) and
of being "frozen with secret sorrows." Electra experiences an up-
surge of *cholē,* bitter anger (l. 183).

Clytemnestra has been awakened by an ominous dream, prompt-
ing her to send offerings to the grave of Agamemnon, by which she
hopes to still the unquiet spirits below the earth that will not let her
rest (ll. 527–34):[39]

Chorus: She told me herself. She dreamed she gave birth to a snake.
Orestes: What is the end of the story then: What is the point?
Chorus: She laid it swathed for sleep as if it were a child.
Orestes: A little monster. Did it want some kind of food?
Chorus: She herself, in the dream, gave it her breast to suck.
Orestes: How was her nipple not torn by such a beastly thing?
Chorus: It was. The creature drew in blood along with the milk.
Orestes: No void dream this. It is the vision of a man.

Orestes goes on to interpret the dream as referring to himself as the
swaddled snake, and as portending that "I turn snake to kill her."

But another ingredient is needed for the brew that will produce
insanity: conflict. The form of the conflict for Orestes is stated quite
explicitly in his speech beginning at line 269. Apollo has charged him
to execute his mother and to avenge his father. If he fails to carry out
the Delphic charge, he must suffer dire punishments:

. . . angers that come out of the ground from those
beneath who turn against men; spoke of sicknesses,
ulcers that ride upon the flesh, and cling, and with
wild teeth eat away the natural tissue. . . .

Note the oral-aggressive imagery, matching the imagery of his
mother's dream.

. . . madness and empty terror in the night
on one who sees clear and whose eyes move in the dark . . .

These punishments of the fathers mimic the punishments that the
maternal avenging Erinyes will mete out. The playwright is quite
clear: Orestes is being crushed between two powerful cosmic forces,
mother right and father right, and will go mad no matter which way
he turns. Further, he faces loss of self-esteem in allowing the citizens
of Argos, and himself, to be defeated by a woman and by a man
with the cowardly heart of a woman—Aegisthus. There is a hint

here, but only a hint, that Orestes has to combat a feminine side of himself. But what is clearly in focus is the sense that Orestes' madness is inevitable.

In an important sense the conflict is an external one, though he may suffer internally because of it. Orestes is caught up in a conflict he did not create. Aeschylus' portrayal of Orestes is different from Euripides' version, where we find that the external conflict between Apollo and the Furies mirrors the inner conflicts between the male and female parts of his character.

For a few brief moments at the end of the *Choephoroi,* Orestes alone sees the Furies, and they are real to him alone. The chorus praises Orestes for his double murder—he has obeyed Apollo and is the savior of Argos (ll. 1046–62):

Chorus: You liberated all the Argive city when
        you lopped the heads of these two snakes with one clean stroke.
Orestes: No!
        Women who serve this house, they come like gorgons, they
        wear robes of black, and they are wreathed in a tangle
        of snakes. I can no longer stay.
Chorus: Orestes, dearest to your father of all men,
        what fancies whirl you? Hold, do not give way to fear.[40]

                            .   .   .

Orestes: Ah, Lord Apollo, how they grow and multiply,
        repulsive for the blood drops of their dripping eyes.

                            .   .   .

        You can not see them, but I see them. I am driven from this place. I
        can stay here no longer.

Note that the onset of the madness occurs when the chorus tells him he has slain two snakes; immediately Orestes hallucinates the snake-wreathed Erinyes. Clytemnestra is a snake, Orestes himself is a snake (and so he has interpreted Clytemnestra's dream). The snaky goddesses, a condensation of his own perception of himself and his mother and a projection of his own condemning and murderous conscience, are now upon him. But in the *Eumenides* the Erinyes are public and observable to all—Orestes is not hallucinating. Clearly the playwright's main interest in this trilogy is not the internal conflict.

The description of Orestes beginning to go mad but not yet hallucinating is instructive both because it is an inner experience and because at the same time it is couched in terms of what is being done to him (ll. 1021–25):

Orestes: I would have you know, I see not how this thing will end.
        I am a charioteer whose course is wrenched outside

the track, for I am beaten, my rebellious senses
bolt with me headlong and the fear against my heart
is ready for the singing and dance of wrath.

Forces out of control are taking over; a drama of madness will begin, in which he is a participant but not an active initiating agent.

Contrast these lines with the succinct statement in Euripides' *Orestes,* when Orestes is asked by Menelaus what disease afflicts him and replies, "The awareness—that I know I have done terrible deeds" (l. 369).

But who are these Erinyes and what do they do? When the Pythia at Delphi first sees them, she is stricken with horror and revulsion (*Eumenides,* ll. 46–59). They are something like Gorgons: they are like disgusting Harpies who snatch and contaminate the food, only they are wingless. They are black and disgusting. Their breath drives one away. Their eyes drip foul ooze, and no human beings would claim them for their own. Orestes has already told us they are wreathed with snakes and dressed in black. They avenge spilled maternal blood by sucking out the blood of the living man (*Eumenides,* ll. 184, 264–66, 365, and passim). Their wombs are filled with fire or poisonous vapors (ll. 137–38) that cause their victim to shrivel and dry up.

But the castration (or impotence) they cause is not only symbolic; they literally destroy and crush the genitalia and the rest of the body. Apollo tells them (ll. 185–90):

It is not fitting you should come to this house;
your place is where sentence is given to lop off heads and gouge out
    eyes,
where murders are, and by destruction of the seed
the manhood of the young is ruined, and there are mutilations
and stoning, and men moan in long lament
impaled beneath the spine.[41]

And, of course, madness is their specialty (ll. 341–46):

Over our victim
we sing this song, maddening the brain,
carrying away the sense, destroying the mind,
a hymn that comes from the Erinyes,
fettering the mind, sung
without the lyre, withering to mortals.

These creatures have another characteristic, however: they too are subject to mental torment and conflict. They must torture others in order not to be themselves tortured by bad conscience and nightmares. Thus the ghost of Clytemnestra reproaches them for sleeping when they should be pursuing Orestes. They are at first tortured in a

nightmare, as if subliminally incorporating into their dream the reproach of Clytemnestra (ll. 155–60):

> The accusation came upon me from my dreams,
> and hit me as with goad in the mid-grip of his fist
> and charioteer strikes,
> but deep, beneath lobe and heart.
> The executioner's cutting whip is mine to feel
> and the weight of pain is big, heavy to bear.

The conflict we might infer is between their need to persecute and
their wish to sleep.[42] They themselves are dubbed insane (*margous*)
by Apollo (l. 67). In fact, the playwright virtually gives us a bona
fide Greek diagnosis of the distress of the Erinyes: they are struck
and hurt "beneath the heart and beneath the liver" and Athena urges
them to "lay to rest the bitter force of your black wave of anger" (l.
832). Pain in the liver is literally hypochondriacal ("beneath the
ribs"), and bitter black anger, turned against the self, is *melancholia*
(blackness plus bitterness).[43] Thus the tormentors have their own
tormentors and torments.

We are also provided with a motive for the melancholia that alter-
nates with their persecution: they are slighted, not given their proper
honors, and will therefore curse and destroy. The male principle
takes precedence over the female: the deck is stacked against them.
No wonder a withering vapor and fire come from the wombs of the
Furies, when the male gods even deny the importance of the woman
in procreation (*Eumenides,* ll. 657–66).

From a psychoanalytic perspective, such material is indeed rich. If
these productions were those of a patient, one could talk of destructive maternal introjects (internal representations of another person).
For example, a little boy views his mother (also sisters, aunts, female
slaves, and so forth) as angry, unsatisfied, demanding, depressed,
and punitive. One could emphasize the redundant oral-aggressive
and oral-sadistic imagery not only in the description of the Furies but
throughout the trilogy (Thyestes eating the flesh of his own children
served up by his brother; eagles eating hares; Clytemnestra's dream
of nursing; her display of her breast to Orestes as she pleads with
him not to kill the woman who gave him suck). These images certainly could have been taken from the dreams, fantasies, and symptoms of melancholics, with their oral-cannibalistic rage, as originally
described by Karl Abraham and Freud.[44] One might deduce that the
references to blood, clots, and foul odors are allusions to menstruation and childbirth. The Furies, then, are the child's introject of an
angry, frustrated, dysmenorrheic mother, at once seeking
gratification from her son, unconsciously punishing him for her own
miseries, and venting upon him her rage at her husband. These

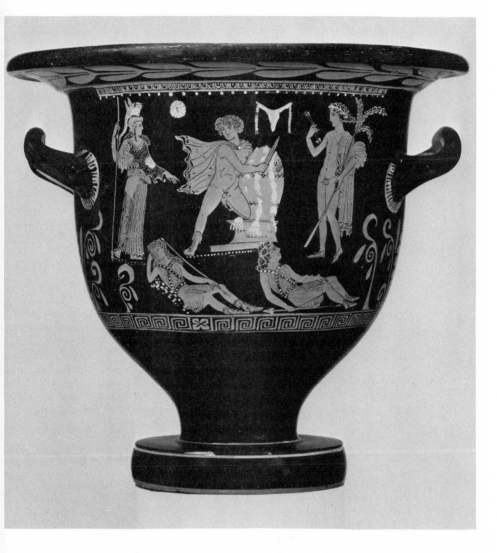

Furies sleeping outside the sanctuary of Apollo at Delphi. Orestes, center, holds the ompha-
los (navel stone) of the oracle. On the right stands Apollo, on the left Athena.
Detail of Lucanian krater, fourth century B.C. CourtesyMuseum of Fine Arts, Boston.

would be the fantasies (or hallucinations) of the male rendered impotent and feeling castrated by overpowering female rage and female desire, fantasies nurtured by the mother and sustained by his own projected rage. These figures also embody a primitive, sadistic superego, which pushes mercy and tenderness aside.

The oral fantasies of nursing, sucking dry, and devouring also carry, in disguised form, the child's wishes to be incorporated inside the mother, to be protected from her wrath and from his own rage by being made one with her. Clinical experience tells us that even the most frightening of persecutory delusions and hallucinations may contain elements of distorted wishes to love and be loved. (Patients who lose such delusions in the course of recovery may experience profound feelings of depression, loss, and inner emptiness.)

I must reiterate that in Aeschylus these conflicts are located in the cosmos and in the society rather than in the individual. Orestes does not work through terrible inner conflicts in order to reach some sort of inner harmony. Rather relief comes by means of a juridical settlement of a battle over which he never had any control. I believe it is fair to say that such plays as the *Oresteia* are a kind of allegory or representation of unconscious mental processes. But in Aeschylus' terms, madness comes from unbearable and conflicting external demands, not from inner ambivalence. These considerations are important to bear in mind as we turn to Euripides' *Orestes.*

The Orestes *of Euripides*

If the atmosphere of Aeschylus' *Oresteia* is that of malignant melancholia—blackness, bitterness, oral-sadistic fantasies—the atmosphere of Euripides' *Orestes* is that of paranoia. Euripides' chorus speaks of Orestes' murder of his mother and his subsequent attempts to justify the murder as examples of "the madness [*paranoia*] of evil-minded men" (ll. 823–24). While the Greek word *paranoia* did not denote a state of persecutory madness, the modern term, especially as enriched by psychodynamic understanding of florid paranoid states, aptly describes the character of Orestes and of his style of functioning.[45]

An ancient summary of the play states that the characters are exceptionally ignoble, and Aristotle said the character of Menelaus was drawn as excessively evil (*Poetics,* 1454a28).[46] But the play would not have been so widely admired in antiquity or so interesting to us today if it were merely a melodrama of villains. On the contrary, not only does Euripides portray a paranoid character but he portrays him with sympathy. We can pity him in his suffering as well as be indignant when he makes others suffer. As in a number of Euripides' plays, the dialogue abounds in the language and imagery of sickness.

At first the nature of the sickness is deliberately ambiguous. It is manifestly Orestes' insanity, marked by dramatic hallucinations of attacks by the Furies. It is almost as if he had fluctuating illness, perhaps malaria, with its intermittent fevers and bouts of mental confusion. He is being nursed and physically cared for. But as the play unfolds it becomes progressively clearer that the sickness entails the entire personality structure of Orestes and the kinds of choices he makes. Several forms of cure are attempted: Electra's tender nursing, the attempts to enlist the help of blood relatives, and an unsuccessful plea to the citizens of Argos to spare their lives. None avail. Electra's love and physical ministrations serve to stir up Orestes' fear of women as well as his incestuous feelings. In contrast to the trial in Aeschylus' drama, here the debate among the citizens ends with a vote to have Orestes and Electra put to death. Finally Orestes, embittered and disappointed with kin and kinship, *philoi* and *philia,* turns to his friend and comurderer of Clytemnestra, Pylades, who himself has been rejected by kin, his father.[47] The two friends now seek to reconstitute (with Electra) a new family, based not on blood but on the spilling of blood. In a kind of manic elation, they throw off guilt and remorse and escape the sentence of death by acting out their own conflicts instead of continuing to suffer with them. Helen is murdered and her daughter Hermione is taken hostage, about to be murdered. Before the play is over, Orestes captures a Phrygian slave and toys with him as he pleads for his life. Orestes taunts him for his effeminacy, a projection of his own effeminate side, and finally deigns to spare his life, finding the man beneath contempt for being "neither man nor woman."

The action crests in the last scene, a nightmare tableau. Orestes, Pylades, and Electra stand on the palace roof, threatening the murder of Hermione, ostensibly to force Menelaus to protect them. Torches are blazing as they prepare to set the palace afire. It is a mad scene of murder and frenzy, yet framed like a wedding. Apollo appears and, by sleight of hand, performs the trick of making everything right. Orestes is to marry Hermione, the hostage he is about to slay— hardly the best beginning for a marriage! Pylades will marry Electra, Helen is deified, Menelaus is to take a new wife, and all's well that ends well. There is a touch of the theater of the absurd here, as Apollo assumes the responsibility but not the blame and almost makes a mockery of the intensity and seriousness of the play. It is not surprising that at the very first performance of the play a famous actor who played Orestes mispronounced a word and turned a line of high seriousness into one that could have been in a comedy by Aristophanes.[48]

Aeschylus' *Oresteia* ends in a triumphant reconciliation of male and female, Olympian and chthonic, civic ties and blood ties, embodying that which is greatest and most creative in Athens. Euripides barely managed to patch the pieces together enough so that the play might end and the audience have some sort of resolution. There has been no transformation, no purification, no catharsis, no learning through suffering.

Certain points of contrast between the two dramatists are of more immediate concern here, namely, those that relate to conflict and madness. Euripides presents a more detailed and vivid clinical picture of the madman than does Aeschylus. In Euripides' *Orestes* we find the equivalent of a case history: for six days, since the cremation and burial of the mother he has murdered, Orestes has suffered from hallucinations and delusions that the Furies are attacking him. At one point he tries to ward them off with an imaginary bow and arrow. The madness first struck at night as he was standing by the pyre to gather his mother's ashes with his accomplice, Pylades. He sees three Furies, women black as night. He has periods of raving, during which he is wild-eyed and foaming at the mouth, leaping off his bed to escape his tormentors. He has periods of exhausted sleep. When not asleep and not hallucinating, he covers himself with a blanket and weeps. He scarcely eats and drinks, and he wishes to die.

This descriptive account is enlivened by interactional and psycho-dynamic detail of a sort that would not commonly be found in psychiatric case histories before the twentieth century. We get a sense that the same conflicts and character traits show up in the actively psychotic Orestes and in the Orestes who appears to be sane.

Orestes has been sleeping, and all are grateful for the respite. Electra has been nursing him physically and morally. He is restless, so she suggests that he try to walk. He assents (ll. 235–36),

> For this would give the appearance of health.
> Better is appearance, even if it is far from the truth.

Orestes is not merely stating a belief that he can be cured by acting healthy. He is making a statement that appearances (here the appearance of health) are better than reality. What is extraordinary is that the same word is used for the "appearance" (*doxa*) of health and for the hallucinations (*doxai*) that are tormenting him.

While his mind is momentarily clear, Electra prepares him for the news that Menelaus has arrived, a hope for salvation, but that he has brought Helen, the whore (ll. 246–87).

Orestes: If he alone had survived [without her], I would be more envious of him. If he brings his wife, he comes bearing a great evil.
Electra: A notorious reproach is the breed of daughters that Tyndareus begat [Clytemnestra and Helen], and infamous throughout Greece.

Orestes: But you now be different from these evil ones. You can. And not only speak differently, but think differently.

Electra: Oh, god, O my brother, your eyes are rolling. Swiftly you have taken on madness.

Orestes: O mother, I beg you, don't urge on against me these bloody-eyed and snake-haired virgins. They—it is they are next to me and jumping upon me.

Electra: Stay, O pitiable one, on your couch; do not shudder; for you see, in fact, nothing of what you imagine you see.

Orestes: O Phoebus, the dog-faced, gorgon-eyed priestesses of those below will kill me, these dreaded goddesses.

Electra: I won't let you go. I shall restrain you with my arms from your miserable wild leaping.

Orestes: Let me go. One of my Furies—that's what you are. And you are holding me back by my waist, in order to hurl me into Tartarus.

Electra: Oh, how wretched am I—what help can I find, now that we have gotten divinity as our enemy?

Orestes: Give me my horn-tipped bow, the gift of Apollo, which Apollo told me to use to ward off these goddesses. When they terrify me with their frenzied madnesses, one of these goddesses will be smitten with a mortal hand, unless she disappears from before my eyes. Don't you hear me? Don't you see the winged arrows, notched, ready to fly— Aha! But why do you delay? Leap high through the air with your wings; blame the oracles of Apollo. Oh, my god—what am I raving at, breathing so hard? Where have I leaped, from off my couch? For now over the waves I see a calm. My sister, why do you weep, with your head covered with your shroud? I am ashamed to so make you share my pains, giving you, a young woman, a burden with my sicknesses. Do not dissolve in tears because of my evils. You agreed to this crime, but the shedding of our mother's blood was my deed. And I blame Apollo, who thrust on me this most unholy deed, encouraged me with words, but not with his deeds.[49]

These lines contain a number of striking points. A man who has just murdered a queen and is now pursued by dreadful goddesses has been restored to sanity by sleep, whom he addresses (l. 213): "O queen, oblivion of sufferings, how wise a goddess. . . . " The poet also adds for us the detail that between hallucinations Orestes weeps. This is a striking clinical observation: many a psychotic, when his delusions are at bay, is profoundly depressed and overwhelmed by helplessness and despair because of a clear realization of the intense and irresolvable conflicts that have brought him into madness. The announcement that Menelaus and Helen have arrived stirs up both hope and the old rages at Helen and Clytemnestra. This news, combined with Electra's touch, activates the intense ambivalence toward the major women in his life—an ambivalence fed by both wishes for revenge and yearnings for tender closeness with caring females. His mistrust of women is profound, as shown in the rapid transformation of Electra from an angel of mercy to a winged persecutor. Dynamically informed observation of psychotics has repeatedly revealed this dilemma, that anyone who comes too close stirs up a defensive withdrawal and a defensive persecutory delusion. Electra, Helen, Clytemnestra, and the Furies are confused and merged. Electra introduces herself as one of three daughters (ll. 22–23), and Orestes hallucinates three Furies. The situation stirs up Orestes' feelings of helplessness, which he equates with femininity. Women are the source of lust, and lust is the origin of all Orestes' difficulties. He suddenly switches from passivity, which he equates with femininity, to a delusional activity. He demands a bow and arrow, the weapons of Apollo, to give him phallic strength; he will shoot down the Furies. Two maneuvers restore him to his senses: the shift from passivity to activity and the thrusting of blame on Apollo, thereby externalizing guilt and responsibility.

As the play proceeds, Orestes' cure, in effect, turns out to be again a switch to murderous action aimed primarily at women (Helen and Hermione). We have, then, a subtle portrait of a man who, when psychotic, feels himself persecuted by malignant females. When "normal" he handles his guilt and ambivalence by externalizing the blame and by destroying women, whom he constantly fears will unman him.[50]

Woven into the fabric of the play, too, are themes of barely disguised sexual attraction to Electra. The physical touching of the nursing scenes finds its culmination in a *Liebestod* fantasy, as brother and sister contemplate the possibility (granted to them by the citizens of Argos) of killing themselves rather than being executed (ll. 1047–53):

Orestes: You will make me melt! I want to reply [to your love] with a loving embrace. Why do I, miserable one, feel ashamed to do that? Oh, the bosom of my sister, oh, a sweet enfolding for me, this is a farewell for us hapless ones, in place of children and the marriage bed.

Electra: Oh, how I wish that same sword, if it is right, might slay us both, and one coffin, crafted of cedar, receive us both.[51]

But Electra becomes safe again as she is made less of a woman. When she proposes to take Hermione hostage and agrees to the slaying of Helen, Orestes is overjoyed and unsexes her (ll. 1205–1206): "Oh, the spirit of a man you have, though very much the body of a woman!" Finally, she will be wed to his friend (and, in effect, brother) Pylades. The incest is negated and then displaced. At the same time, Electra, of course, turns out to be the true daughter of Clytemnestra, another manly woman. (This point is brilliantly made in Sartre's version of the Orestes story, *The Flies*.)

In short, psychodynamic notions about the paranoid character enable us to highlight what is quite prominent in Euripides' portrayal of Orestes. Through either intuition or thoughtful observation of such people or both, the playwright presents a consistent and believable picture of the kind of man who would murder his mother, experience guilt-ridden persecutory delusions, and finally turn again to the murder of women to restore his sanity and save his skin.

This analysis of the character of Orestes illustrates a point made earlier—that Greek tragedy has "psychologized" the traditional myths. While Euripides does not present us with a psychodynamic theory, he does give us a portrait built around an understanding of conflict and defense and their transformations into symptoms and action. His point of view is that the madness not merely is an alien intrusion but has personal, characterological meaning.

Euripides has made abundantly clear a connection between the family history of the house of Atreus and the behavior of Orestes. He views this connection less in terms of a hereditary curse than did Aeschylus, and emphasizes rather the psychological need to repeat the pathological behavior of parents or grandparents.[52]

What of the ending of the play, the *deus ex machina,* Apollo setting all in order and preventing further bloodshed? Critics have disagreed about the meaning of this ending, but my own view is that the playwright intended it to be ambiguous, to leave us with a sense that the world and our fates are not entirely under our control. Both the crime and its resolution are partly in the hands of the gods, partly in the hands of men. The play does not say that all the conflict exists within the protagonists and antagonists. Orestes' action, as in Aeschylus, is embedded in a social and cosmic matrix. Euripides has shown us a man who has internalized the conflicting forces around him, so that he suffers from intelligible human conflicts. At the same time, however victimized Orestes has been, he is capable of choices, including the choice of whether or not to turn victimizer.

The *Bacchae* of Euripides

The *Bacchae,* Euripides' last play, was produced only after his death. It sums up much that he struggled with during the fifty years in which he wrote his dramas. It is the drama par excellence of madness, constantly exploring the question of who is truly mad and who is sane. It is the only extant tragedy in which two main characters are mad, and one may have doubts about the sanity of the others, especially Dionysus. Given the Greek dramatic convention of using no more than three actors, no matter how many roles were to be portrayed, it is possible that the same actor played Pentheus mad at one point and his mother, Agave, mad at another.

It is indeed a drama of confusion. No other play with which I am familiar is so replete with the imagery of dislocation, of the ground and the house giving way, of sudden shifts from vertical to horizontal and vice versa.[53] It is also the drama par excellence of illusion versus reality: one is constantly shifting and being transformed into the other. It is one of the most visual of Greek dramas, both in its imagery and in its preoccupation with prurient seeing and being seen. It is the epitome of dramatic disguise and confounding of identity: a god is disguised as a man, a man is disguised as a woman, and man is confounded with beast.

Of the extant plays, the *Bacchae* is the most closely tied to the setting of ritual and sacrificial feast. It is a grim feast the god demands, as a mother hunts and kills her own son. It is a drama of extreme ambivalence, and nowhere is love more confused with devouring rage, lust with destruction.

At the same time it is a drama of childhood and childish fantasies. "Oh, no, no, no, please don't go, we love you so we'll eat you up," proclaim the Wild Things to little Max in Maurice Sendak's book, and by rotating the axes of the *Bacchae* only a few degrees we can see it as a game in the nursery.[54] It presents infantile theories of sexuality and childbirth. Is sex murder or eating? Can babies be born from a father's thigh as well as from a mother's uterus? Where is daddy in the birth? We only know what mommy does. When and where can I peek at what goes on in private? In the nighttime, in the daytime? Is it safe to look, and can one just look and not participate? Pentheus asks the Stranger (Dionysus) who initiated him into these rites, and the Stranger replies that it was Dionysus himself, the son of Zeus, the same Zeus who wedded Semele. Pentheus continues: "Was it in a night vision or while awake that he forced you?" Dionysus replies: "No, he seeing me and I seeing him he bestows his rituals" (ll. 469–70).[55]

Finally, it is a grandiloquent discourse on reason and emotion, sobriety and drunkenness, ecstasy and orgy, intemperate rationality and temperate insanity. It is an essay on *sōphrosunē,* that great virtue which encompasses moderation, chastity, and sanity. When does change of mind signify an ability to adapt and to stay sane and when is it the cause and manifestation of out-and-out madness? As Pentheus is slipping into madness and Dionysus instructs him how to stride and dance like a Maenad, Dionysus praises him with the ambiguous phrase "You have taken a different stance in your mind" (which may also mean "You have gone out of your mind"), and Pentheus, deluded, asks expectantly whether he can now lift all

Mount Cithaeron on his shoulders (l. 945). Yet all lose. Cadmus, who bent with the wind and suggested acceptance of the fiction of Dionysus's birth—he too is wrecked at the end and accuses Dionysus of cruelty beyond measure.

The *Bacchae* is also a political discourse, concerned with the definition of *sophia* (wisdom) and *sōphrosunē* as collective virtues. The ecstatic group activity of the women of Thebes, an ecstasy shading off into madness, is also a political rebellion.[56] Tiresias and Cadmus argue as eloquently as Socrates in the *Republic* for the necessity of illusion and fiction in the well-governed state. And as in the *Republic,* the fiction that allows civil tranquillity involves the family and birth: Pentheus will not accept the tale that Zeus impregnated Semele. Agave, Pentheus's mother, and her other sisters similarly scoffed at this tale of Semele and her divine consort. Dionysus, in revenge, stirs the women of Thebes into orgiastic frenzy and drives Agave and Pentheus mad.

Dionysus is the god who induces madness, and in some mythic versions was himself driven mad by Hera in revenge against Zeus. Hera is also said to have caused his effeminacy, which is closely related to the theme of madness.[57] As is often the case, we do not know for certain to what extent these other mythic versions were present in the minds of the playwright and audience, nor do we know whether their exclusion from this dramatic rendering of the myth is significant. In any case, the array of myths in which Dionysus drives mad those who oppose him is formidable.

Thus in the *Bacchae,* as in all the other plays about madness, a divinity has been the manifest cause of madness, imposing it as a punishment for infringement of his or her rights. In these later works, in contrast to the Homeric epics, we generally do not find mental activity or mental states manifestly instigated by the gods, but madness is a conspicuous exception, an exception that the *Bacchae* may help to explain. The *Bacchae,* more than any of the other "mad plays," emphasizes that in madness delusion is accompanied by a blurring of the boundaries between the self and the other, a confusion of personal identity. It is clear in the *Bacchae* that Dionysus is a part of Pentheus, a split-off, repressed, and denied portion of him, the embodiment of his unconscious impulses and fears. While *we* may interpret Athena's role in Ajax's madness as a representation of Ajax's feared and wished-for maternal introject, such an interpretation is hardly in the forefront of the dramatic presentation. Euripides' *Orestes* comes closer to showing the Furies as an embodiment of part of Orestes. But in the *Bacchae* we see a detailed interaction of Pentheus and Dionysus, almost an interpenetration. In no other extant play does the plot include an extensive interaction between the agency and the victim. In short, the manifest confusion of inside and outside, of subject and object (in technical language a reprojection outward of destructive introjects), present in many forms of madness renders more plausible the representation of this form of mental activity as directly caused by a god or goddess.

Let us first consider the madness of Pentheus. It is shown step by step to take place in an interpersonal process. Dionysus, the other "person" in this process, embodies the urges for release, the yearnings for ecstatic orgy, the repressed sexuality, and the warded-off, dreaded wishes to be feminine.[58] Further, one sees Dionysus's power not only as he tempts the repressed prurient and voyeuristic side of Pentheus but as he stimulates wishes even more strenuously denied— the wish of the mighty tyrant to be a small baby nursing in his mother's arms or safely absorbed inside the mother. (Note that Pentheus is a man without a father; Dionysus had a father, Zeus, who actually carried him inside himself.) Thus, while most commentators have emphasized the repressed sexuality (the more psychoanalytically inclined can point to the redundant suggestions of a child wishing and fearing to witness the parents' activity), fewer have called attention to such lines as 963–70, where Dionysus takes Pentheus, disguised as a woman, to spy on the mountain Bacchanals.[59]

Dionysus: You and you alone will suffer for your city.
          A great ordeal awaits you. But you are worthy
          of your fate. I shall lead you safely there;
          someone else shall bring you back.
Pentheus: Yes, my mother.
Dionysus: An example to all men.
Pentheus: It is for that I go.
Dionysus: You will be carried home—
Pentheus: O luxury!
Dionysus: cradled in your mother's arms.
Pentheus: You will spoil me.
Dionysus: I *mean* to spoil you.
Pentheus: I go to my reward.

And this is from the man for whom yielding or compromising is womanish, for whom to be bested by a woman is the worst of all possibilities.

"Reaction formation" is an accurate term for the defense that leads to this kind of character structure, but it is pale and prosaic. Dionysus touches off something within Pentheus, but Pentheus appears to experience this as a threat more from without than from within. More accurately, the playwright conveys the sense that Pentheus does not know which danger comes from within and which from without. I believe the palace-miracle scene epitomizes the confusion.

The diversity of scholarly opinion on whether the events take place on stage or in the imagination is an index of deliberate ambiguity on the part of the playwright. The palace is separate from Pentheus, yet it is also Pentheus himself and his family.[60] The toppling palace, the quaking ground, and the fire represent physical and psychical reality. The Maenads have escaped their bonds and Dionysus has escaped Pentheus's prison. Though he knows, as Dionysus reminds him, that the god can easily pass through locks and walls, Pentheus orders his servants to "lock all the towers round the city" (l. 655).

Pentheus is momentarily restored when he hears the messenger's description of the Maenads' activities (ll. 677–774). The messenger's speech, among other things, describes the quiet of the Bacchic women, their peaceful if bizarre occupations (nursing young animals), and the warfare they wage when they feel threatened. They have assaulted villages, routed men at arms, and performed miracles of strength. Pentheus is outraged and yet restored. "Take to arms" is his response, and he arrays his forces. Pentheus looks to his armor and spear to defend himself against *inner* threats, which include his wishes to become a woman among the women and his fears of the Maenads as phallic destroyers.

Dionysus's sadistic "interpretation" to Pentheus is the turning point where Pentheus's will is finally destroyed (l. 810):

Dionysus: Wouldn't you like to see them encamped?
Pentheus: Oh, very much, countless gold would I give to see.[61]

No other Greek tragedy, not even *Oedipus Rex,* makes so much of seeing and not seeing, of seeming to see correctly but really suffering from (or taking pleasure in) an illusion. Pentheus is portrayed as a man of imagination, as many commentators have pointed out. He can visualize what is happening elsewhere, particularly if it has the suspicion of sexuality (ll. 215–25):

> I happened to be away, out of the city,
> but reports reached me of some strange mischief here,
> stories of our women leaving home to frisk
> in mock ecstasies among the thickets on the mountains,
> dancing in honor of the latest divinity,
> a certain Dionysus, whoever he may be!
> In their midst stand bowls brimming with wine.
> And then, one by one, the women wander off
> to hidden nooks where they serve the lusts of men.
> Priestesses of Bacchus they claim they are,
> but it's really Aphrodite they adore.

While he is still manifestly sane, he is told by Cadmus, Tiresias (the blind prophet), and Dionysus that he is mad and neither thinks nor sees correctly. Hence it is altogether appropriate that in the process of going mad he suffers from visual disturbances.[62] He sees Dionysus turn into a bull as he tries to lock him up. As sanity slips further away, he sees double, "two suns, two Thebes." He who is so afraid to look ridiculous and makes fun of the appearance of old Cadmus and Tiresias finally longs to be exhibited, "for I am the only man of these Thebans who dares this" (l. 926).

The imagery of scopophilic impulses blends subtly with the imagery of orality and oral incorporation.[63] In the early stages of the play, Tiresias accuses Pentheus of being unable to see the truth, of being mad, and concludes (ll. 326–28):

> For you are most painfully mad, and you will not
> take cure with any drugs, though
> you are mad because of drugs.

This speech emphasizes the oral aspects of the god: he gives wine, which gives sleep, a balm to all ills, and though a god, he is a libation to the gods. Pentheus is figuratively drugged and blinded by his own evil, and will not be cured because he will not take the medicines that Dionysus offers—wine, dance, ecstasy, and obliteration of self in the group of worshipers.

The madness of Agave, while consistent with the psychological order in which the madness of Pentheus is described, has a different emphasis. Dionysus drives her, too, mad as a punishment, but the process is different. For her the pathway to madness is not through intense personal interaction but rather through the process of absorption into the group. Pentheus refuses to join and, even when dressed as a female Bacchant, wants to look, not participate. Agave not only joins, she is one of the leaders.

The group process of going mad is an extension of the very process of forming the group and conducting the worship of the god. The worship involves dance, ecstasy, the common wish to escape the ordinary (rather limited) life of a woman, and to find another level of experience. The group experience is built around merging of the members with the godhead, the god entering the worshiper (see, for example, l. 298), and the merging implied in the common dance and hymn. We find also the communal hunt, the tearing apart and eating of the animal, and the nursing of young animals. There is union without dissension among the sisters, union of mother and child, and a fusion with the world of nature, animals, plants, and landscape. The play suggests some motivations for these kinds of fusion. As for the unity of the sisters, note that it was the slander of Agave and the other sisters against Semele that led Dionysus to drive the women into Bacchic frenzy and finally into madness. Dionysus, as leader of the women, seems a better father than Cadmus, who is interested only in sons. Their aggression toward their own children leads them to flight and to a compensatory closeness with animal children. At the same time, the aggression is directed toward animals, and the women are identified with the animals they kill. The Bacchantes are themselves fawns escaping the hunter (ll. 862–76), and they are the hunters, who wear the skins of the animals they slay and devour.

The account of Pentheus's madness emphasizes the splitting off of disavowed parts of the personality and the subsequent return of the repressed. The madness of Agave centers more on blissful fusion and merging of the self, which culminates in a destructive, cannibalistic act of absorption of the ambivalently regarded child. (Agave presents Pentheus's head, which she sees as that of a lion, as part of an invitation to a glorious feast.) Euripides, then, captures in dramatic action the psychodynamic significance of ecstatic states and wishes to merge, as they appear in various severe clinical psychoses. The urge toward fusion and ecstatic dissolution of the self gratifies deep unfulfilled longings for a blissful unity of mother and child and simultaneously denies the destructive rage that accompanies the inevitable reality that such wishes must be frustrated. Psychodynamic formulations also point to the wish to merge as a way of dealing with rage at younger siblings who displace the older child at the mother's breast.[64]

Pentheus breaks down because he cannot accept a feminine side of himself which is not oriented toward power (for example, ll. 310–14). He cannot honor the god who is bisexual, honors women, frees them, and invites all to the pleasures that do not demand power and status. (Even Zeus has a "womb" and can accept carrying a baby.) At the same time the god—and this is the dual nature of his temperament—offers to the women the chance to participate in the godhead, to share in his divine power. The women, then, organize around this god because they find an opportunity to express at once their femininity, their nurturant wishes, their wishes to be nurtured, and their wishes to have the prerogatives of men. It is as if they can have the best of both worlds. With their *thyrsoi* (fennel stalks) they are more powerful than bands of armed men. Further, the fusion of male and female in the Bacchic ecstasy is accomplished with ease, without envy, and without malice.

Group ecstasy becomes madness because the Bacchic ecstasy does not, in fact, resolve the underlying conflict. The press to be the male—that is, the hunter—rather than the hunted female or child is too great. We can speculate that because the *thiasos,* the band, is organized around a male leader, there is a continuous reminder of penis, power, and prerogatives that the women do not have. The

women are still dependent upon a male, however effeminate or bisexual he may be.

The play culminates in the meeting of the two madnesses, that of
Pentheus and that of Agave. It is not just a meeting, it is an *agon,* a
contest. Dionysus says (ll. 973–76):

> Agave and you daughters of Cadmus,
> reach out your hands! I bring this young man
> to a great ordeal. The victor? Bromius.
> Bromius—and I. The rest the event shall show.

Agave is deluded into thinking she is the victor along with Bromius
(Dionysus). The messenger presents this grim irony (ll. 1143–48):

> Leaving her sisters
> at the Maenad dances, she is coming here, gloating
> over her grisly prize. She calls upon Bacchus:
> he is her "fellow huntsman," "comrade of the chase,
> crowned with victory." But all the victory she
> carries home is her own grief.

Agave enters, carrying Pentheus's head, but proclaiming it is the
head of a young lion:

> This is the quarry of our chase, taken not with nets nor spears of
>   bronze but by the white
> and delicate hands of women. What are they worth,
> your boastings now and all that uselessness
> your armor is,
> since we, with our bare hands,
> captured this quarry and tore its bleeding body. . . .
> [ll. 1204–1209]

> Now, Father,
> yours can be the proudest boast of living men.
> For you are now the father of the bravest daughters
> in the world. All of your daughters are brave,
> but I above the rest. I have left my shuttle
> at the loom; I raised my sight to higher things—
> to hunting animals with my bare hands.   [ll. 1233–39]

The women have entered the lists of the male contests and defeated the males—but it is a hollow victory, for Dionysus has already
declared that he will be the victor.

Thus the question of how to express both the male and the female
has no harmonious resolution; there is no way to suppress and eliminate elemental rage and envy. What comedy treats as the "battle of
the sexes" is here tragic encounter.[65] Cadmus's wife was named
Harmonia, but the resolution that the god pronounces at the end
hardly sounds harmonious and balanced. She and Cadmus, at whose

wedding the Muses sang, must suffer. Their fate is to perform the very converse of the coming of Dionysus to Greece, he who ostensibly brings joy and ecstasy. They will go into exile and, transformed into serpents, lead a barbarian host that will plunder Greece, even the oracle of Apollo. The thought that at the end they will be made into gods is no consolation to Cadmus. Dionysus promises peace, ecstasy, and harmony, but in fact brings madness and war.

The play has come full circle, as if Euripides has taken characters and situation and slowly rotated them in front of our eyes, so that we have seen the sanity and madness and cruelty and ecstasy in each. Euripides sees the madness as an act far more of divine malevolence than of divine beneficence. Dionysus is revealed as cruel and vengeful beyond measure; gods should be more understanding and forgiving than men.[66] The *Bacchae* is far from a piece in praise of madness.

At the same time, Euripides conveys that it is madness to choke off and deny elemental, pressing human needs. Every god must be given his due. It is madness to resist too much, but it is madness to yield too much to these impulses. This tension makes the *Bacchae* a tragedy—to be human is to fail in making the ideal compromise. It is as if the poet were saying that there is an irreducible quota of cruelty in the universe—in the gods, in the elemental forces of nature, and in the relations between human beings. We can speak prosaically of the language of conflict and ambivalence. We can invoke the poetic truth in Freud's paean to the eternal struggle between Eros and the death instinct. And we can continue to listen to the resonance of the lines of the last and greatest of the tragedians, who has intoned for us a wild dithyramb and the cry of the babe in one and the same symphony.

7

Tragedy and Therapy

Do you not know, Prometheus, that there are words that are physicians for the sickness of wrath?

—Aeschylus, *Prometheus Bound*

Knowledge through suffering.

—Aeschylus, *Agamemnon*

The therapy in the tragedies must be commensurate with the destructiveness of the madness itself. No trifling cures suffice. Words are important but not sufficient; suffering, unless understood and integrated, is meaningless. Action, if unreflective and not aimed toward a new resolution, merely perpetuates the old madness in different forms. In the plays about madness the playwrights have divined that working through conflict is necessary for cure. As various characters try to relieve and cure the madman, treatments that are adequate to the task are contrasted with those that are not.

Is theater therapeutic for the private burdens of the individuals in the audience? Is it therapeutic for the collective or communal ills and the social tensions and conflicts from which all members of the audience suffer? My discussion will turn on the nature of the tragedian's art and the analogous processes in psychotherapy. Finally, I shall explore a hypothesis by means of which we can understand something of the function of madness in drama in the economy of the mind of the playwright who attempts to produce great tragedy.

Let us examine how "cure" or restitution is achieved in several of the plays involving overt madness. We may begin with two instances of incurable illness—the first, in Aristophanes' *Wasps,* is comic; the second, in Sophocles' *Ajax,* is tragic.[1]

The *Wasps* of Aristophanes

The *Wasps* is about an elderly Athenian, Philocleon (Cleon lover), who suffers from a terrible disease that has driven his son, Bdelycleon (Cleon hater), to distraction. The father, though, has little pain and much pleasure and profit from his condition. Two of the son's

slaves are guarding the old man. After some banter about the name
of the disease, one of the slaves proclaims (ll. 88–91):

> He's a JURY-addict! Most violent case on record.
> He's wild to render verdicts, and bawls like a baby
> if ever he misses a seat on the very first bench.
> He doesn't get any sleep at night, not a wink.
> Or, if he closes his eyes a speck, he's in Court. . . .

He details all the other signs and symptoms of the old man's madness.

> In sum, he's insane; the more we reason with him,
> the more he judges everybody else. Absolutely
> hopeless. Incurable.
> 　　　　　　　　So now we've locked him up
> with bolts, and watch to be sure he doesn't go out.
> The son, you see, takes his daddy's disease quite hard.
> First, he tried the Word Cure. Gently he wheedled
> and pleaded with the old man to put away his cloak
> and stay home.
> 　　　Didn't work. So next, the Water Cure.
> Dunked him and dosed him.*
> 　　　　　　　　No dice.
> 　　　　　　　　　　Then applied Religion.
> 　　Made him a Korybant.
> 　　　　　　　　　　Tambourine and all, his daddy
> banged his way into court for more drumhead justice.
> Finally, as a last recourse, he turned to Pure Prayer.
> One night he grabbed the old man, sailed over to Aiginia,
> and bedded him down for the cure in Asklepios' temple . . .
> and up he popped at dawn by the jury-box gate!
> Since then, we never let him out of the house. . . .   [ll. 111–24]
> 　　　　　　.　　　.　　　.
> At last we took these nets and draped them around
> all over the house—and now we keep him in.   [ll. 131–32][2]

We have here a veritable inventory of the Greek methods of dealing with a madman: persuasion with soft words, washing and puri-
fying, Corybantic ecstatic ceremonies that had an explicit therapeutic
aim, and, finally, a trip to the temple of Asclepius for cure by "incu-
bation," a treatment that entailed ritual purification. (The "patient"
spends a night in the temple, and later the priest interprets his
dreams.) The last resort is confinement.

Since none of these efforts has availed, the son contrives a mock
trial at home: the dog is tried for the crime of stealing cheese, and his
father is the jury. Philocleon has momentarily agreed to restrict his

---

Ekathaire, literally cleansed or purged.

trying of cases to domestic affairs, and the dog is first to be hauled before this new stay-at-home courtroom. The father throws himself into the task, but alas, the ploy does not work. The old man tries to sneak out of the house under a donkey, like Odysseus leaving the Cyclops's cave under a ram. The son tries one final approach: convert the father from a crabby old man, whose main pleasures are those of passing judgment and handing out sentences, to a rollicking, frolicking Athenian gentleman, complete with banquets and flute girls. The father's conversion to this new life is the comic counterpart of Pentheus's dressing up as a Maenad and giving vent to previously suppressed impulses. The old man does a complete turnabout, and he likes the new life so well that he is now a different kind of plague to his son. The outcome can be compared to Orestes' fate in the Euripides play. One form of madness has been traded for another. The old man has been turned about but has not mastered his impulses or achieved any true inner understanding.

The *Ajax* of Sophocles

Sophocles' *Ajax* is built on a mythic tradition well known to the Athenian audience.[3] The *Odyssey* (11.541–65) provides a portrait of an Ajax who will never yield in his bitterness: even when, in Hades, Odysseus asks him for forgiveness, Ajax is as unrelenting in his refusal to be reconciled with the man who bested him in the contest for the arms of Achilles as he is unyielding in battle. His suicide may be implicit in this story; it is made explicit, as is his madness, in later epic tradition.

Ajax opens with Athena telling Odysseus that she has driven Ajax mad to prevent him from killing Agamemnon, Menelaus, and Odysseus himself and to punish him for his attempt. To Ajax's mind, Odysseus has been awarded the arms of Achilles unfairly, and he blames the two Atreidae for a dishonest judgment. Ajax has gone to slay these three in the middle of the night, but Athena deludes him into thinking that animals in the flocks of booty are the humans he seeks. Ajax has slaughtered cattle and the guards and has brought some of the animals to his tent, where he has continued to slaughter, torture, and whip them. As the plot unfolds, Ajax comes to his senses, realizes what he has done, and sinks into a state of profound shame and despair. Eventually, ignoring the pleas of his wife and the chorus and the mute appeal of his little son, he kills himself with the sword he once received as a gift from his enemy Hector. The latter part of the play deals with the struggle of his half brother Teucer to obtain a proper burial for him in the face of the bitter refusal of Agamemnon and Menelaus to honor the man who tried to take their lives. In the end, Odysseus, Ajax's rival, prevails upon the leaders of

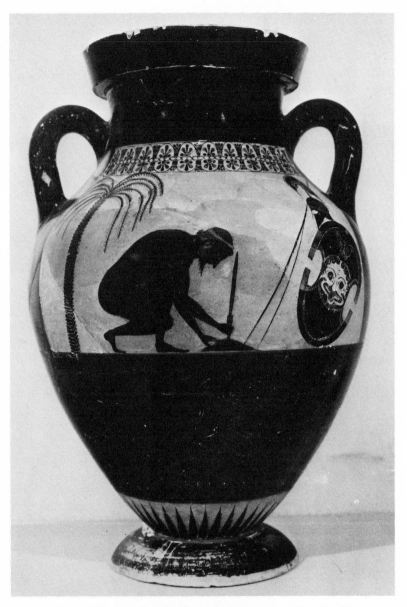

Ajax planting his sword in the ground in preparation for suicide.
Attic black-figured amphora by Exekias, sixth century B.C. Musée Communal, Boulogne-sur-Mer. Photo Henri Devos.

the Greeks to recognize that, even if he was an enemy, Ajax's nobility in life warrants reverence in death.

Ajax's sickness has two phases. First is the delusional state brought on by the cold wrath of Athena. Second is the lucid state of despair and shame, culminating in suicide. Greek popular and medical tradition agreed that Ajax was a melancholic, and the Greek diagnosis probably included both the delusional and depressive aspects.[4] The play, however, gives two conflicting interpretations of the affliction. For the chorus, Ajax has been driven mad by a divinity, and now that the madness is over, he should feel relieved (ll. 262–63, 279–80).[5] But his wife, Tecmessa, articulates Ajax's position:

> Ajax, so long as the mad fit was on him,
> Himself felt joy at all his wretchedness,
> Though we, his sane companions, grieved indeed.
>   But now that he's recovered and breathes clear,
>   His own anguish totally masters him.   [ll. 271–75]

She narrates the wild exultation of his imaginary vengeance on his enemies.

>   Then
> He sprang back in again, and somehow, slowly,
> By painful stages came to his right mind.
> And when he saw his dwelling full of ruin,
> He beat his head and bellowed. There he sat,
> Wreckage himself among the wreck of corpses,
> The sheep slaughtered; and in an anguished gripe
> Of fist and fingernail he clutched his hair.   [ll. 305–310]

> And told him, simply, everything I knew.
> Then he cried out—long wails of shattering pain,
> Like none I ever heard from him before;
> He always used to say such cries were base,
> Marks of an abject spirit.   [ll. 316–20]

> Now, though, quite overcome by his misfortune,
> Refusing food and drink, he sits there motionless,
> Relapsed among the beasts his iron brought down.
> There are clear signs, too,
> That he's aiming to do some dreadful thing; his words
> And his lamentations both somehow suggest it.
> Friends—this was the thing I came to ask of you—
> Won't you come in and comfort him, if you can?
> He is noble and may listen to his friends.   [ll. 323–30]

As the chorus begins to speak with him, Ajax appeals to them to

>   ease my pain.
> For God's sake, help me die!

The chorus cries:

> Hush! Check those awful words!
> Don't seek a worse cure for an ill disease,
> And make your pain still heavier than it is.   [ll. 361–64]

Later, as Ajax, rejecting all pleas, announces his plans for death, he gives their child to his wife and dismisses her:

> . . . no wailing . . .
> Make fast, and hurry!
> It is not for the skilled physician to incant chants for a pain that requires the knife.   [ll. 579, 581–83][6]

We see here two conceptions of sickness and cure. For the chorus, sickness is a divine attack and cure is its remission. For Ajax the delusional sickness is only the first part, and the cure for the entire sickness is no palliative, it is only suicide, "the knife."

At the most literal level, we can see that Ajax believes that the intense disgrace of what he has done in madness requires his suicide. But this is not the stuff of tragedy. The chorus and his wife appeal to him to put aside his personal sense of humiliation and failure, and think of their welfare. They suggest that failure to protect his wife, child, and loyal subjects would also bring disgrace, and that his obligation to them is as great as the obligation "to be always the best and ahead of all the others" (*Iliad*, 6.208). Ajax cannot and will not bend, though for a moment his speech on the subject of time gives hope to the others that he will not kill himself.

The tragedy of the play lies in the fact that Ajax's illness is incurable, because the illness and Ajax are one. This point can be made clear by two considerations, the first a general psychodynamic view of acute psychosis, the second an examination of the famous speech on time.

A psychotic breakdown usually occurs in the face of an unresolvable conflict.[7] A young man, for example, confronts a situation that demands vigorous self-assertion. He has devoted much of his life consciously and unconsciously to disavowing aggression in his makeup, and this new demand is intolerable. Unable to fight or flee, he is overcome by mounting anxiety, guilt, and fear of disintegration. This conflict is the precursor of the actual psychosis, which comes on as anxiety and completely overwhelms his defenses. The acute schizophrenic episode is characterized by confusion, massive anxiety, and a fluctuating array of delusional belief and/or hallucinations. This stage is short-lived, as it is both psychologically and physiologically intolerable, and is followed by a state of psychotic restitution. Here anxiety and pain diminish, and a stable delusional state may ensue. The person is now calm, even happy, for he now "understands" that he is a divinely appointed messenger, preaching a gospel of no aggression, no anger, no self-assertion. In fact, he carries a large knife and is prepared to sacrifice himself or another if the divine message is not heeded. He hallucinates a voice giving him instructions, and he learns the truth by reading omens unintelligible to others. (This stage could be compared to Ajax's exultation at the slaughter of his archrivals. He is joyous. Others feel pain; he does not.) When the psychotic resolution is relinquished, he is left depressed, overcome by hopelessness and helplessness. He can no longer use the psychotic escape and suffers from an awareness of the conflicts that originally led him to his impasse. When the pain proves too great, he reverts to the delusional defense, or he may commit suicide. If he can come to terms with the previously disavowed parts of his self (for example, if he ceases to feel an intense need to deny all aggression) and can understand why his conflicts were intolerable, he achieves a significant cure, in the sense of working through his conflicts, not merely suppressing them or translating them into behavior that repeats the conflict.

This psychodynamic formulation embodies a view of human life as tragic, in the sense that conflict is inevitable and that cure entails coming to grips with that conflict. These ideas highlight the conflicting conceptions of cure in the *Ajax*. At the end of his delusional episode, Ajax is in despair not only because of his shame at what he has done but because he knows that he has come to this pass largely because of the kind of person he is. Pride and fear of humiliation and ridicule (as both internal and external pressures) did not allow him to accept the awarding of the arms to Odysseus. He could not bend, acquiesce, or compromise, and indirect revenge is just not his style. After his acute delusional attack, he knows that he cannot continue to live honorably. He sees himself as unable to return home to his heroic father, having achieved less honor than he. How can he return in absolute disgrace? He has lost too much face to be able to face the important people in his life. He is not the kind of man that Odysseus is, not just because Odysseus is unscrupulous but because Odysseus can yield, change, and modify.

At this juncture, let us turn to Ajax's speech on time, uttered just before he goes off to kill himself. He announces to his wife and the chorus that he will yield to their entreaties and forgo suicide.

> Strangely the long and countless drift of time
> Brings all things forth from darkness into light,
> Then covers them once more. Nothing so marvelous
> That man can say it surely will not be—
> Strong oath and iron intent come crashing down.
> *My* mood, which just before was strong and rigid,

No dipped sword more so, now has lost its edge—
My speech is womanish for this woman's sake;
And pity touches me for wife and child,
Widowed and lost among my enemies.
But now I'm going to the bathing place
And meadows by the sea, to cleanse my stains,
In hope the goddess' wrath may pass from me.
And when I've found a place that's quite deserted,
I'll dig in the ground, and hide this sword of mine,
Hatefulest of weapons, out of sight.

                 .   .   .

From now on this will be my rule: Give way
To heaven, and bow before the sons of Atreus.
They are our rulers, they must be obeyed.
I must give way, as all dread strengths give way,
In turn and deference. Winter's hard-packed snow
Cedes to fruitful summer; stubborn night
At last removes, for day's white steeds to shine.

                 .   .   .

                              . . . Shall not I
Learn place and wisdom?* Have I not learned this,
Only so much to hate my enemy
As though he might again become my friend,
And so much good to wish to do my friend,
As knowing he may yet become my foe?   [ll. 644–81]

Most commentators, while noting its ironies (such as "I'll hide my sword," l. 692), have considered the speech only as a piece of conscious deception on the part of Ajax. He dissembles, pretending that he has found inner peace and his friends can now rest easy. Bernard Knox, however, has argued convincingly that the speech in fact reveals most poignantly Ajax's motives for suicide.[8] Ajax is not for this world, for he cannot conform to the world as it is; he is the snow that cannot melt and the night that cannot yield to day. He cannot allow his sword to become dulled, but must rather kill himself with it. He cannot learn the lessons of compromise; hence, with the shattering of the simple world of the heroic ethos, he cannot survive. To bend is to become impotent or, even worse, a woman. He must kill himself because he sees no way out of the impasse that originally led him to go mad. His dissimulation is actually an explanation of his suicide. The play is all the more tragic because the resolution takes place only after his death; only then do the sons of Atreus yield their implacable hatred to the arguments of Odysseus.

---

*Sōphronein, to be moderate, to be sane.

Only then does Odysseus convince them that to change one's mind is not weak.

Other suggestions in the dramatic portrayal of Ajax's character are in harmony with this view of the speech and of the play. In brief, one could construct an argument that Ajax has to be *monos,* the loner, the only one.[9] He cannot accept help. He committed an act of *hubris* against Athena by proclaiming that only weaklings need divine help (ll. 749–59), and he cannot accept help from wife or supporters. He cannot envision his parents helping him in his defeat, only reminding him of his disgrace. He has no less difficulty in dealing with rivals. We catch overtones of Ajax as a kind of "only child" who goes beserk when his rivals get more than he does.[10] He has lost to Odysseus in the contest; Athena used to be his protecting goddess, but she has always preferred Odysseus. Even Ajax's moving speech to his son (ll. 550–52) contains a note of envy.

In sum, the theme of Ajax as one who needs to be alone, to be unique, and to be recognized as special is interwoven with the theme of Ajax as the man who cannot bend and cannot yield. Sophocles' art has made Ajax not an obstinate man or a spoiled brat but a hero who arouses our sympathies. His quest for honor and the honorable appeals to something in our own ideals. The poet has simultaneously portrayed a sickness that has no simple cure and a hero who must die because he can accept nothing less than a definitive cure.

The *Heracles* of Euripides

A comparison of the *Ajax* with Euripides' *Heracles* is instructive. Heracles, driven mad by Hera's malevolence, kills his wife and three sons, and almost slays his father. Like Ajax, he wishes to die when he becomes aware of what he has done. Unlike Ajax, he comes to a resolution that allows him to continue living.

The *Heracles* is the earliest of the three extant Euripidean dramas of madness.[11] I have argued that in the *Orestes* and *Bacchae* madness is interwoven with character; in the *Heracles* it comes from divine caprice and is cured by divine intervention. No character in this play suggests that Heracles' madness is anything but a terrible external affliction.

The structure of the play poses problems that have bedeviled critics, for it seems to be composed of either two or three discrete parts. Those who admire and are deeply moved by the play have argued for its intrinsic unity, while its detractors have focused on its obvious discontinuities. I am convinced that those discontinuities are part of the message of the play and help to convey the poet's view of the causes of Heracles' distress.

The play opens as Heracles' family—his wife, Megara; their three young sons; and his aged father, Amphitryon—are huddled around an altar in Thebes. They have found temporary sanctuary. Lycus, an upstart who has slain Megara's father, Creon, and has taken over Thebes, intends to kill them all. But where is Heracles? He is, as far as they know, in Hades, where he has gone to help his friend Theseus after having completed his twelve labors. By now his is presumed dead, and virtually all hope for the family is gone. We learn that he has embarked on his heroic labors in order to help regain his father's lost kingdom of Argos. His great labors have helped to civilize, or tame, all of Greece; he has carried a great burden, made literal when he held the earth for Atlas. At last he appears, just in time to slay the tyrant Lycus and save his family. This part of the play verges on the melodramatic and is relatively stiff and stereotyped.

The second part begins with a dialogue between Lyssa (madness) and Iris in which the two deities announce their intention to drive Heracles mad as part of Hera's jealous revenge. Lyssa is reluctant to do her part—Heracles is a great hero and this affliction is not deserved— but she must yield to Hera. Lyssa and Iris begin the mad music and dance that make this scene the most chilling and awe-inspiring in Greek tragedy. The attack of madness begins as the whole family is gathered at the sacrificial altar for a thanksgiving offering. Heracles suddenly begins to foam at the mouth and go berserk, beginning an imaginary journey and hunting down his own wife and children, slaughtering them as though they were his enemies, and barely sparing his father. His attack, and this part of the drama, ends as Athena heaves a great stone at his chest, knocking him unconscious.[12]

The third part consists of the awakening of Heracles, his gradual realization of what he has done and his wish to kill himself, and finally the arrival of Theseus. The dialogue with Theseus leads to a resolution of the horror of the murder.

William Arrowsmith has offered the most compelling arguments for the unity of the play.[13] For him, the discontinuities bespeak a deliberate effort of the playwright to express a discontinuity in the world of the hero, a stark contrast between a world of received and conventional conduct and a world where "tradition is dumb and conduct uncharted." Heroes know how to come to the rescue of beleaguered friends and family and how to slaughter their enemies—the first part of the play. The madness is a "wrenching dislocation" that moves the hero to a new problem—how to come to terms with his own frailty.[14] How does the man of action behave when he finds himself the enemy of his own family, when he cannot solve the problem simply by destroying an external foe? "Tradition does not give a clear answer, and the received, traditional heroic reality must be transfigured. The dissonance between the two realities is itself a madness."

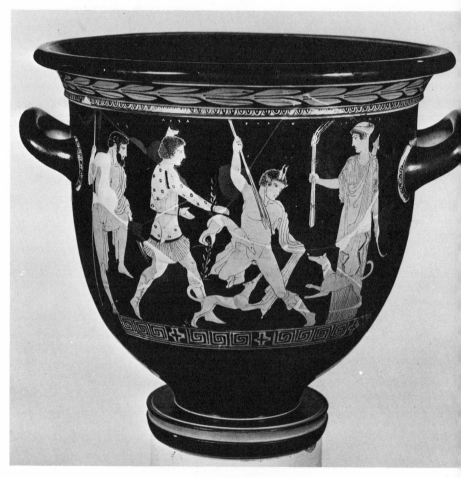

Lyssa and Actaeon. In this unusual version of the myth, Lyssa has driven either Actaeon
the dogs mad. The central figure is Actaeon, shown as he turns into a stag and is attacke
his hounds. To the left of Actaeon stands Lyssa (spelled Lysa in the inscription) with a
head atop her own. At the far left is Zeus; Artemis is at the extreme right.

Attic red-figured krater, fifth century B.C. Courtesy Museum of Fine Arts, Boston.

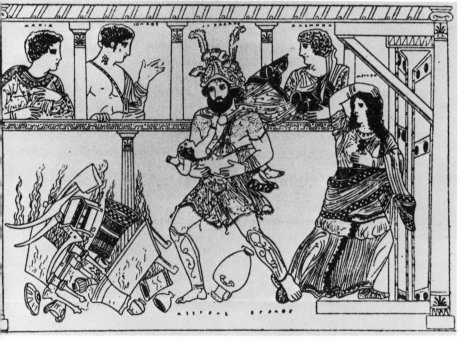

The madness of Heracles. The scene probably illustrates a version of the story other than Euripides'. Represented, from left to right, are Mania, Iolaos (Heracles' nephew), Heracles, Megara (his wife), and Alcmene (his mother).

Detail of Attic red-figured krater by Asteas, fourth century B.C., in the Museo Arqueológico Nacional, Madrid. Sketch from Euripides, *Hercules Furens,* ed. E. H. Blakeney (Edinburgh: Blackwood and Sons, 1904).

The change from the heroic and mythic ethos to the more tragic and existential permeates and unites the parts of the play. Consider Euripides' use of the dual paternity of Heracles—Zeus is the immortal father and Amphitryon the mortal. Early in the play Amphitryon begins to denounce the formal paternity of Zeus, which contrasts with Zeus's lack of care for his own son (ll. 339–47). By the end of the play, Zeus as father has become irrelevant. Amphitryon's paternity is established by virtue of the love between him and Heracles, and by his capacity to suffer with his son.

Other characters echo the theme of the inadequacy of the heroic-mythic outlook. Megara describes her meager efforts at comforting her children (ll. 73–79):

> First one, then another, bursts into tears,
> and asks: "Mother, where has Father gone?"
> "What is he doing? When will he come back?"
> Then, too small to understand, they ask again
> for "Father." *I put them off with stories:*
> but when the hinges creak, they all leap up,
> to run and throw themselves at their father's feet.

Amphitryon still holds out some hope (ll. 96–99):

> My son, your husband, still may come. Be calm:
> dry the living springs of tears that fill
> your children's eyes. Console them with stories,
> *those sweet thieves of wretched make-believe.* [15]

Having a wandering epic hero for a father is, in fact, small consolation; "Bye baby bunting, daddy's gone a-hunting" is not a soothing lullaby in the face of a brutal reality.

Later in the play, after the madness and murder, Theseus attempts to console Heracles, blaming the disaster on Hera's caprice (ll. 1313–16):

> My advice is this: be patient, suffer
> what you must, and do not yield to grief.
> Fate exempts no man; all men are flawed,
> and so the gods, unless the poets lie.

Heracles does not believe him and says that he will accept fate and prevail against death not with weapons but with inner strength. [16] But hardest for him, the hero who has relied on his strength, is the fact of tears. Heracles says to Theseus (ll. 1351–56):

> I shall prevail against death. I shall go
> to your city. I accept your countless gifts.
> For countless were the labors I endured;

> never yet have I refused, never yet
> have I wept, and never did I think
> that I should come to this: tears in my eyes.

Even Theseus, who offers him everything of friendship and material support, balks at Heracles in tears.[17] He responds to Heracles' wish to take one last look at his slain children and once again to embrace his father (ll. 1410–17):

Theseus: Have you forgotten your labors so far?
Heracles: All those labors I endured were less than these.
Theseus: If someone sees you as a *female* he will not praise you.
Heracles: I live: am I so low? You did not think so once.
Theseus: Once, no. But where now is famous Heracles?
Heracles: What were you when you were underground?
Theseus: In courage I was the least of men.
Heracles: Then will you say my grief degrades me now?[18]

Earlier in the play, Heracles describes his children clinging to him and following like little boats in tow behind a larger one (ll. 631–32). At the end of the play, as he leaves with Theseus, he himself is a little boat in tow (ll. 1424–27). As he can identify with weakness—childhood weakness, female weakness, all human weakness—he is transformed.

In comparison with the *Ajax,* the *Heracles* is a play infused with tenderness. Words with the root *phil-* (love) abound.[19] Tenderness between parent and child and between friend and friend are important. *Philia* connotes both the feeling appropriate to those bound by blood ties or by other socially defined obligations and tenderness or love per se. In this play it is a human, not a divine, attribute. Heracles, for example, is a man capable of playing with his children (ll. 462–75). He can express his deep paternal affection (ll. 630–36):

> Here, I'll take your hands and lead you in my wake,
> like a ship that tows its little boats behind,
> for I accept this care and service
> of my sons. Here all mankind is equal:
> rich and poor alike, they love their children.
> With wealth distinctions come: some possess it,
> some do not. All mankind loves its children.

Human tenderness is set off against the vindictiveness of the gods.

At the same time, this drama suggests an intense ambivalence of parents toward children. Heracles saves his family as it is about to be immolated at the altar by Lycus, but ends up himself slaughtering his children at the altar. Artistically, the ambivalence is marked by the device of the split between a divine parent, who is callous, and a human parent, who is loving. Where, then, does madness come in? In terms of the play, it does not arise out of any *hamartia* (tragic flaw)

of Heracles, or because of any crime he has committed. It is a gratu-
itous affliction, an expression of Hera's cruel jealousy and desire for
revenge against Zeus. Madness represents the violent disjuncture between the divine and the human. A crucial figure in the onset of
madness is Lyssa: she bridges the gap between the cruel mythic
world and the human world where pity and love can prevail. She
balks at her assigned task and argues with Iris (ll. 845–856):

> My functions make me loathsome to the gods,
> Nor do I gladly visit men I love.
> And I advise both you and Hera now,
> Lest I see you stumble, to hear me out.
>
> I advise you; renounce these wicked plans.
>
> I would place you on the better path: you choose the worse.

Conflict and ambivalence are connected with madness, but they are
not explicitly localized within Heracles himself. It is as if the madness
is in the universe, in the order of things, or rather in the *disorder* of
things. If the playwright wishes to say anything about Heracles and
his madness, it is that the order of the mythic-heroic world is only an
illusion. In psychodynamic terms, it is an order dependent on the
acting out of parental ambivalence toward children. Such a realization
is associated with madness and suicidal despair.

When one begins to take seriously the ruthlessness implicit in the
heroic ethos, it proves gravely unsettling. Madness is part of the
moral world being turned upside down. Heracles' own unintended
cruelty, however, turns out to be the beginning of a new basis for
the relationship between parent and child—a true identification between the two. Further, only such *philia* could be the basis for a
relationship between gods and men—or so Heracles proclaims.

Strictly speaking, we cannot speak of therapy for Heracles' madness but rather of therapy for the despair that follows. Ajax cannot
deal with his despair except by one last "epic" act: suicide. Heracles
can deal with despair because *philia* and his newly found capacity to
identify with the weak prevail. A new notion of heroism is defined
in the *Heracles,* a heroism that incorporates rather than disowns the
suffering and enduring that are the lot of the old, the child, and the
woman (for example, l. 1350).

The process by which this therapy takes place is in itself dramatic.
It is both an inner drama, as the hero struggles toward new realiza-
tions, and a drama enacted between the hero and those around him.
Here it is important to consider a paper by George Devereux, "The
Psychotherapy Scene in Euripides' *Bacchae,*" and its applicability to
the *Heracles.*[20] The "psychotherapy scene" is the one in which Agave

appears with the head of Pentheus and proudly proclaims it to be the head of a lion she has slain. Devereux emphasizes that Cadmus gently helps her to accept consciously the repressed knowledge that she has killed her own son. The scene is an elegant piece of careful, empathic psychotherapy, where step by step Cadmus allows Agave both her wish to deny and her wish to know. As she relinquishes her delusion, she is overcome by deep despair. She comes to some acceptance of the horror, neither disowning her deed entirely by proclaiming herself a victim of the gods nor totally assuming a crippling sense of guilt. Devereux, contrasting that dialogue with the scene of Heracles' awakening, makes the important point that Heracles genuinely does not know what has happened. His knowledge of his murderous deeds comes as new information; Agave recognizes what she has done. In both instances, however, something therapeutic, something akin to verbal psychotherapy, ensues.[21]

The pathway to resolution of Heracles' despair is consonant with his character and represents some working through. He moves from the ability to play heroic, imperial games with his children (ll. 463–71) to the ability to suffer like and understand a little child. In the dialogues, first with Amphitryon and then with his friend Theseus, Heracles begins to overcome his shame and despair and to choose life over death. The contrast with the unsuccessful therapeutic dialogues in the *Ajax* is noteworthy.

While both Heracles and Ajax are strong-minded men given to immediate physical expression of their rages and discontents, Heracles clearly has the greater capacity to endure and to suffer. He has gone through terrible labors, but even as he emerges from his madness (and in his madness) he is willing to continue to toil. There are two striking images of eternal toil and suffering in the *Heracles,* namely, Sisyphus and his stone (l. 1103) and the moving comparison of Heracles to Ixion (l. 1297): "I am like Ixion, bound forever to a wheel."[22]

First, both Ajax and Heracles can fight, even toil, but Heracles, however guilt-ridden, is prepared to endure.[23] Second, both Heracles and Ajax proclaim that they have nowhere on earth to go, that they have no recourse but suicide. But even here (compare Ajax's speech, ll. 457–80, with Heracles', ll. 1279–1310), there is a difference in tone: Ajax's feeling of hate and bitterness is far more intense than Heracles'. One can note the difference in tone between the two in another scene: the madman slowly comes to his senses and asks a loved one to tell him the truth about what has happened. In the *Ajax,* according to his wife's account, Ajax threatened her (ll. 311–13):

> Then finally he spoke those fearful, threatening words—
> What should befall me if I failed to say
> What had befallen him.

Heracles not only does not threaten Amphitryon in demanding to know what has happened but even responds to his father's tears (ll. 1111–12).

This difference is consonant with the way Ajax and Heracles view their parents. As Ajax sees his parents, they are figures before whom he must be disgraced and who will reproach him (ll. 459–66). In his view, they will only add to his sense of shame and disgrace. (His wife, Tecmessa, tries to remind him to have reverence for [*aidesai*] his father and mother and not kill himself—his mother is praying for his safe return. She chooses the wrong word—*aidesai* is related to *aidos*, shame, and comes too close to Ajax's overwhelming sense of shame.)

Heracles, by word and deed, conveys far more trust in his father— a father who, indeed, declares his unconditional love: "O child, even in your misfortune you are mine" (l. 111). The two playwrights have achieved a remarkable psychological consistency: Heracles, the character who is able to accept help from a friend, is the one who sees his father (and fathers in general) as loving. Heracles has an indifferent or even cruel father, Zeus, but clearly he also has a loving and forgiving father. (With a patient as bitter and depressed as Ajax, a therapist would have to work hard to make available to him giving and forgiving images of his parents.)

Euripides portrays Theseus as friend, helper, and a kind of therapist. First, Theseus is able to shift roles: he comes leading a military expedition (ll. 1163–77) in response to the news that Heracles' family is menaced by Lycus. His military help is not needed, but he is able to deal with a different kind of war, a combat to save Heracles' life with love and generosity as his weapons. Further, Theseus is willing to risk personal danger—the risk of pollution (*miasma*) by touching and helping the man who has murdered his wife and children: "There is no avenging curse to loved ones from loved ones" (l. 1234). In this remarkable line, overturning a deeply held Greek belief,[24] Theseus proclaims that such pollution is not automatic, even if the blood of loved ones is shed. Love—from a friend to a friend—can overcome the traditional awesome curses on one who has shed blood or one who even touches the murderer. In the *Oresteia*, a new divine order and a new legal order must be instituted to remove Orestes' pollution. Here the pollution is cleansed by the ability of one man to offer all he has to another and the ability of the other to accept his offering.[25]

The dialogue between Heracles and Theseus has other important nuances. Theseus is able to shift his tack when one line of argument does not work. At one point, his emphasis on Heracles' bad behavior (*duspraxia*), in not simply understanding that a man must accept what the gods give, drives Heracles more deeply into despair. Theseus then shifts to emphasizing Heracles' heroism and bravery, and this approach is more successful in mobilizing hope and the will to live. The resolution of Heracles' despair does not involve a complete and total transformation. This is not a case of Saul turned Paul. Heracles can take away with him something of his past as an epic hero. He decides he will take his bow and arrows with him, even though each time they knock against his ribs he will remember the murder of his wife and children (ll. 1376–85). He will carry them in order not to be left naked before his enemies, but will wear them unhappily. Finally, to complete his labors, he asks Theseus to help him take Cerberus to Argos.[26]

The Greek audience, of course, viewed this dialogue not as psychotherapy but as a species of rhetoric, the art of persuasion. The *Heracles* illustrates that if rhetoric is to be therapy, the speaker must have a very special caring relationship to the person he addresses— without the intense concern of the speaker, rhetorical devices and even sophistic logic cannot avail.

If we depart for a moment from the language of treatment and cure, and speak in the language of individuation, of maturation, we again find an instructive contrast between *Ajax* and *Heracles*. In the *Ajax,* as in other Sophoclean plays, the hero, by his behavior, defines a certain type of individual—one who achieves his distinction by following his inner light, who acts according to inner conviction, no matter what the consequences. The Sophoclean hero gradually learns the details of what he must endure in order to carry out what he knows is right, as exemplified by Oedipus in *Oedipus Rex.* He will not flinch from the truth, and proceeds to uncover the whole story. He learns who he is both by uncovering the facts of his identity and by persevering in what he knows he must do. Ajax grows in stature by the strength of his resolution, by his unwillingness to compromise merely to save his own skin.[27]

The *Heracles,* like other Euripidean plays, presents another ideal of individuation and maturity. One must live with the ambiguity and moral disorder of the universe and thereby come to know what it is to be human, able to feel for and with another person's plight. This is hard-won knowledge—it goes beyond mere pity. Here are two different forms of tragic knowledge: Sophocles emphasizes a certain kind of knowledge of oneself, such as the price one is willing to pay to carry out the dictates of one's own sense of what is right. Euripides emphasizes the pain of knowing and recognizing what others endure and suffer. Both playwrights, then, have enriched our awareness of what it is to be truly and fully human.

Catharsis and Psychotherapy

The hope that drama could be a form of therapy for mental distress has a long history. Witness the mock trial of the dog that stole the cheese in *The Wasps*. In later Greco-Roman medicine we find suggestions for staging little dramas built around the patient's delusions and hallucinations, dramas intended somehow to shock the person out of his madness. We also find recommendations for reading and seeing plays as a way to distract the melancholic from his morbid preoccupations. In eighteenth-century France, at the asylum of Charenton, and in postrevolutionary America under the aegis of Benjamin Rush, the use of drama as adjunct to the treatment of madness was suggested. In the twentieth century we have the psychodrama movement, which aims to exploit various aspects of writing and enacting dramas for a number of purposes (not primarily the cure of florid psychosis). In a modern play about the use of theater to cure madness, Pirandello's *Henry IV,* the protagonist has gone mad in the midst of enacting a historical pageant, killed a man, and remained mad for twenty years. As the play opens, the characters are planning to stage a new drama to cure Henry IV of his madness, but this new drama similarly ends in murder. Pirandello has here captured the crucial point about drama as therapy: it is palliative, it does more for the therapists than it does for the patient.

Here I have been speaking of drama as a treatment for florid madness. What about the power of drama to relieve grief, to help give shape and name to the conflicts within individuals in the audience? I have spoken of Hesiod's notion of the bard as a healer of private woes. Here too, while a few may have achieved some important insight, some crucial realization in the course of seeing or reading a drama, the effects tend to be transitory. It is surely neurotic to look to tragedy for therapy for neurosis rather than for its particular form of pleasure (Aristotle's *oikeia hēdonē*).

Finally, we must consider drama as a form of collective therapy for collective ills, for major tensions endemic in the life of a society. If, as I shall argue later, classical Greek culture was marked by particular tensions around male–female and parent–child relations, did the staging of dramas of parricide and incest act in any kind of mass therapeutic way? The god of theater, Dionysus, was also called *eleutherios,* the liberator, and *lusios,* the loosener, and under his sway the unutterable could be spoken and the unthinkable could be staged. Emotions and thoughts previously pent up could be released, presumably in socially acceptable ways, on the stage, when they could not be in real life.

As we consider these diverse issues, the notion of the cathartic effect of tragedy keeps recurring. It is my purpose in this section to explore the concept of catharsis in theater and in therapy and to show that it is an inadequate model for either the artistic effects of drama or the healing power of psychotherapy. The metaphor of a good bowel movement hardly does justice to either theater or therapy.

Let us first examine the origins of the modern use of the term "catharsis" in relation to theater and to therapy. By an interesting and important confluence of circumstances, soon after catharsis was introduced as an important term in discussions of the effect of tragedy, it was incorporated into both the popular and technical vocabulary of psychotherapy.

Aristotle's characterization of tragedy as effecting "a catharsis through pity and terror" (*Poetics*, 1449b27–28) has become one of the most controverted passages in all of Greek literature. As Pedro Laín Entralgo points out, the ten words of the passage have served as a projective test, with each author and each age finding there the meaning that each needs to see.[28] The precise meaning intended by Aristotle will probably never be known.

The modern interpretation of catharsis as a medical—that is, not a moral—term, implying a purgation of unhealthy emotions, had its antecedents in the works of various critics over the ages, but originates primarily in the writings of Jacob Bernays. First appearing in 1857, Bernays's views gained wide circulation about 1880. He defines catharsis as "a designation transferred from the somatic to the affective in order to designate to the treatment of a sufferer a treatment with which the endeavour is not made to transform or repress the aggrieving element but to excite and foster it in order thus to bring about the relief of the sufferer."[29]

Soon thereafter, the notion of tragic catharsis as the elimination of unhealthy emotions became extremely popular in the artistic and intellectual milieus of Germany and Austria.[30] As a catchword, it was used to explain anything and everything about theater. (Compare the way such terms as "identity crisis" and "alienation" have entered contemporary popular usage.)

In the early 1890s Freud, in collaboration with Breuer, introduced the term "catharsis" into the realm of psychotherapy as a description and explanation of a process of hypnotic cure for hysterical symptoms. The method entailed having the hypnotized patient first recall and then relive the circumstances under which the symptoms first appeared. In their experience, such a procedure resulted in a dramatic expression of painful emotions, after which the patient seemed relieved of symptoms and of the accompanying subjective distress. They characterized this process as abreaction or catharsis, the former term implying a heightened repetition of the hidden painful emotions and the latter their expulsion. Their choice of the term "catharsis" was facilitated by its availability in popular intellectual usage, and both Breuer and Freud had received good classical gymnasium educations. Moreover, Jacob Bernays was an uncle of Martha Bernays, Freud's wife, and the Freud and Bernays families moved in the same social circles of Vienna.

One must consider, however, the details of the case of the now famous patient "Anna O.," who was the subject of the report in which Freud and Breuer first used the term "catharsis." Breuer had treated this young woman for multiple hysterical afflictions during the years 1880–1882 and had discussed the case with Freud. Anna O., it seemed, readily entered into spontaneous autohypnotic states, in the course of which she would recall the particular event, with its attendant feelings, that seemed to be the beginning of a particular conversion symptom. The recall-and-affect storm seemed to lead to a remission of the symptom in question. The patient referred to this process as "chimney sweeping"—getting out the material clogging up the pipes (a decidedly anal metaphor). The doctors, in effect, translated chimney sweeping into Greek and called the process catharsis. Both patient and doctors lived in the intellectual and cultural ambience where the term "catharsis" was in vogue. This patient apparently had a long-standing interest in theater and was also involved in a rich fantasy life, which she called her "private theater." Thus a confluence of personal and cultural factors allowed the doctors to use the term "catharsis" to explain the effects of a specific type of psychotherapeutic technique.

For Freud, catharsis was an early and preliminary formulation of the process of cure. By 1895, when *Studies in Hysteria* was published, he was beginning to have misgivings about the range of effectiveness of catharsis as an explanation and of abreaction as a procedure. Within the next few years Freud began to discard catharsis as a major explanatory concept. The technique of psychoanalysis that he developed relied little on the abreaction of pent-up pathogenic emotions and memories. By 1940, the date of Freud's last publication, one could scarcely have guessed that the notion of catharsis had ever played any role at all in psychoanalysis. As W. Binstock has cogently pointed out, however, the idea of the great value of catharsis (or such modern equivalents as "letting it all hang out") persists in our culture.[31]

In brief, the idea of the curative value of catharsis has long since been discarded by psychoanalysis. Euripides' account of the resolution of Heracles' despair comes much closer to contemporary notions of the complexity of psychotherapy than does the term "catharsis." "Tragic knowledge" and "knowledge through suffering" bespeak a view of therapy that is antithetical to the implications of catharsis.

Further, as several modern critics of Aristotle's *Poetics* have argued, however Aristotle may have meant his catharsis passage to be interpreted, catharsis is at most a relatively minor element in his larger view of the construction and enjoyment of great tragedy.[32] These trends in modern approaches to the *Poetics* emphasize as its central theme the intricate use of knowledge and craft to produce a play that is both intellectually and emotionally satisfying to the audience. As a corollary, one can then argue that the connotations of the term "catharsis" are in fact quite complex and that the process Aristotle is trying to describe is a subtle mixture of cognitive and affective responses.

There is a confluence, then, between these views of what Aristotle is saying about the art of tragedy and what contemporary ego psychology says about the nature of psychoanalysis and the complex ways in which it effects its cure. The views of such classicists as Gerald Else and Leon Golden can be termed ego-psychological approaches to Aristotle. One of the pioneers of psychoanalytic ego psychology, Ernst Kris, in fact suggested (in most compressed form) just such an understanding of Aristotle on catharsis.[33]

With these considerations at hand, we can now move the discussion of theater as therapy into a different framework, that of the similarities between what one derives from drama and what one derives from psychoanalytic insight.

The patient and the theatergoer mobilize and expand their ability to make an empathic identification with other human beings, especially ones who suffer. In theater, this implies not only that we identify with the protagonist, or the "good guy," but that we see something of the plight and viewpoint of even those we may not ultimately like or admire. (Aristotle's *philanthropia* is relevant here.) Anyone who has had the experience of repeated rereading or reviewing of a great tragedy at different points in his life is aware that such a play allows for empathic identification with several characters, who may be completely at odds with each other within the drama. Similarly, we should expect a variety of rearrangements in the loves and hates of the patient in the course of therapy as he enlarges his understanding of the viewpoints of significant others in his life. The patient may, for example, come to see that someone he has hated with a great passion in fact embodies the most unaccaptable and hated parts of himself.

Some inner turmoil must attend the rearrangement of thoughts and feelings in both therapy and theater, not merely a calm confirmation of all the person has thought and felt. Therapy that proceeds in an absolutely straight line, without turmoil and surprise, is analagous to the play constructed without any dramatic reversal, without *peripeteia*.

Both therapy and theater should give an enhanced awareness of the tragic dimension to human life.[34] Within human institutions, especially the family (and Aristotle certainly makes clear the concern of Greek tragedy with the family), guilt, ambivalence, and tragic misunderstanding are inevitable. An awareness of this inevitability, while sobering, does not necessarily lead to rigid pessimism or unwillingness to reduce or eliminate those sources of suffering that can be dealt with. If anything, the tragic hero serves as a model of striving to do, even in the face of the undoable.

Affects and emotions become more refined, more differentiated, and in a way more discriminating. Pity and terror are not purged, but transmuted and integrated into a new level of response and understanding. In this respect, I believe Aristotle's notion of catharsis has been misunderstood to mean a primitive kind of purging. The Oedipus plays of Sophocles illustrate the movement from primitive dread of pollution because of unspeakable deeds to a more refined and focused sense of moral responsibility. Terror and madness are not made to disappear; they are refined and integrated in the dramatic resolutions.

Related to the changes in the experience of emotions is a reshuffling and reintegretion of thoughts and emotions. "Tragic knowledge" implies that by the end of the play the characters and the audience know things they did not know before, and know them in a way they have not experienced before. If we consider Aristotle's notion of the pleasure that tragedy provides, we find that a scale of pleasures is implied. The pleasure of tragedy is of a higher order than the more undifferentiated desires and lusts of humankind. Tragedy, too, must in some ways stir up the body as well as the soul; but Aristotle's views of the highest forms of pleasure, including that of tragedy, assume an increasing differentiation of the bodily appetites and responses along with more discriminating cognitive responses. One is thrilled by a well-constructed play, but decidedly not in the same way one may shudder at an unadorned scene of terror, destruction, or sexuality.

Finally, tragedy should bring some altered and new sense of what one is and who he is in relation to those around him. The tragic figures in the plays struggle with their relationships and obligations to those in their past, present, and future. The audience acquires a new sense of the possibilities in being human and in coming to terms with the forces that are more powerful than any one individual. In therapy we also expect an enlarged view of the possibilities that are open in relationships to the self and to others.

Thus good therapy and good theater have in common a set of inner processes. Theater is not, and was not for the Greeks, primarily intended to be therapy for especially disturbed or distressed people. It was expected to provide a certain form of pleasure, even in Greek culture, and was an integral part of the *paideia* (education in the broadest sense) of each Athenian. Therapy, in contrast, is addressed to people who complain of difficulties; it can help provide a new understanding of those difficulties and increase the patient's awareness of what must be done over the long term. In fact, the patient who enjoys each session as if it were a great theatrical performance is probably not wholly committed to the more prosaic and painful task of implementing the lessons of his therapy day by day. This is not to say that therapy is a pleasureless or joyless experience, or that it may not at times reach dramatic heights. The patient, however, in contrast to the theatergoer, cannot rest content after he leaves the performance, but must on his own be playwright, actor, and audience in his own life.

I have the impression that insofar as good drama can enable an individual to undergo some of the inner rearrangements here described, theater can initiate or advance a therapeutic process. The experience of intense emotionality alone, especially if one fails to reflect and to experience intellectual integration, is likely to produce no important change.

In Chapter 13, "Hysteria and Social Issues," I shall discuss some important tensions in Athenian society, particularly tensions between men and women. Philip Slater has used the themes of myth and tragedy as a basis for important hypotheses about such tensions within the Athenian family.[35] Briefly, he argues that the suppression of women has particular consequences for the rearing of male children. Little boys would presumably be raised by angry and resentful women, who would either displace their anger at husbands, fathers, and brothers onto their sons or rear their sons to be instruments of revenge against the men in their lives. Greek myth and tragedy are, of course, replete with the theme of mothers who kill their sons (Clytemnestra, Medea) or use their sons to get back at their husbands.[36] The male child of such a mother would, in turn, grow up to fear women and mistrust female sexuality. If Slater is correct in his surmise that such tensions, including male fear and depreciation of women, were rife in fifth-century Athenian family life, can we say that tragedy represented some sort of therapy for this kind of distress? To the extent that tragedy exemplifies and expresses such conflicts, we may consider it diagnostic, perhaps a necessary prelude to therapy. In the sense that tragedy succeeds according to the criteria we have just considered (for example, enlargement of one's empathy for other human beings), then it can be potentially therapeutic as well. To the extent that the actual conditions of family relationships are unalterable within the society, however, no therapy could be effective against these malignant male–female conflicts. I believe that Euripides goes the furthest of the three tragedians in expressing these conflicts and in suggesting that a new kind of *philia*, or love, must arise in families. As a tragedian, however, his emphasis seems to be on the inevitability of such conflict and the impossibility of a resolution that does not involve tragic disaster.

Madness and Theater

I have argued that the representations of mind and its disturbances in the Homeric poems are reflections of the mind that is needed to create and perform an oral epic poem. This thesis, with appropriate modifications, can be extended to mind as portrayed in tragedy and the mind necessary to create a tragedy. Mental life is a more interior process in the tragedies than in the Homeric epics, and concomitantly, the process of creating a tragedy involves a more private and internal form of activity. The epic poet created and composed with his audience in full view; the tragic poet created and composed in writing alone, his audience only in his mind's eye.

In this section I shall develop a hypothesis, even more speculative, that connects the portrayal of madness with the task of poetic creativity. It is through the madman that the poet makes his statement— however disguised—of his struggles as creator and craftsman. I believe that this hypothesis is particularly relevant to Euripides, the most experimental of the three great tragedians. Accordingly, the discussion deals primarily with Euripides, and in particular with his last play, the *Bacchae.* I propose that we consider this drama as a play about plays.[37]

In the *Odyssey,* we find poems within a poem, examples of the poets at work. Is there an analogue in tragedy, a play within a play? In Shakespeare's *Hamlet,* in James Barrie's *Peter Pan,* and most of all in Pirandello's major works, we find the formal device of a play within a play. While Greek tragedy provides us no such examples, I believe that the representation of madness is a form of play within a play. Thus in Aeschylus' *Choephoroi,* the onset of Orestes' madness is compared to a song and dance, a choral presentation (ll. 1024–25), while in the *Heracles,* Lyssa and Iris almost literally orchestrate the madness. The mad scenes themselves are works of the imagination, dramas portrayed with only a few props. Heracles' madness could be titled "Another Journey of Heracles on His Labors," or "Heracles Murders the Children of His Enemy Eurystheus." Orestes, in Euripides, wages an imaginary battle with the Furies. In the *Ajax,* Athena is both playwright and producer, as she invites Odysseus to witness the madness of Ajax. The chorus, as audience to these dramas, experiences the emotions that Aristotle ascribes to the audience in the theater. Finally, in Euripides' *Bacchae,* which is full of illusions, theater and madness are joined in the person of Pentheus dressing up as a woman. He does on stage what a typical Greek male actor playing a woman must do offstage—get his costume just right, ask for help in final adjustments, and get last-minute coaching on how to walk and hold himself as a woman. In sum, the play within the play is the creation of madness, and in those scenes of madness the playwright can express something of his struggles in artistic creation. For madness is ultimately unbalanced, unharmonious drama, and only the consummate skills of the great playwright can render the madness with *sōphrosunē.*

There are three areas in which we can fruitfully compare drama and madness and explore the hypothesis that the madman is a dramatist manqué: (1) illusion and reality; (2) the rational and the irrational (and the question of the role of inspiration and reason in creating plays—"poetic madness"); (3) tradition or stereotype versus innovation. Good theater strikes the right balance of these three concepts, and madness fails to achieve that balance.

Illusion and Reality

Theater, no matter how realistic the staging, must always evoke in the mind's eye sights that the physical eye cannot see. Beyond this level of theatrical illusion there is Coleridge's "willing suspension of disbelief," the ability of the viewer to know and not know at the same time. The man who cannot allow himself this suspension of his faculty for testing reality cannot enjoy the theater, and the person who allows it too completely is a madman. In the *Bacchae* Pentheus starts out at one extreme—he will brook no illusions or convenient fictions. By the end of the play, this insistence on brute reality has turned out to be quite brittle, and he gradually goes mad. The boundary between reality and madness is marked by the scene in which he dresses as a woman, deluding himself that he is not deluded.

It may well be, as E. R. Dodds has suggested, that Dionysus is a god of illusion, and as such eminently suited to be the god of theater.[38] Clearly in this play he is the master of illusion, and Pentheus is his prime victim. Dionysus as stranger, Dionysus as bull, Dionysus as inside the palace and outside at the same time—all these incongruities are certainly designed to drive Pentheus mad. As the Stranger, Dionysus reports Pentheus' confusion in the courtyard (ll. 629–31):

And then the Lord of Thunder made, or so I think—I give you guesswork here—a phantom in the courtyard. And the King rushed at it in passion and tried to stab bright vapour, thinking that he spilled my blood.[39]

The theatricality of these illusions is striking, in that a reality, "a phantom," is made out of thin air. But Dionysus can play with illusion; Pentheus must grimly suffer from the imbalance between reality and illusion.

The *Bacchae,* so concerned with ritual, touches upon another crucial issue in theater: the degree to which one becomes immersed in the illusion. Theater demands a certain degree of absorption, while ritual demands a much greater degree of relinquishing the self, of being participant and not spectator. Pentheus cannot strike a balance here either. He begins wishing no involvement in the spectacle of the Maenads, except to stop it, but ends up as prurient spectator quickly turning into unwilling participant in the ritual. Agave too has crossed the boundary from theatrical illusion to madness. In the terms of the play, she has taken the ritual too literally and has been unable to content herself with even its gorier symbolic displacements, killing an animal instead of a man.

For the Greeks, imagination was closely tied to visualization, and the Greek stereotypes of madness emphasize visual distortions. In Aristotle's writings, three groups, ecstatics, maniacs, and melancholics, define a continuum from mild abnormality to extreme madness, but all of them share in the power to visualize and to interpret visual images (as in divination). In mild or controlled form, imagination is useful for poetic creativity, but in extreme form it is part of madness.[40]

Another aspect of the overlap among illusion, theater, and madness is Euripides' concern with the phantom (*eidolon*), or double. The theme appears in his early, middle, and late plays, and is especially important in the *Alcestis* and the *Helen*. The *Bacchae* refers to a double of Dionysus, and the *Hippolytus* contains several references to copies of a real person. This interest in the double is integral to Euripides' concerns *qua* dramatic craftsman, for is not this the work of the dramatist—the creation of phantoms?

Much suggests that the Greeks themselves had a keen sense of the role of illusion in enhancing and enriching reality. One can see this in the remarks of Aristotle about artistic imitation of reality (e.g., *Poetics,* 1448b4–5), in the interest of Greek artists and architects in optical illusion, and in remarks such as those of Gorgias, the fifth-century orator and sophist: "Tragedy, by means of legends and emotions, creates a deception in which the deceiver is more honest than the non-deceiver, and the deceived is wiser than the non-deceived."[41]

In modern times several psychoanalysts, especially Geza Róheim and, later, D. W. Winnicott, have emphasized the vital importance of illusion in human life. Winnicott coined the term "transitional objects" to describe what he felt were the first illusions in the life of the infant.[42] The infant's blanket is the prime example, for it provides a continuous presence, such as even the mother cannot provide, yet it is reminiscent of the mother. It is transitional in the sense of allowing the child to move from the symbiotic tie to the mother to relative autonomy. Winnicott speculates that much of human culture, such as art, religion, and drama, is related to the early experience of creating a mothering presence out of a mundane object, such as a blanket. Winnicott also argued cogently for the importance to mental health of the ability to play. Other writers have pointed out that psychotics, particularly schizophrenics, often demonstrate little ability to play, to take temporary roles, and even to fantasize and daydream.[43] Such considerations argue that the capacity to develop illusion is a hallmark, if not a guardian, of sanity. The playwright allows us to keep illusion and reality in balance, a juggling feat that the madman cannot easily perform.[44]

The Rational and the Irrational

If madness is a failure to balance reality and illusion, it is even more a failure to achieve a compromise between the rational and the irrational. The modern view of psychosis includes the idea that the suppression of instincts and passions, an excessive rationality, can be the matrix from which frank psychosis develops. We have seen (in the discussion of Ajax) how an eerie rationality and sense of "now I understand" may pervade the delusional state of the psychotic.

The great dramatist, in contrast, must find just the right balance between order and chaos, reason and passion, skill and inspiration. Within himself he must find an Archimedean point somewhere between cold sobriety, controlled ecstasy, and a frenzy bordering on madness. If he is successful, his audience can enjoy the play and feel moved and even enobled, experiencing an intense emotionality that is shaped by reason and judgment. The *Bacchae* seems to bring all of these issues together, some more explicitly than others. It is the play that deals most explicitly with wisdom, *sophia,* sanity and temperance, *sōphrosunē,* and out-and-out madness.[45] The action hinges on the issue of who is mad, and Tiresias and Cadmus urge Pentheus to consider that being too rational is itself a form of madness. Because Pentheus lacks the *sōphrosunē* to admit the strange and irrational, he will go completely mad.

At the same time, it is a play of such intensity and power that many students of the play have assumed it must be an intensely personal statement of Euripides. Speculations about its meaning hinge on the fact that he wrote it in self-imposed exile in Macedonia, where presumably his life was more elemental and less intellectual than it had been in Athens. My own guess is that Euripides not only was trying to come to terms with the role of the rational and irrational in human life—a preoccupation of almost all of his plays—but was also crystallizing a new understanding of the poetic craft, of the balance between madness and skill needed to write about the most disturbing aspects of human life.

Lacking intimate biographical information about Euripides, we can never prove or disprove such an assertion. At least one other reader of the play, however, has come to a similar conclusion. Reginald Winnington-Ingram, in his magisterial work *Euripides and Dionysus*,[46] has also connected the preoccupation with *sophia* and *sōphrosunē* in the *Bacchae* to the problem of the role of poetic skill and balance in the composition of the play. *Sophia* as poetic skill in this case, must include a sensitive sympathy with its subject matter. Winnington-Ingram concludes that "the personal quality of *sophia* which enabled him to write his play and the contribution of *sophia* which he makes in it are, in the last analysis, one and the same thing."

As for the question of audience reaction to such a play as this, we can guess that the *Bacchae* must have reached the outer limit of the audience's tolerance for the horrible, for the raw and instinctual. The text suggests that the dismembered body of Pentheus is to be brought onto the stage, with the actors handling various parts. If so, this is a uniquely gruesome scene in the extant tragedies. Antiquity is silent on audience's response, and Euripides may have remained within the limits of artistic *sōphrosunē*.

Greek culture, I believe, stood in awe of the creative process much as it stood in awe of overt madness. Both gave some sense of an external agent at work. While poets and audiences certainly knew full well that the creation of great poetry required hard work and considerable skill, some allowance was always made for a divine source. In the centuries from Homer to Plato and Aristotle, however, the emphasis seems to have shifted from divine to inner human sources.[47] Madness is similarly rendered as having both a divine and a human component, with over the centuries a shift in emphasis from outside to inside origins. But even the medical author of the fifth-century treatise on epilepsy called *On the Sacred Disease* left some room for divine causation of disease.

The *locus classicus* for the discussion of the relationship between madness and poetry is found in Plato's *Phaedrus*, where Socrates speaks of the four forms of divine madness, from which our greatest blessings come: poetic madness, Bacchic madness, prophetic madness, and the madness of love. These four are distinguished from madness as a disease brought on by natural causes. The implication is that these madnesses occur in a controlled or modulated form, and that most people could easily distinguish these cultural syntonic forms of "possession" from extreme cases, in which neither poetry, ritual, prophecy, nor love was adequately served.[48]

The situation in Aristotle is complex, and his position appears to have changed in the years between his earlier and later writings. In his earlier work, he emphasized the divine element in such activities as ritual (Corybantic) ecstasy, divination, and perhaps artistic creativity. Later on, he relied more on physiologically based theories to explain these phenomena as well as certain character types and their propensities. "Why is it that all those who have become eminent in philosophy or politics or poetry or the arts are clearly melancholics?"[49] reflects the most extreme view to be found in Aristotle and his followers on the connection between genius and madness. The basis of the character that is associated in milder forms with creativity and in more extreme forms with madness is a temperament of black bile. In terms of poetry and drama, Aristotle's interest seems to have shifted over time from the question of the nature of poetic inspiration to a more detailed consideration of the talents needed to produce a good play.

In the *Poetics* (1455a30–34) Aristotle states some reasons that "the poetic art is an enterprise for the gifted [*euphues*] rather than the 'manic' individual."[50] The former is sensitive but adaptable, the latter eccentric and unbalanced, though the two types exist on a continuum. Both the gifted and the manic have a physiological constitution dominated by black bile, and both have an unusual ability to visualize. The gifted, however, of whom Homer is the best example, are the recipients of a divine gift that allows them to control their "ecstatic" powers and channel them into balanced creativity. The manics (related to ecstatics and melancholics) have less control over their more irrational powers. That these themes are present in the *Poetics*, a handbook on how to produce the best kind of drama, suggests that the playwrights themselves were concerned with issues of art and madness, and that such concerns might well be reflected in their plays.

Modern theories on creativity, especially psychodynamic theories, have dropped the idea of divine inspiration but kept the notion that somehow a touch of madness is associated with creativity. Detailed psychodynamic investigations of the lives of creative artists have illuminated some of the motives that drive creativity—such as the need to master psychic trauma, especially traumatic separation and loss. On the whole, it is fair to say that the nature of the creative process or processes has yet to be adequately elucidated.

Tradition and Change

Greek tragedy took as its subjects the traditional myths of its culture. Apart from transformations wrought by the great tragedians in the form and content of some of the myths, new tensions and meanings were introduced into the old stories. The tragedies mirror the fundamental change taking place in Greek life, and at the same time they were undoubtedly agents of some of that change. In a profound sense, the tragedies took up the issues of continuity and change by reshaping the time-honored myths. Again, of the three great tragedians, it is Euripides who most clearly echoed the theme of change. The madness of Ajax, of Euripides' Heracles, and of his Orestes is set in the context of conflicting and shifting values.

Great tragedies, whether Greek, Elizabethan, or modern, take myths that have meaning for their cultures and translate them into the idioms of contemporary tensions and issues. Nevertheless, it can be argued, at the least, that the madman of great tragedy, whether Orestes or Lear, is uniquely suited to express these painful cultural transformations and conflicts.

Moreover, there is a particular kind of transformation that the Greek tragedians, especially Sophocles and Euripides, effected for the portrayal of madness. They began not only with the traditional and received myths, but also with the culturally held stereotype of the madman's nature and behavior. They transformed these relatively two-dimensional images of the madman into individualized portraits, which at the same time, by virtue of the tragedian's art, became a kind of classic figure. In short, they moved from a general stereotype via an individualized portrait to a new level of more general description. (It is my impression that later Greek and Roman authors tended to use the madmen of classical drama as a new stereotype. Horace, in his *Ars Poetica* [ll. 123–25], advises the poet to "let your Medea be wild and unconquerable, Ino weeping, Ixion perfidious, Io wandering, and Orestes sad.")[51]

What was, as far as we can reconstruct it, the Greek stereotype of the madman? First there are the physical signs: raving, roaming around or running wild, eyes rolling, sweating, drooling, foaming at the mouth. There is greater emphasis on visual disturbances than on auditory ones: terrifying visual images cause or accompany madness. Also, madmen do things that are contrary to all good Greek custom, such as deeds that are harmful to their friends and helpful to their enemies.[52]

Stoning was a stereotyped method of handling the dangerous madman in Greek culture.[53] It seems to have had ritual associations and probably had at its root a magical attempt to heal and get rid of the danger of contagion that the madman posed. Note that Euripides' Orestes is sentenced to death by stoning in the *Orestes* and is stoned by the shepherds in *Iphigenia in Tauris*. Ajax is afraid of death by stoning if he does not kill himself, and Heracles' bout of madness is interrupted when Athena throws a heavy stone at his chest; later tradition called it "the sanity stone."

The Greek playwrights of the fifth century were in general reworking tradition, innovating, and yet trying somehow to stay within a recognizable traditional framework. Their innovations affected the content of stories, the subtlety of motivation described, and the form of the play. They experimented with plot structure, introducing more and more complicated reversals and complex scenes of recognition. The numbers of actors increased and the role of the chorus changed, along with the accompanying music and dance.

Euripides developed intricacies of recognition scenes that went far beyond those of his contemporaries and predecessors (with the notable exception of Sophocles' *Oedipus Rex*). His ability to devise complex sequences of *peripeteia,* reversal, reached dizzying heights, as exemplified in his *Orestes.* [54] The madness of Orestes, with its sudden onslaughts and remissions and transformations, is well suited to parallel the labyrinthine twists and sudden starts and stops in the plot structure. Aristotle's *Poetics* devotes much space and effort to describing, classifying, and prescribing different kinds of recognition and reversal. He tried to develop a taxonomy of plot structures that would correlate with the degree of pleasurable audience response.

To a great extent, then, the playwrights experimented and thereby took considerable risks. They had to strike just the right balance between satisfying the audience's need for an old tale well told and for the excitement of innovation. The audience had to enjoy its own variety of *anagnorisis,* recognition, by recognizing the old in the new and suddenly seeing the new in the old. Contemporary comedy (Aristophanes) and later traditions about fifth-century drama amply document the fact that Euripides did not consistently find popular favor and usually did not win first place in the contests. Not until Aristotle, who had a keener eye for the historical development of the dramatic form and who realized that there had been continuous artistic innovation in the fifth century, was Euripides adequately defended (in the *Poetics*).

The madman exemplifies what can go wrong in the difficult task of moving from old to new. The madman, like the other tragic heroes, does not necessarily consciously proclaim that he has a new doctrine or a new message; in fact, he may be appealing to even older values than those supported by his antagonists or friends. Again, it is well to recall that the *Bacchae* is a play about old and new—manifestly Dionysus is new, but, Tiresias argues, he is really old and authentic in many respects. Cadmus argues for tradition, as does Dionysus, yet he himself is a really "new man," only a few generations removed from the sown men of Thebes.[55] Pentheus sees himself as trying to maintain certain established values, but he is also protecting his own authority, something that is not per se timeless.

In sum, madness, as transformed from stereotype to classic (that is, the individualized portrait that still represents something universal), is well suited to represent the dramatic problem of tradition versus innovation. This problem in turn is part and parcel of the social task of the tragedians, namely, to document, interpret, and render into classic form the tensions and torments of an age in transition.

III

THE PHILOSOPHICAL MODEL

8

Plato's Concept of Mind
and Its Disorders

I saw Socrates [in Hades] and he seemed to be in love with Hyacin-
thus—at least he was refuting him most.

—Lucian, *True History*

And now we come to Plato. Our discourse must be in quieter tones,
our arguments more reasoned. Passion, yes, but the passion must be
for argument and for truth. We must put behind us the pity and the
terror, for the philosophic Muse speaks in dialectic, and dialectic
cannot be heard amidst the cries of the chorus and the anguish of the
tragic hero. There is a late tradition that Plato, "the dramatist of the
life of reason," had written dramas in his youth, but when he discovered philosophy he burned them all.[1] Nursed by Homer, taught
by the great tragedians of fifth-century Athens, he nevertheless proclaimed the poets obstacles to the truth and banned them, with re-
gret, from his polity, the true Republic. It is thus apparent that he
struggled within himself and proclaimed one part of himself the
enemy of the other. He knew his inner war had to end with the
victory of reason and the grudging surrender of passion, the victory
of philosophy over poetry. This was the man who divided the soul
into parts, who separated psyche from soma and assumed that one
must be master and the other slave. He dreamed that philosophers
could be kings and kings philosophers, but when he tried to make
Syracuse into his Republic, dream became nightmare. He was one of
those men whose dream was to endure though the reality perished.
Among his lasting monuments was a school, the Academy, that
existed from the early fourth century B.C. to the sixth century A.D.,
almost a thousand years. Had he been able to see the long history of
his school, he would have been disappointed, though not surprised,
that philosophy had failed to transform the world. More enduring
are his dialogues, though here too he failed, never achieving the
ultimate truths for which he so devoutly yearned. The forms of the
true, the good, and the beautiful eluded even him. His true immortality, then, rests not in the particulars of his questions and answers

but in the idea of philosophy, the idea that men must enter into dialogue with each other and within themselves in order to find the truth. From the perspective of the history of ideas about mind and mental illness, we can epitomize Plato as the man who took the distinction between mind and body very seriously indeed, and who equated the activities of the mind with sanity and the impulses of the body with madness. Only sane men can philosophize, and only philosophy can make men sane.

Plato lived from 427 to 348 B.C. and wrote a large number of dialogues, beginning at about age forty and probably continuing until his death. These dialogues all purport to be conversations of his master, Socrates; Plato himself never speaks. Almost all of our information about both Plato and Socrates derives from the dialogues, and it follows that it is often extremely difficult to specify what was Socrates' opinion and what was Plato's own.[2] I shall not attempt to make a sharp distinction between Platonic and Socratic positions.

Almost any statement about what Plato said on a particular major issue in one dialogue can be controverted with a passage from another dialogue. My working assumption is that there is a considerable coherence and unity to Plato's thought, but that as a creative thinker who wrestled many years with important and vexing issues, he was bound to try different tacks and come up with different answers. Though most of the dialogues can be classified as written early, in the middle, or toward the end of his career, unresolved problems of dating remain. Hence it is often difficult to speak with certainty about the "evolution" of his thought, and often one must make *a priori* assumptions about the development of his thought in order to date some of the dialogues. Accordingly, I shall focus on what appear to be the main issues and the principal kinds of answers in the dialogues. When we take up what seem to be recurrent unconscious fantasies in the dialogues, we must keep in mind that of necessity we are analyzing the products of the man's efforts and can speak only tentatively about what manner of man Plato himself was.[3]

The Discovery of the Mind: The Pre-Socratic Background

In the sixth and fifth centuries, at various places in the Greek-speaking world, a number of thinkers who have come to be known as the pre-Socratics appeared. Among the more famous names are Thales, Anaximander, Anaximenes, Heraclitus, and Empedocles. Anaxagoras, Democritus, and Parmenides were contemporaries of Socrates, and hence not strictly pre-Socratic. What did this heterogeneous group of thinkers have in common? Histories of philosophy, beginning with Aristotle's sketches of the development of philosophy down to his day, have tended to discuss the pre-Socratics from the viewpoint of the *contents* of their teachings, their doctrines. These men have properly been regarded as the first philosophers in the Western world, but the emphasis on their doctrines rather than on their language and on their attempts to formulate a new approach to discourse has obscured the sense in which they are truly pioneers.[4] Recognizing that this is one of the most controversial and problematic areas in classical scholarship, I shall summarize what I believe to be the implications of the activity of the pre-Socratics for the history of mind, particularly as it relates to the later activity of Plato.

1. They began to develop the basic abstract and definitional vocabulary of all later philosophical, psychological, and physical thought.
2. They defined "mental" and "mind" and characterized the latter as that which organizes and abstracts.
3. They distinguished two modes of thinking, or two modes of discourse—the physiological ("natural science") and the mythological.[5]
4. They asserted the superiority of the physiological mode of discourse, called the language of awareness, of true being, and equated the mythological with sleeping, dreaming, becoming, and perishing.
5. They asserted the superiority of those who think abstractly and of the abstract mode of thought. The philosopher, the one who "abstracts," is superior to the poet.

The following fragment of Anaxagoras (ca. 500–428 B.C.) illustrates the novelty of language and of emergent concepts in the writings of the pre-Socratics:

All other things have a portion of everything, but mind alone is without boundary and self-ruled, and is mixed with nothing, but is all alone by itself. . . . Most pure, it has all knowledge about everything, and the greatest power; and mind controls all things, both the greater and the smaller that have life.[6]

Mind, *nous,* is separate from all the things of which it also is a part. In this and related passages, Anaxagoras is developing a view of mind as a powerful, organizing, and creating force in the universe. Note that it is not Zeus, but rather mind per se. Such a text accords an importance to a disembodied mind that differs radically from the mythopoetic notions in the Homeric epics. One can sense here a language that is straining to define the contrast between the abstract and the concrete. Abstractions (from the Latin *abtrahere,* to pull away from) are terms "pulled away from" concrete instances, and I believe this process is what Anaxagoras is groping to describe.

While *nous* in Homeric usage is one of the more "mental" words in Homer's vocabulary of mental life, particularly in the *Odyssey,* this passage goes far beyond the Homeric in its ascription of uniqueness to mind, as well as in its account of the activity of mind. This fragment can be seen as a way station toward Plato's use of *nous* and its cognates as terms denoting the intellectual, abstracting, and defining activities of the psyche.[7]

A related movement from the Homeric use of *psuchē* to the Platonic can be seen in Heraclitus' statement "The boundaries of *psuchē* you will not find in travelling, though you traverse every road."[8] Psyche is thus no longer the *eidolon,* the double, or the ghostly survivor of the living man, but is without dimensions, not a physical, measurable entity.

Another fragment of Heraclitus forcefully demonstrates the shift from the Homeric view of a god as the cause of irrational behavior to the Platonic view of man as an agent responsible for his own deeds. "*Ēthos anthrōpō daimon*" (Character is the demon for a man).[9] In Homer, a deity or *daimon* can bring bad luck to a person. The exclamation "*Daimonie!* " is used to mean "You're crazy!" and can be rendered as "What demon has gotten into you?" For Heraclitus, that demon is the man himself.

The pre-Socratics, then, began to define the uniqueness of mind, transforming such traditional terms as *nous* and *psuchē.* They also located this mind and its activity within the person. In defining two modes of thinking, a superior and an inferior, they laid the groundwork for some of the central issues in Platonic thought. One of these issues is how to understand man as a creature capable of both abstract, sophisticated, logical thinking and impulse-ridden, fantasy-dominated thinking. The second is the issue of how to control this creature, whether to educate, to persuade, or to coerce him. Plato, indeed, shared with the other great thinkers of his day an intense concern with issues of individual and collective impulsiveness and restraint. Let us turn to Plato and begin with an examination of the psyche as Plato portrayed it.

The Representation of Mental Activity in the Platonic Dialogues

The Greek term *psuchē* remained in use from Homer to all later Greek philosophical and religious thought. It is the core *psych*ological and *psych*iatric term in Plato, which is to say that the term is the main carrier of Plato's notions about mind in both ordinary and disturbed states. Its translation poses major problems, for to translate it with any one common English term is to narrow prematurely the range of connotations in Plato. It is most commonly translated as "soul," though if one had to choose a single term, "mind" would be preferable.

It appears that the term retained much of its Homeric coloring down to the time of Socrates. Such passages as that quoted from Heraclitus ("the boundaries of *psuchē*") seem to herald a radically different usage, but it was not until Socrates and then Plato that the word became radically transformed.[10]

Foremost among the changes effected by Plato is the suggestion that the psyche is equivalent to the self. The new usage of psyche may well be part and parcel of the task of defining this elusive notion called the self, a term without equivalent in classical Greek. In Plato we find extensive use of phrases involving "itself" or "himself" but not "the self."

The self that is implicitly associated with or defined by psyche thinks, decides, initiates, and is conscious of what it does. Havelock is correct in suggesting that psyche in Plato is equivalent at times to consciousness. Plato also clearly asserts that the psyche is an ethical aspect of the self, the self as moral agent.[11]

This conception of psyche as the thinking and deciding self is striking in some of the earlier Platonic dialogues. In the *Apology*, Socrates defines his mission as to continue philosophizing and questioning as long as he still has breath in him. His purpose is to point out to the Athenians the supreme importance of attending to their psyches (30A–B; 36C). Similarly in the *Protagoras* we find Socrates reproaching a young man who turns up at the door of the visiting sophist Protagoras (313B):

But when it comes to something which you value more highly than your body, namely your psyche—something on whose beneficial or harmful treatment your whole welfare depends—you have not consulted either your father . . . or any of us who are your friends on the question whether or not to entrust your psyche to this stranger who has arrived among us. On the contrary, having heard the news in the evening . . . here you come at dawn, not to discuss or consult me on this question of whether or not to entrust *yourself* to Protagoras, but ready to spend both your own money and that of your friends.[12]

Such a usage of psyche and "self-" words contrasts with the opening lines of Homer's *Iliad*: "[The destructive wrath of Achilles] sent the psyches of many brave heroes down to Hades, while themselves [*autous*] were left as prey to the dogs of the field and birds of the air." Plato argued that the self is not synonymous with the body. While it is not clear if Plato himself would have said that the psyche equals the person (or that psyche is the definition of the person), a spurious Platonic dialogue (*Alcibiades I*) makes that assertion.[13]

In the early and middle dialogues Plato strives to clarify "the thing itself," whether the "thing" be piety, virtue, temperance, love, or justice. While a technical term for "definition" was probably not available to Plato, the language in these dialogues is replete with phrases involving "itself," "the selfsame," and the personal reflexive pronouns "myself," "himself," and "yourself." Plato's characterization of the psyche as the essential part of the man thus appears alongside his effort to find the essential characteristics, or definitions, of things in the world.

While the earlier dialogues emphasize the connection between psyche and "oneself," the middle ones introduce the idea of the psyche as a structure and as an organization. As a structure it is not material, neither a vapor-like existence (as in Homer) nor a physical substance (a view found in Democritus and the medical writers).[14] One finds psyche compared to physical objects, such as a wax tablet or an aviary (*Theatetus*, 191D and 197D), but these analogies are introduced to emphasize the idea of the contents of the psyche. The most famous analogies of psyche as an organization are those between psyche and state in the *Republic* and psyche and body in the *Timaeus*.

Another major contrast between Homer and Plato is suggested by a vocabulary of *activity* (in place of the passive receptiveness in Homer) in descriptions of psyche. The psyche exercises control over incoming stimuli, digests them, and determines their fate inside the mind. If it were otherwise, the mind would soon be filled up with sensations, as if it were a Trojan horse full of warriors (*Theatetus*, 184D). (See also *Philebus*, 39A, and *Theatetus*, 191A–E.)

Psyche is not moved but moves itself (*Phaedrus*, 245C–D).[15] "Management, rule, deliberation, and other such tasks [*erga*]" is one epitome of the activity and activities of psyche (*Republic*, 353D; see too 518B).

Plato emphasizes the uniqueness of mind and mental processes in a variety of ways, most prominently with metaphors drawn from mathematics. Mathematics provides some sort of model for nonmaterial, nonanthropomorphic discourse about mind. This need may be one reason for the central role that Plato assigns (in the *Republic*) to arithmetic and geometry in the education of the philosopher kings. In the *Meno* one finds Plato using the notion of an "irrational number,"—for example, the square root of 2—side by side with the idea of a radically different notion of virtue. Plato seeks a virtue that is not the simple addition or ratio of particular virtues, but the definition of virtue, virtue in the abstract.

The idea of immortality of the psyche, obviously rooted in Homer, serves Plato as a way to emphasize the uniqueness and separateness of psyche. Psyche is only temporarily linked to the body.

The psyche must apprehend material things but it must do so by nonmaterial means. The knower is different from the object of knowledge. Repeatedly Plato emphasizes that what mind apprehends is nonphysical: "the very being with which true knowledge is concerned; the colorless, formless, intangible essence, visible only to rational mind, the pilot of the soul" (*Phaedrus,* 247C). We can thus understand Plato's work as a further extension of the efforts of the pre-Socratics to coin the terms of abstract discourse. Side by side with an evolving notion of mind as unique, radically separate, and nonphysical is a notion that the *objects of knowledge* are to be similarly described. Plato has several terms for these "intangible essences": true being, ideas, forms (for example, the idea of the good; the form of justice). Havelock contends that ideas or forms should be seen as way stations toward abstraction and definition, terms not available to Plato. "Definition" as a technical philosophical term first appears in Aristotle.[16] Rather than merely categorizing Plato as an idealist philosopher, we can see him as the one who struggled to describe and understand the relationship between things and their definition. Plato helped discover the abstract, and was still uncertain where the abstract belongs—to use later terms, does it have a logical or ontological status?

Thus psyche is associated with the self, it is a structure and has organization, it is active, it works in nonmaterial ways, and it apprehends nonmaterial objects. It is clearly associated with the self as moral agent as well as with the self as philosopher.

The earlier dialogues (for example, the *Phaedo*) deal with psyche as unified and as contrasted with the body. The middle and later ones shift to one or another schema of the psyche as divided into parts, ideally cooperating, but actually in frequent conflict. The earlier view raised some serious epistemological problems, particularly in relation to the question of a nonphysical entity, mind, apprehending physical objects. More important, however, was the need for a richer and more complete account of man in conflict with himself. The Socratic position on the phenomenon of man's acting against his own best interests was that no man errs knowingly (the *Protagoras*). Plato must have felt the inadequacy of that model to deal with the conflicts engendered by the strength of appetites and passions, and turned to a model that included reason, passion, and appetite as parts of the psyche.[17] The language of this model becomes almost unabashedly anthropomorphic, depicting a struggle among persons within a person, contending parties within the commonwealth of the psyche. Process language and mathematical formulations of the mind must yield to anthropomorphism when conflicts involving reason and appetite must be discussed.[18]

In the *Republic,* Plato divides the psyche into three parts: the rational (*logistikon*), the spirited-affective (*thumoeides*), and the appetitive (*epithumetikon*). In this scheme, the highest (rational) part is typically in conflict with the lowest (appetitive) part. The middle part, the *thumoeides,* has energy and passion that can be enlisted on the side of either the rational part or the appetitive part. The rational part represents the claims of the highest mental functions, knowing, dissecting, managing, and abstracting (though the latter term is not found in Plato). The appetitive part represents the person's imperative demands, such as the bodily lusts and appetites, but also other varieties of peremptory urge, such as monetary greed (to achieve one's other desires). It is the animal, or the wild animal, within the person, the imperative, childish, demanding part. One image of the tripartite psyche is of a beast with three parts, corresponding respectively to the appetitive, the spirited-affective, and the rational. The first part is a multi-headed Cerberus-like creature, sprouting forth heads of both wild and tame animals, heads that fight with and devour each other. Second is a spirited lion, and third, much smaller than the lion, is a man. The whole creature is then molded in the exterior likeness of a man.[19] In general, the ratio of reason to impulse declines as we move from the rational to the spirited-affective to the appetitive. Each part has its particular pleasures, desires, and governing principles (580D). They are likened to three different kinds of men: the lover of wisdom (*philosophos*) corresponds to the rational, the lover of victory (*philonikos*) to the spirited-affective, and the lover of gain (*philokerdes*) to the appetitive (581C).

Each of these three parts has its characteristic way of knowing and its characteristic objects of knowledge. In general, throughout the middle and later dialogues the baser parts of psyche are assumed to be suited to apprehend the baser parts of the world. The appetitive part apprehends sensory perceptions, sensual demands, and concrete, particular, mortal objects. The rational part is capable of knowing the most general and the most abstract, the timeless, the nonbodily, as epitomized in such terms as "forms" (ideas) (*Timaeus,* passim; *Republic,* passim; *Phaedrus,* 247C). "Becoming" versus "being" is another expression of this contrast.

The contrasting attributes of higher and lower forms of mental activity may be summarized as follows:

Baser Parts of Mind	*Higher Parts of Mind*
The appetitive	The rational
The somatic	The psychic
Begetting, being born, and perishing	True being
Opinion (*doxa*)	True knowledge (*episteme*)
The pictorial, illusory	The intellectual
Shadow	Sun
Sleep, dreaming	Awareness

Child	Adult
Imitation	Abstract understanding
Flux	Stability
Conflict	Harmony
Heterosexuality	Homosexuality and asexuality[20]

In some dialogues, principally those touching upon child rearing (the *Republic* and the *Laws*), Plato assumes a natural development from childhood to adult life in the capacity to use the higher parts of the psyche. Another way to describe the relation between higher and lower parts is provided by Plato's idea of innate knowledge and later recollection (*anamnesis*) (e.g., *Phaedo*). In the *Phaedrus* (246–56) Plato presents, in poetic and mythopoetic language, the story of the previous existence of the psyche, or its contact in that existence with the forms or ideas of the true, the good, and the beautiful.

Recollection, however, also serves as a kind of transforming factor—an examplar of the way the mind converts what it receives into something truly mental, not simply passively registered. The recollection of these forms, under the proper circumstances, converts sensory representation (*doxa*), the lowest form of mental life, to true knowledge (*episteme*).[21] In the *Meno* (97D–98B) Plato compares thoughts (*doxai,* mere opinion) to little mechanical wind-up men that can wander in all directions. Memory ties up these little figures so that they cannot run loose. Memory converts opinions into true knowledge by a process of binding (see *Theatetus,* 197–98). The metaphor of mobile thoughts and bound thoughts appears centuries later in Freud, who uses it to characterize the difference between the energies of primary process (primitive thinking) and secondary process (rational thinking).

The picture of one part of the psyche binding and controlling another part raises the question of both conflict and cooperation between the parts of the divided psyche. Plato split off intellect from appetite, reason from passion, and then wrestled with the problem of how to put them back together again. When he comes to issues of political control and, most important, education, he is painfully aware that reason cannot dispense with either emotion or appetite. The philosopher must be a lover of wisdom; he must lust after wisdom, not merely seek it. Plato seems to have offered two major theoretical constructs to bridge the gap between intellect and appetite, namely, the middle part of the psyche, the *thumoeides,* and the idea of *eros.*

In the *Republic* Plato takes great pains to introduce and defend the notion of the middle part of the psyche, the *thumoeides,* the spirited-affective. It can be an ally of either the highest or the lowest part. It is compared to a lion—that is, a magnificent and regal animal, powerful and potentially destructive, better to have as a guardian than as an enemy. It is capable of anger, and one hopes its anger is righteous. It is the part that "loves honor" and "loves victory." It corresponds to the class of the guardians, good fighters in the service of the state. In short, it describes an ideal of the good Greek citizen, a man motivated by the classic aristocratic ideals of honor and victory won through courage and competitive excellence.[22] It is a type of citizen that Plato realized was indispensable for the survival of the state. As such, the middle part adds an important measure of effectiveness to the activity of either the highest or the lowest part. Neither philosophy nor pure appetite could survive without this kind of ally. The spirited-affective fulfills a certain theoretical function, the need for some agency that supplies an effective driving force to psychic activity.

Eros similarly appears to be a transferable energy, available either to reason or to appetite. The *Symposium* states the problem of how to get men to love the true, the good, and the beautiful. The *Phaedrus* poses the problem of harnessing persuasive power to the quest for truth. In the *Symposium, eros* is the energic force for all human activity from the base to the sublime. *Eros* drives us to love and lust, it drives us to want to procreate children and create other forms of posterity (institutions, governments, works of art, poetry).[23] It also drives us to want to know, to learn, and to approach the forms of the true, the good, and the beautiful. What is the origin and nature of this love? Is it originally from and of the body, or did it come from the higher spheres and become corrupted? In Socrates' part of the discourse about *eros,* he invokes a number of mythlike and allegorical statements that point to the intermediate and mediating nature of *eros.*[24] It is neither human nor divine; it is the child of Plenty and Poverty. These statements suggest that Plato does not wish to assign this force to the sphere of either the mind or the body, the higher or the lower, but rather wishes to leave it as an energic term, sharing in the operations of either and both.

Much more in Plato's notions about normal mental functioning could be profitably discussed. Issues of pleasure and pain, the nature of the forms, the Platonic virtues, the relationship between the state and the individual, all are crucial to the understanding of Platonic psychology. Time and space, however, compel us to bypass these issues and move on to the diseases and disorders of the psyche, and the problem of their cure.

Disturbances of Mind

For Plato, philosophy must be in the service of the rational against the irrational. Like a general who needs careful intelligence about a wily enemy, Plato scouted and explored the territory of the irrational.[25] He learned to respect its power and to expect its protean forms. He described it so well, however, that we begin to suspect he spoke from deep firsthand knowledge. A rationalist par excellence, he never fully relinquished a certain admiration for the irrational, as evidenced by the Socratic pronouncement that "our greatest blessings come to us through madness."

Plato clearly knew of those forms of madness that were associated (or thought to be associated) with disorders of the body, but these were of interest to physicians of the body. As a physician of the psyche, he was concerned with the diseases of misunderstanding wherein lie a man's true interests, the madnesses of immoral decisions.[26]

He must have seen many of the great mad plays of the Athenian dramatists, but felt that the madness on the stage was as nothing compared to that of the state divided against itself. For Plato, the madness of the individual and the madness of the state go hand in glove.

His *Republic* elaborates his thesis that the structure of the psyche and the structure of the state are parallel, that we can look to the state to find the parts of the psyche writ large. While he seems to give priority to the psyche as the source of the "forms and traits" of the state, he has no doubt about their interdependence.[27]

In Book 4 he develops the analogies between the rational part of the psyche and the philosopher kings, between the spirited-affective and the guardians, and between the appetitive and the common citizens (including artisans).

His definitions of madness and sickness of the psyche are spun out over the whole course of this dialogue by means of the interweaving of psychology and political theory. In brief, justice is health, in both the psyche and the state, and injustice is disease. But what is justice? In the early books of the *Republic* that very question is debated, and in Book 4 the Platonic answer emerges. Justice in the state occurs when everyone goes about his own business, sticking to the task appropriate to his class, deliberating or guarding or working to support the state. Justice in the psyche occurs when each part performs its own function, with the *logistikon* as ruler. Only thus is the man a unit, "one made out of many, self-controlled and harmonized" (*hena genomenon ek pollōn, sōphrona kai hermosmenon*) (443E). *Sophia*, philosophical wisdom, is the knowledge (*epistemē*) *that can direct this process of unification*. *Doxa*, seeming, mere opinion, and *amathia*, ignorance, threaten to overthrow the proper balance. "Self-controlled" is the rendering of *sōphrōn*, which denotes temperance, sexual modesty, and sanity. Injustice is *polupragmosunē*, the performing of more than one function by any one part.

The equation of justice and health, injustice and sickness, becomes explicit (444D–E):

But to produce health is to establish the elements in a body in the natural relation of dominating and being dominated by one another, while to cause disease is to bring it about that one rules or is ruled by the other contrary to nature. . . . And is it not likewise the production of justice in the soul to establish its principles in the natural relation of controlling and being controlled by one another, while injustice is to cause the one to rule or be ruled by the other contrary to nature?[28]

Ordered rule is the definition of justice and of health in the psyche, and conflict is the definition of injustice and of sickness. Indeed, it has not generally been noticed that Plato here effects a subtle transformation of contemporary Greek medical notions.[29] Hippocratic medicine emphasizes health as the proper balance of the basic bodily humors (and/or qualities), but the domination of any one humor can lead to sickness. For Plato, balance and harmony mean *domination* of the inferior part by the superior.

"Sickness of the psyche" as a metaphor for undesirable disturbances of the psyche runs throughout Plato, though it is not always used in precisely the sense implied in these passages from the *Republic*. In the *Sophist* (227E–28E), sicknesses of the psyche are equated with vice, and vice is equated with discord. "Cowardice, intemperance, and injustice . . . all alike are forms of disease in the psyche." These three vices are the opposites of three of the four cardinal Platonic virtues—courage, temperance, and justice (wisdom is the fourth). The opposite of wisdom is ignorance, and in the *Timaeus* we find ignorance specifically labeled a disease of the psyche and intimately related to madness. After concluding his discussion of diseases of the body, Plato moves to consider diseases of the psyche (86B):

Such is the manner in which diseases of the body come about; and those of the soul which are due to the condition of the body arise in the following way. We must agree that folly [*anoia*] is a disease of the soul, and of folly there are two kinds, the one of which is madness [*mania*], the other ignorance [*amathia*]. Whatever affection a man suffers from, if it involves either of these conditions it must be termed "disease"; and we must maintain that pleasures and pains in excess are the greatest of the soul's diseases.[30]

Thus two themes are interwoven in Plato: sickness of the psyche as discord, and sickness of the psyche as ignorance.

A species of ignorance, perhaps the most pernicious kind, is ignorance of oneself, self-deception. Repeatedly Socrates is portrayed as proclaiming his own ignorance, or rather that his wisdom consists of knowing what he does not know. Xenophon, a less philosophical follower of Socrates than Plato, epitomized the Socratic position:

Madness [*mania*] he called the opposite of wisdom—though he certainly did not equate ignorance with madness. Nevertheless, he did think that not to know oneself, and to imagine that one knows things that he knows he does not know, is the nearest thing to out-and-out madness. [*Memorabilia, III, IX, 6*][31]

Ignorance and knowledge form a central polarity within Plato, and they undergo a change in emphasis over the course of the dialogues. The earlier (Socratic) emphasis is on "know thyself." In the middle and later dialogues, knowledge of the abstract, the rational, the universe of the ideas becomes an ever more prominent ideal. This knowledge is the moral good. Ignorance is equated with (or caused by) the temporal, the illusory, the bodily, and the sensual. Excess passion, overwhelming pride, the drive for power—these may interfere with the acquisition of knowledge and are in themselves kinds of madness. Excess pleasure and excess pain are specifically cited as the causes of ignorance or intemperance (for example, *Republic,* 402E–403).

The portrait of the despotic man (the tyrant) in the *Republic* is drawn with the aid of metaphors of incontinence, unbridled lust, and madness (573A–C).

Why then this protector of the soul has madness for his body guard and runs amuck, and if it finds in the man any opinions or appetites accounted worthy and still capable of shame, it slays them and thrusts them forth until it purges him of sobriety, and fills and infects him with frenzy brought in from the outside. . . . And again the madman, the deranged man, attempts and expects to rule over not only men but gods. . . . Then a man becomes tyrannical in the full sense of the word . . . when either by nature or by habits or by both he has become even as the drunken, the erotic, the maniacal [*melancholikos*].[32]

As part of the portrait of the tyrant, Plato, as if by free association to the theme of madness, details the wishes of the wild and irrational part of the psyche. Among these wishes he includes the forbidden oedipal wish.[33] In dreams, while the rational part of the psyche sleeps and relaxes its guard,

the beastly and savage part, replete with food and wine, gambols and, repelling sleep, endeavours to sally forth and satisfy its own instincts [*ēthē*]. You are aware that in such cases there is nothing it will not venture to undertake as being released from all sense of shame and reason. It does not shrink from attempting to lie with his mother, [so it thinks], or with any one else, man, god or brute.[34] It is ready for any foul deed of blood; it abstains from no food, and, in a word, falls short of no extreme of folly [*anoias*] and shamelessness. [571C–D]

There exists in every one of us, even in some reputed most respectable, a terrible, fierce and lawless brood of desires, which it seems are revealed in our sleep. [572B]

In one stream of Platonic thought we find the implication that sanity is the highest rational form of thinking and madness is anything less. The forms (ideas) are stable, unchanging, "being," while all the rest is "becoming." The universe of *doxa,* opinion, is born and perishes, subject to great swings and variations.

This fear of excessive flux, too wide a range, too much variation (and too much excitement) permeates Platonic thought. In more cosmological terms, as in the *Timeaus,* the contrast between regular, organized, periodic motions and wild, erratic motions is intertwined with the contrast between *psuchē* and *sōma,* between ideas and sensibles. Irregular motion equals physical, moral, and cosmic disorder (for example, *Timeaus,* 43–44; *Laws,* 897C).

Representations of this concern with wild flux versus order are seen in the discussions of music and drama (for example, *Republic,* the whole of Book 3, especially sections 392–403). Socrates speaks of musical modes and of dramatic presentations that are calm, have small gradations, and are more or less uniform. No violent emotions or sudden cacophonies are allowed. He condemns rhythms that are "appropriate to illiberality and insolence or madness or other evils" (*Republic,* 400B). Music must not be too licentious or too provocative.

In contrast, among Plato's highest values are harmony, symmetry, and temperance (*sōphrosunē*). Here Plato expands upon a fundamental Greek value, as expressed, for example, in the Delphic maxim "Nothing in excess." This concern with harmony and balance is the other side of the coin of Plato's preoccupation with conflict, particularly conflict among the parts of the psyche. The rule of the rational is the most harmonious.

If one follows the Platonic conception of mental health and sickness, then most men are mad. The philosopher alone can claim to be sane, and the men who can be philosophers are precious few (see *Republic,* 491B). Only Socrates, in fulfilling the dicta of "Know thyself" and "Nothing in excess" (except philosophy, of course!), in his search for the truth, and in his willingness to die for the belief that "the unexamined life is not worth living," was sane.

The Origins of Madness

But what is Plato's diagnosis of the source of human evil, sickness, and madness? In his mythic account of the creation of man and the cosmos, the *Timaeus,* Plato betrays a profound disappointment with human nature. The demiurge, the craftsman who molded man, was limited in what he could accomplish. The emotions, "terrible and irresistible," constituted this limitation.

[Those agencies that created man] received . . . the immortal principle of the soul; and around this they proceeded to fashion a mortal body, and made it to be the vehicle of the soul, and constructed within the body a soul of another nature, which was mortal, subject to terrible and irresistible affections—first of all, pleasure, the greatest incitement of evil, then, pain, which deters from good; also rashness and fear, two foolish counsellors, anger hard to be appeased and hope easily led astray; these they mingled with irrational sense and with all-daring love according to necessary laws, and so framed man. [*Timaeus*, 69C–D][35]

What "psychological theory" in Plato is equivalent to this mythological version? In brief, to judge from Plato's suggested reforms in the *Republic*, it is because of the family as it is that we ordinarily develop into the imperfect creature called man. Plato's proposals for the abolition of the family in favor of the guardian class reveal a profound but perverse understanding of the crucial psychological role of early family relationships for the growing child. His discussions of myth as a pernicious force in child rearing and of drama and poetry as destructive in adult life are based on an awareness of the power of *mimēsis*. *Mimēsis* in Plato seems to designate a combination of imitation and identification, both crucial ingredients in child rearing. His recommendations for the censoring of the gory nursery tales told to Greek children reveal a knowledge of forbidden childhood wishes and their accompanying terrors: cannibalism, parricide, castration.

Plato's view of the origins of human imperfection seems to include the fact of sexual differences between men and women and the relation between intercourse and birth. Certainly sexual differences represent for him conflict rather than harmony. In the extended myth in the *Statesman*, one sees that sexual intercourse and sexual propagation are features of that part of the human cycle in which the god is *not* at the helm, and motions are wild, erratic, and impulsive. During the period when the god is in control and the motions lead to good and perfection, birth does not follow sexual intercourse. Rather men arise from the earth as old, and grow progressively younger. In the *Republic*, Plato devises the "noble lie" that he claims is necessary to teach the community, especially the guardians: the guardians were not born of women, but from the earth, who is their common mother.[36]

We can carry the analysis a step further. If we review the lists (pp. 164–65) of the characteristics of the baser and higher parts of mind and now consider the last proposition—Plato's denigration of sexual differences and of intercourse as a method of begetting and creating—a rather simple but remarkable construction occurs.

Consider the items in the list: shadow; flux; sleep and dreaming; conflict; begetting, being born, and perishing; and heterosexuality—do these add up to any one simple unifying construct? I propose that they do, and that we can best see that unity by thinking in terms of a particular childhood experience and its fantasy concomitants—a *primal scene* fantasy. For all these terms can be easily matched with the conscious fantasy versions of children and the persistent unconscious fantasies of adults of the experience of witnessing or overhearing parental intercourse. Such a construction brings together many diverse themes in Plato and adds an important dimension to our understanding of the meaning of ignorance and madness in Plato. The discussion is also designed to illustrate a hitherto neglected aspect of the history of psychiatry, namely, the exploration of the unconscious fantasies about madness that may flourish in any culture or epoch. Clinically, when a patient says, "I'm going crazy," we are prepared to listen for the idiosyncratic meanings of that statement for the patient. For one person it means to lose his intelligence, for another to lose control of murderous rage or of forbidden sexual impulses, and for still another to give up and surrender to infantile helplessness. Thus, by analogy, we shall listen to images and motifs recurring through the dialogues which suggest a particular meaning of madness.

What is meant by the terms "primal scene," "primal scene trauma," and "primal scene fantasy"?[37] In the course of the psychoanalysis of some adults, Freud discovered memories, dreams, conscious fantasies, and bodily experiences that, when analyzed, seemed to refer back to the patient's childhood experience of witnessing or overhearing parental intercourse, the primal scene. From time to time such psychoanalytic reconstructions of the childhood experience have been verified by some independent information. A most striking instance is that of Princess Marie Bonaparte, one of Freud's analysands. Freud had surmised that though orphaned young, she had been repeatedly exposed to adult intercourse, but she had no such memories and deemed it unlikely. She later learned from the old coachman that on a number of occasions she had been present in the room where he and her nursemaid were having intercourse.[38] More often the reconstruction depends on material provided only in the course of the analysis, and the conviction of the truth of the reconstruction rests both on its therapeutic effect and on its overall cognitive and affective plausibility.[39]

From time to time people enter analysis who are quite aware of having been repeatedly exposed to their parents' (or other adults') sexual intercourse. Such people teach us about the correlation between certain adult fantasies, defenses, and character traits and the childhood traumatic experience.[40] These people are more likely to develop strong defensive reactions to the repeated exposure and may present evidence of strong visual fixations, powerful exhibitionistic needs, a variety of perversions, and occasionally massive pseudostupidity. Sleep disturbances and fear of dying may be other symptoms.

Undoubtedly the parental motives for exposing the child to intercourse play an important role in shaping the nature and extent of the trauma. In much of the world where whole families sleep in the same room (or even the same bed), parents expose their children to their sexuality more out of necessity than out of unresolved sadistic or exhibitionistic needs. The parents who can have privacy but *choose* to include their child in the parental bedroom are more likely to do so out of their own conflicted needs, and these conflicts must play a part in the meaning of the experience to the child. It is unlikely that repeated (or even occasional) exposure has *no* effect on the child. However, details of the social setting, the parental motives, and the opportunity the child is legitimately given to discharge his own excitement may act to make the scene less traumatic, neutral, or perhaps even positive (though we rarely hear any evidence to affirm this last possibility).[41]

In the course of psychoanalysis of most, if not all, patients, material emerges in the form of fantasies, dreams, and behaviors which has the stamp of primal scene exposure, but it is not possible to reconstruct a particular exposure or series of exposures. For this group, we speak of primal scene *fantasies* rather than primal scene *trauma,* the latter term strictly applying to patients who definitely witnessed the scene, either occasionally or regularly. We call them *primal scene* fantasies because they greatly resemble the fantasies of people who can provide evidence or strong indications of actual primal scene exposure. Primal scene fantasies are extremely common, perhaps universal, but their importance in mental life is highly variable. While we are not certain about the origins and significance of these fantasies, we can surmise that they incorporate childhood theories about birth and intercourse. They probably build on the bits and fragments of exposure to adult sexuality which the child has experienced, and are elaborated with age-appropriate fantasy. Thus childhood knowledge and desire are simultaneously expressed in primal scene fantasies.

What are the main features of primal scene fantasies, whether or not they have arisen from primal scene exposure? The scene may be experienced as a sadistic attack of one partner on the other, or of both on each other. The child may be confused as to which sex is which, who has a penis, and who is doing what to whom. The immature mental apparatus of the child, the condition of darkness, a state of drowsiness, mild delirium due to sickness—all these factors may facilitate such confusions. There may be a confusion of boundaries between the child and parents in the scene he is observing, a confusion probably enhanced by mounting excitement in the child which he may not be able to understand or cope with. A sense of extreme loneliness and exclusion is a frequent concomitant of the primal scene experience, and with it a heightening of possessive and jealous feelings. The scene may prove alternately overwhelming and fascinating—the child cannot look, and yet, immobile, must stare. The child often has a sense of immobility and at times sensations of dizziness or floating. His excitement sometimes culminates in loss of bowel or bladder control, perhaps nausea and vomiting.[42] (These bodily events may also represent childhood symbolization of the parental sexual activity. One little boy explained how his parents made babies: they put on their pajamas and go into the bathroom, where they eat a lot of candy and then get sick and vomit.) Such fantasies often involve a show, a performance, an arena.[43] Finally, the scene may be understood as having some relationship to the begetting of siblings. Primal scene fantasies may appear in the course of a discussion of rivals or new arrivals. The confused, dark, aggressive scene of parental intercourse is thus associated with the unwelcomed arrival of other children who steal the parents away.

We can now restate our hypothesis: the core unconscious meaning of madness in the Platonic dialogues is the wild, confused, and combative scene of parental intercourse as perceived by the child. We may take this inference from the imagery and the total context of the dialogues in which madness is discussed. This equation embraces the two main aspects of madness in Plato, unbridled impulse and ignorance. The wildness of the primal scene is associated with lack of restraint of impulse and appetite, and the frightening yet fascinating aspect of the scene is associated with blindness and ignorance. The appetite cannot be controlled or the veil of ignorance lifted unless the primal scene can be controlled or abolished. Philosophy provides new ways of looking and new objects of contemplation and thereby liberates men from their blindness and madness.

Another aspect of the psychology of the primal scene is crucial in Plato: the primal scene as focus for feelings of exclusivity, possessiveness, and jealous rivalry. Plato's conscious desire to minimize these emotions because they are impediments to political sanity and philosophical inquiry is a reflection of an unconscious preoccupation with the primal scene. Fraternal love can replace fratricide only if primal scene sexuality can be made unimportant.

Admittedly this extended hypothesis is speculative, especially if we wish to make statements about the author of the dialogues, Plato himself. While we cannot *prove* its validity, we can demonstrate its utility in explicating numerous aspects of Platonic psychology, epistemology, and political theory.

I have alluded to Plato's apparent discomfort with the idea that procreation depends upon sexual intercourse; the full extent of his disdain for and mistrust of all intense sexuality, including homosexuality, is worth considering. Heterosexuality, for purposes other than controlled procreation, is a necessary evil. Only in the more rarefied expressions of sexuality in his visions of mystic union with the forms, the ideas, is there any sense of sexuality as a good. The true philosopher must transcend even homosexuality if he is to reach the highest levels of truth.[44]

Plato's *Symposium* contains a myth that represents a *happy* primal scene fantasy, and this myth is rejected by Socrates. I refer to the myth of the origin of sexual desire which is narrated by Aristophanes (189E–190A), a myth shrewdly analyzed by Noel Bradley as a primal scene fantasy:[45]

The sexes were not two as they are now, but originally three in number; there was man, woman, and the union of the two, having a name corresponding to this double nature, which had once a real existence, but is now lost, and the word "androgynous" is only preserved as a term of reproach. In the second place, the primeval man was round, his back and sides forming a circle; and he had four hands and four feet, one head with two faces, looking opposite ways, set on a round neck and precisely alike; also four ears, two privy members, and the remainder to correspond. He could walk upright as men now do, backwards or forwards as he pleased, and he could also roll over and over at a great pace, turning on his four hands and four feet, eight in all, like tumblers going over and over with their legs in the air.[46]

The confusion of sexual and personal identity, the odd placement of limbs and genitals, and the sense of rolly-polly rapid movement support Bradley's interpretation. We are reminded of the "beast with two backs," Shakespeare's description of a copulating man and woman; this creature has two fronts. Primal scene fantasy material includes just such representations of the copulating parents as hybrid monsters. While such composite monsters as the centaur, sphinx, and chimaera are ubiquitous in Greek mythology, we find Plato devising still another, the psyche of man. (See above, p. 164; *Republic*, 588B–589A.)

Another piece of Platonic psychology falls into place here, the dislike of conflict and the associated definition of injustice as *polupragmosunē*, doing and being many things at once. Consider Plato's denunciation of tragedy (to be discussed later): he singles out the dangers of *mimēsis* (imitation or imitation–identification) and gives the following example of an undesirable situation on the stage (395D–E):

[We will not allow the young men of the Republic] to play the parts of women and imitate a woman young or old wrangling with her husband, defying heaven, loudly boasting, fortunate in her own conceit, or involved in misfortune and possessed by grief and lamentation—still less a woman that is sick, in love, or in labour.[47]

Plato's fear of such a confusion of sexes in the state is reminiscent of the confusion of male and female found in primal scene fantasy.

Let us turn to a consideration of the structure of the *Republic* as a whole. I believe that an important *unconscious* aspect of Plato's design for his ideal state is the wish to protect the elite and the guardians from primal scene trauma and its consequences. This unconscious wish unifies Plato's views about how to deal with conflict both in the psyche and in the state. The dialogue takes place on a festival day in the Athens of 410 B.C. The festival celebrates a deity relatively new to Athens, the goddess Bendis.[48] Her Thracian cult must originally have been orgiastic, and, like other such cults, had been tamed by the Athenians. The allusions to orgiastic religion help set the stage for the dialogue—the problem of reason versus passion, and how to blend the two. After the daytime festivities, Socrates is induced to stay for the night-long (*pannuchida*) celebration, and the dialogue takes place over the course of the night. Scattered throughout are numerous references to night, including night terrors (330E), gods who go around in disguise at night (381E), and battles at night (520C–D). In all, there is a flavor of underlying concern about things that go bump in the night. (See also 377, 379–80.) One of the central allegories in the work, the myth of the cave, is, of course, built around the contrast between shadowy darkness and bright light. References to sleep and dreams are scattered liberally throughout the work as well.[49] (Consider the unlawful desires that emerge in dreams.)

Interwoven with the imagery of night are the imagery and theme of sexuality. Even before the introduction of the central question of the first half of the dialogue, "What is justice?" the topic of sexuality is introduced by Cephalus, an old man (329B–C).

I remember hearing Sophocles asked by someone, "How goes it, Sophocles, with your sexual lusts [*aphrodisia*]? Are you still able to get together with a woman?" "Be quiet, man," he said, "I am most pleased to have escaped this thing, as if I had escaped from a raving [*luttōnta*] and wild master."[50]

Discussions of sexuality and random allusions to sexual desires, especially illicit ones, also appear. An important argument about morality is presented by means of the myth of Gyges. Gyges, a shepherd, found a ring that made him invisible and with its aid seduced the queen, slew the king, and took possession of the kingdom (359D–360D).[51] The most famous discussions of sexuality and procreation, of course, are found in Book 3, on the "noble lie," and in Book 5, on the sexual and marital arrangements for the guardians, leading to the abolition of the nuclear family.

In Book 3 Plato proposes that the rulers tell their subjects the "lie," "a kind of Phoenician tale" (because Phoenicians are presumed to be liars). All their previous lives had been but a dream (414D). They were not born from the union of man and woman but were formed complete with armor inside the earth, their mother, and were then born from her (note the similarity to the myth of Cadmus and the sown men). In Book 5, Plato proposes that the rulers allow the guardians to mate infrequently and for eugenic purposes only. Children must not know their biological parents. All children born at about the same time (presumably the dates of mating would be regulated) would be considered brothers and sisters. A child born from intercourse outside the state-regulated matings would be illegitimate, "a child conceived in darkness and dire incontinence" (461B).[52] All the adults who cohabited at the time of conception of a certain cohort of children would be considered the mothers and fathers of all of those children. Unions between those two groups of parents and offspring would be regarded as incestuous, though no special mention is made of unions between the "brothers and sisters" as incestuous. Here we have the most dramatic kind of confirmation of our hypothesis about an unconscious primal scene fantasy in the *Republic.* Ordered, regulated intercourse, not "in the dark," is the aim, and as far as possible, intercourse should be dissociated from biological and social parenthood.

The method in the madness becomes clearer if we consider the political aims of these reforms, namely, to minimize jealousy and rivalry and maximize allegiance to the state. Plato sees sexuality as an acquisitive appetite, and permanent liaisons lead men to regard sexual partners (wives) as a form of property. For the guardians and the philosopher rulers, all property must be held in common, hence wives and children cannot be regarded as one's own. Private property is associated with jealousy and ultimately with civil strife. Fratricide will inevitably replace fraternal love if any brother thinks another has more or better than he. Implicit in Plato's discussions of the evils of Greek politics is the notion of fratricide. (The *Republic* is one of the two dialogues that involve Plato's brothers.) The state is the mother who treats all her children exactly alike.[53]

The unconscious element corresponding to these conscious arguments is reflected in the imagery of conception and birth in the dark. The nature of the child's experience of the primal scene is such as to consolidate feelings of intense possessiveness. Further, as the child comes to sense that intercourse leads to the birth of siblings, the primal scene experience is an important focus of the rage aroused by both the sibling and the parents who begat him.

Finally, we must consider the central allegory of the *Republic,* the allegory of the cave (514A–C). Here the contrast between light and darkness is crucial to the exposition of the pedagogic, philosophical, and political aims of the *Republic:*

> Next . . . compare our nature in respect of education and its lack to such an experience as this. Picture men dwelling in a sort of subterranean cavern with a long entrance open to the light on its entire width. Conceive them as having their legs and necks fettered from *childhood,* so that they *remain* in the *same spot,* able to *look forward only, and prevented by the fetters from turning their heads.* Picture further the light from a fire burning higher up and at a distance behind them, and between the fire and prisoners and above them a road along which a low wall has been built, as the *exhibitors of puppet shows* have partitions before the men themselves, above which they show the puppets. . . . See also, then, men carrying past the wall implements of all kinds that rise above the wall, and human images and shapes of animals as well, . . . some of these bearers presumably speaking and others silent. . . . A strange image and strange prisoners. *Like to us* . . . for, to begin with, tell me do you think that these men would have seen anything of themselves or of one another except the shadows cast from the fire on the wall? . . . And if their prison had an echo, . . . do you think that they would suppose anything else than the passing shadow to be the speaker? . . . Then in every way such prisoners would deem reality to be nothing else than the shadows of artificial object. . . . Consider, then, what would be the manner of the release and *healing* from these bonds and this *folly.* [54]

It would be difficult for these prisoners to emerge from the cave and at first they would be blinded by the bright light. As they gradually became accustomed to the sunlight, they would realize they had been living in a world of illusion. Now it would be difficult to get them to return to the cave, but return some of them must, the philosophers who become kings, and they will instruct those still in the cave.

My contention, then, is that this scene can also be understood as a primal scene fantasy: children in the darkness of the bedroom, seeing the shadows and hearing the echoes of parental intercourse. The prisoners are fixed, they cannot even turn their heads away (corresponding to the immobility and staring of the child experiencing the primal scene). They see a shadow play, a puppet show. [55] They see shadows of animals, objects, and people. These prisoners (who are we ourselves) can be freed and released from *aphrosunē,* folly and madness. [56] Ignorance and madness are thus states of misapprehension of things that go on in shadow and darkness. Farther on (518C), Plato labels the spectacle in the cave as "the world of being born" (*tou gignomenou*), in contrast to the objects of vision outside the cave, the world of true being, the world of forms. The cave and the sunlight thus correspond to the thinking of the lowest part of the psyche and the thinking of the highest part, respectively.

The allegory continues with an account of the visual ascent of the psyche to the *noeton topon,* the realm of pure intellect. Note how the imagery of bright light, sanity, and birth and procreation are interwoven (517B–C):

In the realm of pure intellect, the last thing to be seen, and then only with great difficulty, is the idea of the good. Once we have seen it, we must conclude that the idea of the good is the cause of all that is right and beautiful in everything. In the realm of the visible, the idea of the good has given birth to light and to the master of light. In the realm of pure intellect, the idea of the good itself is the provider of truth and intelligence. Anyone who is to act sanely, in either private or public life, must eventually see the idea of the good.[57]

The discussion then turns to politics, the government of the ideal state, the Republic. Those who have ascended from the cave into the light must go down once again into the cave and instruct the dwellers in darkness and lead them into the light. These are the political leaders, who must take proper control of the Republic: "So our city will be governed by us and you with waking minds [*hupar*], and not as most cities now which are inhabited and ruled darkly as in a dream [*onar*] by men who fight one another for shadows and wrangle for office as if that were a great good" (520C).[58] Propagation in the dark and the shadows leads to rivalry and civil war; propagation in the light leads to cooperation and suppression of individual pleasures for the common good. For Plato, the way the cities of Greece are governed (that is, by democracy or mindless, hedonistic tyranny) is equivalent to copulation and birth in the dark.[59]

In a way, such a formulation should come as no surprise to students of totalitarian political theory. Whether imaginary (*Brave New World, 1984*) or real (Hitler's Germany, the early years of the Soviet Union), totalitarian governments have seen a link between the maintainance of tight political control and the state regulation of copulation and birth. Democracy tends to be described in the language of chaos, a mad carnival, endless dissent, and as totally libertine.

Thus, our analysis of the themes and images of birth and copulation and death in the *Republic* leads to a frightening primal scene fantasy, which seems to be the substrate from which arise the Platonic notions of evil, madness, and that special brand of madness which is political rivalry and civil war. If only we could devise, so Plato yearned, new modes of sexuality and birth that would eliminate the possibility of children's watching parents copulate in the dark, we could eliminate this whole host of evils.

In the next chapter, I shall discuss Plato's attempt to devise new methods of looking and new objects for contemplation. In brief, we come to the problem of education, which is at the heart of Plato's understanding of therapy for the sicknesses of the psyche. What is Plato's prescription for turning men away from the world of illusion, madness, begetting, and perishing to the world of truth, sanity, and true being?

9

The Philosopher as Therapist

> . . . for you will do me much greater good by putting an end to
> ignorance of my psyche than if you put an end to an affliction of
> my body.
>
> —Plato, *Hippias Minor*

If madness is ignorance, if sickness is discord, what is the treatment?
How can we begin to stabilize the staggering psyche, drunk with lust
and appetite and consorting promiscuously with every sensory impression? The answer is philosophy. Philosophy alone is the *therapeia*
for sickness of the soul.

From Plato's perspective, all the traditional Greek modes of therapy can be reduced to one or another variant of poetry. The songs of
Homer, the great tragic presentations, and the croonings of a mother
to a child—these are what the Greeks have used as relief for sorrow
and a restoration from injury.

E. A. Havelock, in *Preface to Plato,*[1] has penetratingly examined
the complex of reasons behind Plato's antagonism toward the entire
Hellenic poetic tradition. In the *Republic* Plato declares that "there is
an old quarrel between philosophy and poetry" (607B). The quarrel
cannot be too old, for philosophy was not very old in Plato's day.
But the fragments of some of the pre-Socratics (Xenophanes, for
example) seem to indicate that the rise of philosophy was associated
with a denunciation of the predominant place given the poets as the
teachers of Greece.[2] In the *Republic,* Plato launches a two-stage attack
on poetry. The first stage begins with a discussion of myths and
nursery tales (Book 2) and culminates (Book 3) with Plato's denunciation of only "bad poetry." At this stage he attacks both content, a
harmful theology, and the alleged deleterious effects of drama.
Drama is too emotional, too erratic, and as such inconsistent with his
moral aims. He fears the contagious effects on audience and actors of
a show of cowardice or cruelty by one of the characters. He is
distraught over what he sees as the contradictions and inconsistencies
in the portrayal of character and the fact that the great tragedies must
portray all the complexities of a character and a situation. In short,
he rejects everything in the works of Homer and the tragedians

which make them great art as opposed to propaganda or sermonizing. One can compare Plato's view to arguments raised in modern times by totalitarian governments—art must conform to "socialist realism" and the like.

Plato, Havelock argues, correctly saw that a crucial element in the way poetry and drama exert their influence is *mimēsis*. This term, as Plato uses it, seems to subsume both conscious forms of imitation, such as the actor's role playing, and processes involving actors and audience which might be termed unconscious identification. Plato's discourse makes it clear that he tends to equate transient role playing with permanent identification—hence his fear that evil behavior on the stage will inevitably lead the audience to become evil. Plato's view of the power of *mimēsis* must be juxtaposed with his notion of justice, each man doing his proper job and only one job. Plato attacks *polupragmosunē*—doing many things at once—as a form of evil, injustice, and madness. The poetic performance, however, fosters a number of identifications; Homer makes many chords resonate within us. (See Chapter 8 on *polupragmosunē* as an aspect of the primal scene fantasy.) Other aspects of Plato's rejection of poetry at this point in his argument concern the emotionality of the poetic experience and the passivity of the audience (and even the passivity of the poet, who is inspired by the Muse). In his *Ion,* Plato characterized the performance of the rhapsode as out-and-out madness, of great destructive potential to the audience. He will allow nothing that might stir up excessive emotion.

In Book 10 of the *Republic* Plato returns to his attack on poetry and drama (and even on the plastic arts) and dismisses them all from his state. This global condemnation of literary and dramatic art is based on a total rejection of *mimēsis* as a principle of learning, for *mimēsis* is the *modus operandi* of the lower parts of the psyche. The highest part learns by *epistemē*, by *noēsis*, processes that rely on intellect, logic, and dialectic, rather than on imitation and identification. Even the epistemological discussion of Book 10 contains hints that *mimēsis* is rejected because of some connection with sexuality and reproduction. *Mimēsis* is "a cheap woman, having intercourse with a cheap man, and giving birth to cheap offspring" (603B). *Mimēsis* is a whore. Thus the *Republic* moves from state regulation of the dramatic and musical arts to a ban on all art forms.[3] Only with radically new forms of education, those outlined in the *Republic,* can the state be safely and properly governed.

Plato's attacks on poetry and *mimēsis* are attacks on the Greek educational tradition. Poetry entails the system and values of oral communication, that is, face-to-face transmission of knowledge, be it ethical or factual, and the overriding value of continuity of tradition and authority from generation to generation. Plato, in effect, dismisses the very essence of the notion of "classic," which is to find the best model and then to imitate it. Plato's notion of the forms (whether the form of the good, of the beautiful, or of the table or chair) seems to incorporate the ideal of the classical. But he moves the ideal beyond any exemplar of a true idea or beautiful body. Anything less than the form itself is a copy—man is a copy of the form of man, and a poet who "imitates" a man in his writing is merely producing a copy of a copy.

Philosophy as Countercharm

Plato wished to replace poetry with philosophy. As we have seen, he redefined mental distress and mental illness as species of ignorance resulting from the excessive power of the appetitive over the rational. Ignorance of what? Ignorance of oneself is the Socratic answer; ignorance of the forms is the Platonic expansion of the Socratic definition. But Plato has not only made his own definition of madness and disturbance of the mind; he has also moved in the direction of labeling the old method of treatment, poetry, as itself a source of illness. "Bewitchment," "charms," and "sorcery" are some of the words Plato uses to characterize the effects of poetry; philosophy must provide a "countercharm" (608A).[4] But even Socrates enjoys and profits from poetry, "we ourselves are bewitched by it."[5] The philosopher's duty, however, is clear (608A–B):

As long as she [poetry] cannot give a good argument for herself, let us pay attention to the reasons we have given, chanting them as a countercharm, being careful lest we fall back again into this love, which is childish and belongs to the masses. For we perceive that we must not take such poetry seriously as a way of touching the truth, but that he who pays attention to it [poetry] must be careful, fearing for the city-state within him, and must listen to what we have said about poetry.[6]

The allegory of the cave provides an entry into an understanding of what lies behind this rejection. Inside the cave a dramatic performance takes place, a "puppet show" (*thaumatopoia,* making wonderful spectacles). The inhabitants of the cave witness a shadow play, staged by people who parade between the fire and the backs of the spectators.[7] Thus, for Plato, the world of opinion or seeming is not totally random: it is to some extent purposefully organized, though the purpose is not clear to the spectators. Plato equated drama and epic poetry with this parade of images. These images, in effect, are those of the Hellenic culture, the myths and traditions as they are represented in poetry. According to my analysis of the cave allegory, myth and poetry are equivalent to primal scene sexuality.

I have argued that tragedy, in particular, does not merely present myths, but *represents* them in such a way as to give them a new meaning. From Plato's perspective, however, poetic interpretations are inadequate.[8] They are neither explicit enough about the connection between past and present nor sufficiently shaped by articulated abstract thought and principles. They are liable to be abused, and each playwright, in principle, could come up with his own interpretation of the significance of a particular myth. Plato, in effect, regards the tragedies and epic poems as a psychoanalyst regards dreams and neuroses. The psychoanalyst views the dream as a form of matching up and condensation of images and feelings from the past with ones from the present. The neurosis, similarly, is a restatement in symbolic form of a part of the patient's past, a mythic, imagistic reenactment, as it were, of an earlier drama. But, from a psychoanalytic perspective, the dream that is not interpreted is a distinctly limited kind of statement about the relationship between past and present. A neurosis that is not understood and interpreted has the *potential* for revealing the connection between past and present, but in actuality is only a monotonous reenactment, inchoate and ill understood. Plato considered tragedy a shadow show, a mute reenactment, not an explicit interpretation.

What is this countercharm that is philosophy, and how does it work? In the *Phaedrus,* Socrates, in the course of rejecting as a waste of time attempts at naturalistic explanations of myths, outlines what for him is the essential task of philosophical inquiry: "I must first know myself, as the Delphian inscription says; to be curious about that which is not my concern, while I am still in ignorance of my own self, would be ridiculous: . . . am I a monster more complicated and swollen with passion than the serpent Typho, or a creature of a gentler and simpler sort . . . ?" (229E–230A).[9]

What is the method by which a man can come to know himself, or to know himself in relation to ideas and to the world of true being? The method is first *dialogue* and finally *dialectic.*

Dialogue and Dialectic

Dialogue is conversation. In the earliest Platonic dialogues (which scholars agree present the most accurate picture of Socrates) we find Socrates engaged in philosophical conversation. He not only adduces logical proofs for his arguments; he charms, persuades, seduces. He ridicules, confounds, and forces his opponent to feel uncomfortable. He is the gadfly and the electric eel. In the *Charmides,* Socrates describes his mode of discourse (his *logos*) as "magic charms," as if the words themselves had a certain potency. In this dialogue Socrates' discourse has a Homeric flavor: he tells a story. Thus in the earlier dialogues we see not so much the delineation of a general philosophical method (though its beginnings are present) as the portrayal of Socrates questioning. The method is the man at work.

In the middle and later dialogues Plato develops and refines a general method, the dialectic. The dialectic is grounded in dialogue but is certainly not synonymous with it. Dialectic is a method of questioning and answering—dividing, defining, categorizing, and abstracting. As we see dialectic in Plato—and probably in other contemporary thinkers—certain ground rules determine the form of the inquiry. Questions are frequently posed to allow only a yes-or-no answer. Typically, a *reductio ad absurdum* ends a line of argument. Its aim is to arrive at a certain fixity and clarity, to define the various and changeable aspects of the phenomenal world, the world of becoming. Dialectic is the tool by means of which one moves from becoming to being, from opinion and appearances to true knowledge (see the list on pp. 164–65).[10]

Dialectic involves laying down hypotheses, using them as stepping-stones on which one advances toward the conclusions that ensue from the hypotheses, and then determining whether or not the hypotheses have led to contradiction. If contradiction has resulted, the path must be retraced, the hypotheses reexamined and either discarded as leading to logical contradiction or restated so that another pathway may be followed.

Dialectic is radically different from dialogue in that the latter relies heavily on some of the techniques of rhetoric: persuasion, seduction, pandering to irrational fears and an appeal to identification with the speaker. Dialectic aims to discover and uncover truth, not to persuade or cajole. It contrasts with rhetoric and with eristic—the art of verbal contention with the aim of overcoming an opponent's arguments.[11] Rhetoric seeks to win elections; dialectic seeks truth.

Dialectic, however, clearly does not operate independently of emotions. The emotions associated with dialectic differ from those associated with rhetoric. The former include surprise, frustration over a knotty problem, shame at not knowing, the discomfort that comes from discovering contradictions in one's own beliefs, and the pleasure that comes with solving a problem. To coin a phrase: these are the academic emotions as opposed to the rhetorical ones.

Although they are academic, or pedagogical, they are hardly weak. For Plato, they are a necessary aspect of the active struggle of the soul as it strives for truth. The attainment of truth must not be a passive experience, and it must produce discomfort; dialectic and philosophy are not soothing and comforting—as in Hesiod's account of the therapeutic effect of the bard—but disruptive and irritating. Plato hopes that when men are truly involved in the dialectical process, they will "grow angry with themselves and gentle toward others" (*Sophist,* 230B). This kind of turmoil is the sine qua non for genuine change (see, for example, *Republic,* 518A–B). Thus in the transition from dialogue to dialectic in Plato's writings we see an attempt to move away from poetry toward philosophy as the method of treatment of ignorance and confusion.

Though the distinction between dialectic and dialogue (or between poetry and philosophy) underlines a problem, it hardly solves it. Plato was very much concerned about the proper balance between affect and intellect. He was profoundly aware that men resist knowing the truth, and that the appetites are at the base of this resistance. At the same time, what would motivate one to lust for knowledge rather than for power or sexual gratification?

In seeking an answer to this question, let us turn to the *Phaedrus* (244) and the theme of "the blessings of madness." Socrates states that some of our greatest blessings come through madness, provided it is a divine madness and not one caused by human disease. He lists:

1. Prophetic madness (as in the Sibyl at Delphi).
2. "Telestic," or ritual, madness (as in the Dionysiac rituals).
3. Poetic madness ("inspiration").
4. The madness of love.

As Dodds has observed, it cannot be that "the father of Western rationalism here praises madness over sanity, and the irrational over the rational."[12] Indeed, there is never any question that philosophy is superior to even these kinds of divine inspiration.

This section becomes intelligible in relation to the central issue in the *Phaedrus:* the question of the relationship between "carnal love" and love of knowledge. The problem that Socrates struggles to solve is that of devising a method of seeking and transmitting truth which can really "write in the hearts of men" (278A). Only dialectic is adequate to the task, not rhetoric and sophistry. These forms of madness fascinate Socrates and are relevant to his problem. If he could only borrow some of the enthusiasm and ecstasy of these madnesses and combine them with dialectic, he could be surer of success. Dialectic must produce a radical, permanent, and *qualitative* change in the way men think, feel, and act. Syllogism alone does not suffice.

Along with "divine madness" one must consider Plato's use of "myths" (such as the myth of the cave, the myths of immortality of the soul, the description of Eros in the *Symposium* and in the *Phaedrus*). Plato's use of myths and of mythlike allegories is a concomitant of the transition from dialogue to dialectic.[13] Particularly in the middle dialogues (for example, the *Republic*) one can see, *pari passu,* the evolution of the idea of a dialectical method, the rejection of Homer and the mythopoetic modes of thought, and the deliberate introduction of Platonic myths. The later dialogues, where the dialectic is on somewhat surer footing, have less "mythology," but in the last work, the *Laws,* we find the balance has again shifted to "reason for the few and magic for the masses."[14] The masses are to be treated as children.

But the balance between emotion and reason is delicate. Philosophy and dialectic are potent drugs, and "philosophic madness," is a distinct danger. Dialectic is heady stuff, and the young must not drink of it prematurely (*Republic,* 537C–539D). And to the world at large, the true philosopher, such as Socrates, appears mad (*Phaedrus,* 249D; *Republic,* 499C). By a reversal of conventional values, this madness must be considered a divine inspiration, and philosophers must rule as kings. The final proof of the risks of dialectic is to be seen in the life and death of Socrates. The Athenians who tried and sentenced him did not distinguish between his aggessiveness in the cause of making men see the truth and his aggressiveness toward his fellow Athenians as such. Not everyone welcomed the unsettling effects of philosophy, and Socrates was executed.

Socrates died in accordance with the beliefs by which he had lived. Philosophy, then, can serve as a way to put a man in touch with his true self, and truly help him to know himself. This is the sense in which the Socratic ideal comes closest to ideals held up by various schools of psychoanalysis and psychotherapy—ideals of an integrated awareness of the self, of one's own past, present, and future, and of the relationship between oneself and one's group.

I believe that this point, or something like it, is at issue in the last book of the *Republic,* which begins with the attack on poetry. The book concludes with the famous myth of Er, the tale of the way souls are rewarded and punished after death and of their opportunity to choose the lives they will lead in their next incarnations. All of the psyches except Odysseus' are unable to choose lives that are substantially better than their previous ones, and instead choose lives that constitute endless repetitions of their previous misery (or of their miserable characters). Ajax chooses to become a lion; Thersites, the buffoon, becomes an ape. Consonant with the argument of Book 10, the superiority of philosophy over poetry, the myth of Er affirms the difficulty of understanding one's past life in order to change that life. Only Odysseus seems to have acquired the practical wisdom to change.[15] The message is clear: only philosophy allows a man to escape from the endless cycle of fruitless repetition of his past. Only philosophy will lead us to the point of becoming one rather than many.

But is dialectic an instrument of the pursuit of truth which the true philosopher will apply to anyone and anything, including himself

and his own beliefs? Suppose dialectic were to uncover some contradictions and inconsistencies in either the life or the work of the
philosopher. Evidence in Plato's writings is insufficient to answer
this question, but it suggests that dialectic might be used in the
service of questioning even the most fundamental tenets of the philosophic method and beliefs. For example, in the *Parmenides,* a much
controverted dialogue, Plato applies the dialectical method to the
theory of the forms, the relationship among the forms, and the relationships between the forms and their particulars. It appears to many
scholars that Plato arrives at a contradiction in the theory of the
forms as stated in the dialogue. Even if Plato does not intend to let
the contradiction stand, the flavor of the discussion is certainly one of
relatively impartial inquiry that may lead where it will.[16]

The Sōphronisterion

Another side of Plato, however, is heavily invested in keeping
tight political control of his polity and does not allow unbridled
dissent. How literally does Plato take his equation of madness and
ignorance? Where dissent within the state is concerned, we find evidence of an ominous turn. In the *Laws* (a dialogue in which Socrates
does not appear), Plato proposes penalties for those who do not
accept his program of belief in gods. If they are atheists and ill
behaved besides, they are to be put to death. But if they are mistaken
in their beliefs and are not actively doing injustice to their fellow
citizens, a curious treatment awaits them. Plato devises an institution
called a *sōphronisterion* (from *sōphrosunē,* temperance), a kind of jail
and reform school, a "house of temperance." *Sōphrosunē,* it will be
recalled, is actually the Platonic antonym for madness.

. . . let those who have been made what they are [i.e., atheists] only from
want of understanding, and not from malice or an evil nature, be placed by
the judge in the *Sōphronisterion,* and ordered to suffer imprisonment during a
period of not less than five years. And in the meantime let them have no
intercourse with other citizens except with members of the nocturnal council
and with them let them converse with a view to the improvement of their
souls' health. And when the time of their imprisonment has expired, if any
of them be of sound mind let him be restored to sane company, but if not,
and if he be condemned a second time, let him be punished with death.
[*Laws,* 908C–909B][17]

The translation, though not literal, captures the flavor of this passage by its choice of the words "health," "sound mind," and "sane
company." The implication is that this particular form of dissent is a
kind of madness (certainly a kind of ignorance and intemperance),
and that the appropriate treatment is segregation in an institution
where attitudes and feelings are reformed through persuasion and

coercion. Plato verges on making a political and moral definition of madness. One sees a precedent for coercive reeducation of those with undesirable ideas—certainly an unseemly reverse to the coin that has dialectic as its obverse.

When this institution is examined, a new notion emerges: health in the psyche is not merely analogous to health in the state, it becomes contingent upon it. The healthy state will make healthy the psyches of its citizens and at the same time designate what is healthy and what is sick.[18] These, as we shall see, are the premises of social psychiatry, and both its shame and its glory.

Since "sickness of the soul" is equated with the basic conflictual nature of the human soul, we are all, to one degree or another, mad. Plato proposes radical treatments intended to bring harmony, order, and self-control. Dialectic produces sanity by profoundly disturbing the individual and causing him to reexamine his ideas and values. Philosophy, for Plato, alienates a man from the world as it is by not allowing a mere passive acceptance of conventional values. *Per contram,* his programs of radical political and social change aim at promoting the maximum degree of integration of the individual with the state. For Plato the tension between these two aims, the alienation of the philosopher from the world and the integration of the state and the philosopher, is never fully resolved. Though Plato himself never labels these aims contradictory, it is also clear that he cannot produce—even in utopian fantasy—a wholly satisfactory solution to the problem of how to make men sane.

The Craft of the Philosopher and Its Institutional Setting

Plato's Academy was the great compromise between these two contradictory trends in his thought. On the one hand, philosophy should be content to build "the republic that is within the man" (*Republic,* 608B); on the other, both the philosopher and the world need a republic in which the philosopher can be king. The Academy was the meeting ground between the life of contemplation and the life of action, a place in which men could pursue philosophy and dialectic, and from which they might foray into the world of Greek politics (and to which they might beat a hasty retreat). The contents of Plato's philosophy were also taught, and at various times its members must have been active in research, particularly in mathematics and astronomy.[19]

In order to appreciate the significance of the Academy and the connection between its structure and function and the Platonic model of mind, we must review its cultural context. This context, broadly speaking, was the crucial transition from a culture that was based primarily on oral communication, on face-to-face teaching of skills and values, to one that increasingly relied on reading and writing. Specifically, the context was the conflict and crisis in Greek educational values, in which Plato and Socrates were participants. Their activity was both a reflection and a cause of this problem in education.

The Platonic model of the psyche, as divided into a cognitive and an appetitive or somatic aspect, was intimately related to the philosopher's perception of his own activity in relation to the society around him. His position as teacher and then as mediator between the older and newer methods of teaching and learning was intimately related to his account of the role of the rational part of the psyche. The thesis of an underlying primal scene fantasy in Plato's writings is also relevant here, for that fantasy indicates Plato's perception (however exaggerated and distorted) of what is entailed in the older methods of oral communication.

The Rise of Literacy in Classical Greece[20]

In the centuries between Homer and Plato, the use of writing gradually spread. It is likely that the Homeric epics were composed either under the influence of the new technology or with its aid. In the seventh century, writing was used in the composition and/or the preservation of poetry, as well as in inscriptions. By the sixth century, writing was used more commonly for private and public inscriptions and for coins, and was scratched onto pottery to indicate the maker, recipient, owner, and mythological characters in the vase paintings.

The use of writing in these contexts does not mean, however, that the habits of oral communication of information had been replaced by those of written communication. The available evidence suggests that literacy took hold only gradually, and that teaching by oral presentation and by memorization and recitation remained the core of the educational experience well into the fifth century. (Education, in this sense, was primarily for the upper classes.) Music, gymnastics, and some reading and writing were being taught at "schools." The heart of the education of the aristocratic young man remained his intimate involvement with an older man who taught him the necessary arts and crafts of being a citizen of the polis.[21]

There are suggestions that sometime in the latter half of the fifth century sons were becoming more literate than their fathers. If this is true, it raises the intriguing possibility that the audience that first watched Sophocles' *Oedipus Rex,* a play about blindness and seeing (about 430 B.C.), was composed of fathers who were marginally literate and sons who were significantly more literate.[22]

Extended prose writing first appears in the fifth century. The histories of Herodotus (perhaps completed soon after 430 B.C.) still bear the earmarks of a work designed as much for reading aloud in company as for private reading. Thucydides' prose (ca. 402 B.C.) is far more compact and analytic. The pre-Socratics seem to have written either in verse or, if in prose, in gnomic, epigrammatic form. Plato's dialogues (composed after 390 B.C.) are purportedly reports of dialogues, but clearly were composed in writing and intended for careful reading and study. By the second half of the fourth century one could write a prose treatise with none of the trappings of oral communication.

In view of what we know about the spread of literacy in Europe and the admixtures of written and oral communiation in many contemporary societies where literacy is limited, this picture of the gradual spread of literacy in Greece is quite plausible. What may have been unique to the Greek situation was the *use* to which the Greeks put this confluence of the oral and the written modes. They not only used writing to record their classics but exploited its potential for new genres of material, particularly expository and analytic prose. We can speculate that the Greeks achieved a creative synthesis of the oral and the literate, and cannot specify too much beyond that.[23]

Plato and the Impact of Literacy

Havelock contends that Plato was a pivotal figure in the transition from an oral to a literate culture. Plato's work was an indication of this transition and at the same time was considerably influenced it. The clearest indicator of both Plato's awareness of the change and his role in further promoting the change is his attack on poetry and the poets. By arguing that philosophers must replace poets as the teachers of Greece, he was both documenting and fostering the change from an education based on oral, face-to-face communication to education based on organized, systematized, written communication.[24]

The rational psyche as presented by Plato, Havelock argues, functions according to the premises of literacy, not according to the premises of an oral culture. As for the "self" that emerges from the Platonic effort, it is a thinking self.

The "personality," as first invented by the Greeks and then presented to posterity for contemplation, could not be that nexus of motor responses, unconscious reflexes, and passions and emotions which had been mobilised for countless time in the service of the mnemomic process. On the contrary, it was precisely these which proved an obstacle to the realisation of a self-consciousness emancipated from the condition of an oral culture. The *psyche* which slowly asserts itself in independence of the poetic performance and the poetised tradition had to be the reflective, thoughtful, critical psyche or it could be nothing.[25]

The thinking, calculating, and abstracting self is in marked contrast to the self that is implied in the epic poems, which is defined by the social nexus. The contrast between the activity of the bard and that of the philosopher illustrates Havelock's point about the autonomous psyche. The bard sees himself as operating in a traditional manner and as transmitting traditional information to his audience. He teaches and reinforces what the culture already knows and values. He functions in a close, continuous, and intimate relationship with his audience. That relationship is an aspect of the larger social intimacy and close personal interdependence characteristic of oral and tribal cultures. Such intimacy and continuity are ideals as well as facts, and the culture may well have a strong vested interest in acting as though the ideals were always factually true. The poet does not see himself as separated or radically different from his audience. His sense of individuality rests only on his craft as a poet, a maker of tales. He has the gift of song from the gods, just as other craftsmen have their gifts.

By contrast, consider the relationship between the philosopher and his audience. First we have the portrait of Socrates at work (especially in the earlier dialogues) confronting in the agora one kind of audience, Athenian citizens who are not yet disciples of any particular philosophical system or method. He is questioning, arguing positions, and forcing his hearers to examine the meaning of the traditional values. While he appears to share these values with his interlocutors, such values as piety, justice, courage, and temperance, he demonstrates the inadequacy of the traditional views. In some instances he reaches an impasse, *aporia,* but in others he moves in the direction of radical new definitions of the conventional terms. The gap between audience and philosopher is highlighted and even exaggerated, especially in the *Apology.* Socrates clearly says things that his audience does not wish to hear, and says them in a manner neither familiar nor comfortable.

But what was so disconcerting in the Socratic manner? A reading of the dialogues in general and the *Apology* in particular conveys the impression that it must have been his argumentativeness, his ability to irritate, that stirred up so much antagonism. Certainly it should come as no surprise that one of Socrates' accusers, Anytus, had earlier been quietly cut down by Socrates. In the *Meno* (89E), Socrates addressed him as the son of a noble and virtuous Athenian and then proceeded to demonstrate that virtue cannot be taught, even by an Athenian gentleman to his son.[26] Such is the stuff of which smoldering resentment is made, resentment that can easily be rationalized as requiring prosecution for the good of the state.

But contentiousness and love of argument, even ad hominem, hardly seem uncogenial to the litigious Greeks. In the long run, what proved most alien and discomfiting about the Socratic method was that it was, in fact, not primarily an ad hominem attack. Its very impersonality stirred up anxiety and then antagonism. Socrates' method of inquiry placed a heavy burden on the cognitive, rational faculties and downgraded the emotional and the pleasurable. The prime task of the philosopher is to tame instincts and passions by means of abstract, rational tools of inquiry—always the same tools, whether the philosopher is addressing his colleagues or governing a polity.

In the poet–audience exchange that produces the epic poem, the distinction between thought and feeling is not emphasized. Rather thought and feeling must be combined to produce the sensuous and soothing effect of the poetry. Philosophy is an irritant, hardly suited (except for the very few) to calm the troubled psyche and reassure us about our worst fears. In brief, the split between the rational and appetitive portions in the Platonic psychology parallels the split between the philosopher and his audience. The philosopher emphasizes the autonomy and the internalization of thinking and assumes that the mind is an active, synthesizing, and regulating agency. The audience, be it a part of himself, a part of the psyche of other philosophers, or "the masses," is the repository of emotion and appetite.

The *Republic* provides the clearest examples of the connection between the philosophical craft and the philosophical model of mind. It is explicitly built around the proposition that the divisions of the psyche correspond to the divisions of the state (that is, the ideal state of the *Republic*). The philosopher king corresponds to the *logistikon,* the rational, abstracting, and defining part of the psyche, the part that knows and learns by dialectic. Implicitly the *logistikon* is also analogous to the philosopher or dialectician (Socrates) at work, trying to guide the participants in the dialogue to the truth.[27] While the various characters in the dialogue are not equated with the parts of the psyche, there is some correspondence between them. In the *Republic,* Socrates, especially as he engages in the dialectical process, corresponds to the *logistikon,* while Thrasymachus, who says that justice means "the strong do what they can and the weak suffer what they must," is an exemplar of the lowest part, the *epithumetikon.* Glaucon comes closest to representing the activity of the *thumoeides,* insofar as he is the eager and "erotic" young man who must be enlisted on the side of dialectical inquiry.[28]

In the *Timaeus,* the dramatic follow-up of the *Republic,* the rational part of the psyche (*nous*) is analogous to the brain, the spirited-affective to the heart, and the appetitive to the liver and other organs below the diaphragm including the genitals. The body is analogous to the body politic; the philosopher is the brains of the organization.[29]

In sum, while I have construed a model for the activity of the mind to be implicit in the societal view of the craft of the bard, the analogous construction, that the mind described in philosophy is akin to the activity of the philosopher, is made explicit by Plato. At times the philosopher is viewed as the equivalent of the rational part of the psyche, while all the rest of mankind is viewed as equivalent to the lower parts. At other times the emphasis seems to be on the separation of the philosophic part of the philosopher's psyche from the sensory and appetitive parts. Similarly, the opposition of psyche to soma may be viewed as analogous to the role of the philosopher vis-à-vis the world, or to the role of the rational faculties of the philosopher versus the tugs and pulls of his own body.

Plato and the Academic Revolution

What was Athenian education like in the fifth century? As far as we can reconstruct the situation, at least the upper classes were given what may be called elementary schooling, which began in early adolescence and consisted of some reading and writing, memorization of poetry (especially Homer), music, and gymnastics.[30] This schooling was one stage in the grooming of the young man to be a competent, knowledgeable, and well-spoken Athenian citizen. It was not designed to foster independent thinking, but rather to impart traditional knowledge, morality, and civic virtues. The emphasis was on learning by example; various Homeric heroes were presented as models of one virtue or another. Certain important kinds of civic learning must have taken place in associations of youths of the same cohort, as in military training. A crucial part of a boy's education, however, involved an intimate association with an older man. The man might be a relative or a friend of the father. He was the boy's mentor, teaching him the practical skills of public speaking, proper behavior in such social settings as the gymnasium, and something of practical economics and finance; and no doubt he imparted the particular political viewpoints of the extended household. Often, though we do not know how often, such a relationship would involve an overt homosexual relationship, with the older man being the *erastes,* the lover, the younger the *eroumenos,* the beloved. This arrangement appears to have served to deflect a certain amount of tension and conflict from the father-son relationship. The father in upper-class families was often perceived as a somewhat remote figure, not always intimately involved in the family, and certainly not in the rearing of young children.[31] The older man may have offered intimacy seldom available in father-son relationships.

Sometime in the second half the fifth century, individuals who came to be called sophists began to appear in Athens, offering, for money, specialized instruction in various skills, especially forensic and political rhetoric. Their teaching was admixed with various new philosophical and scientific ideas, implying moral values that came to be viewed with more or less suspicion by Athenians of all classes. Several of the Platonic dialogues involve conversations, real or imaginary, with particular sophists (Gorgias, Protagoras), and the *Sophist* attempts to give a definition of the word. In one sense, these men fulfilled an important need in Athenian society, that of providing more intensive and "sophisticated" education for youths in a society that was growing more complex and becoming progressively more involved in the intricacies of governing a large empire. In another sense, they came to be viewed as threats to traditional Athenian education, for implicitly they presented a notion of knowledge as relative, and also relatively impersonal. The sophists probably began the use of lectures and tests. They offered a logical supplement to the training of a young Athenian gentleman, but what they had to offer seemed to upset the particular social and personal balance that a gentleman was to maintain.

Socrates tried to distinguish himself from the sophists. He did not accept money for teaching, and he insisted that he did not offer any particular kind of knowledge, only the knowledge of his own ignorance. Nevertheless, what he did was a continuation of what the sophists had begun. Socrates and then Plato developed methods of teaching, learning, and discovering new knowledge that tended to be independent of the processes of learning by imitation of models. This latter kind of learning is close to what Plato denounces in the *Republic* as *mimēsis*. The establishment of the Academy, a school with prerequisites ("Let no one enter here without geometry") and a curriculum, imparted an even greater degree of impersonality to the body of knowledge. While much oral teaching must have taken place, still there were now texts to be studied, lectures to be given, and new texts to be written.

In some ways, as teaching becomes institutionalized, the overt expression of sexual impulses (and of certain aggressive ones too) become inimical to learning. In particular, the learning of abstract material and of abstract thinking tends to go along with teaching that is abstracted from the intensely personalized and sexualized bond between teacher and student. In reality, of course, as Plato himself recognized, there can be no learning without passion, but the pedagogical problem is how to develop a passion for learning rather than a passion for the teacher.

Havelock has argued that the Athenians tried and executed Socrates because they saw him as a threat, both real and fantasied, to the traditional system of education.[32] As we shall see, even their fantasies had a kernel of truth. Even the Athenians who brought him to trial and convicted him, however, appear not to have fully articulated for themselves the nature of the system he was threatening and the nature of the threat. They accused him of "corrupting the youth," whereas in refraining from the use of sexuality as a dialectic tool he avoided the corruption of youth.

The *Symposium* illustrates the kind of puzzlement that Socrates must have induced in many Athenians. The topic is *eros,* for the Greeks certainly homosexual as well as heterosexual love. The setting is a drinking party, which traditionally would include conversation, drink, and sexuality. At this symposium, however, the proportions of the mix turn out to be quite different from those expected. Ultimately the discussion moves toward Socrates' definition of the various grades of *eros,* from heterosexual love to homosexual love to love of beautiful bodies to love of the beautiful, the highest form of *eros.* To underline Socrates' seriousness about the kind of *eros* that should be valued, Plato introduces the drunken and licentious figure of Alcibiades.[33] The dialogue concludes with Alcibiades' grudging affirmation that even he has not been able to seduce Socrates. Nothing in this or other dialogues implies that Socrates was uninterested in or ignorant of the pleasures of the flesh. Rather, the love of the abstract and philosophical involves a gradual movement away from the love of the carnal. It is as if Socrates had proclaimed, "I'm not averse to having sex with my students, in fact I'd really love it, but first things first. Philosphy comes first."

Aristophanes' *Clouds* reveals much about the fears and fantasies that Socrates and the Socratic method must have stirred up. It was performed (in two different versions) around 423–420 B.C., some twenty years before the trial and execution of Socrates and at least thirty to forty years before the founding of the Academy. A father, Strepsiades, is distraught over the debts his horse-loving son has run up. He decides to enroll his son in Socrates' school, the *phrontistērion,* a think tank. There he will learn "newthink,"[34] the Socratic-sophistic ways of arguing; armed with that kind of perverse logic, he will be able to argue his way out of all the debts he has incurred. The son refuses to go, so the father enrolls, hoping to learn some of these skills himself. After a grueling encounter with Socrates, in scenes that are caricatures of philosophical and sophistic teaching methods, Strepsiades is converted, even though he has proven too dense to master the method. At the suggestion of the Chorus, Strepsiades again tries to enroll his son, who is still most unwilling. He has the son witness a mighty debate between "just discourse," the traditional Athenian educational method, and "unjust discourse," the new educational method.[35] To Strepsiades' delight, the son learns the Socratic method and becomes a first-rate sophistic logic chopper. But the denouement is that the son turns on the father, starts to beat him, and justifies the beating with all the new Socratic tricks he has learned. The play ends as Strepsiades, outraged, burns down the Socratic school.

First we find the theme of a son disobeying and beating his father, which, as Dodds has pointed out, is prominent in fifth-century literature.[36] While the son was disrespectful and disobedient to the father before either of them had anything to do with Socrates, the experience in the school encouraged the son to feel free actually to beat the father and then justify the act as conforming to both good logic and the laws of nature. (Incidentally, the play makes plain at the outset that the schism between father and son had been fostered by the mother, an insight also seen in Plato's description of the origin of the "timocratic" man in the *Republic*, 549C.) This reversal of traditional values is one of the dire consequences of the new education (see *Clouds*, l. 911).

Related to the disturbance in the father-son relationship is the disturbance in the proper balance of homosexual love created by Socratic teaching. As in all things Greek, a certain modesty and moderation were expected in homosexual behavior. There were ground rules for courting and for being courted. Homosexual relationships that were too obvious or too promiscuous were ridiculed. Aristophanes emphasizes this sense of male *sōphrosunē*, modesty (ll. 979–80): "Toward their lovers their conduct was manly: you didn't see them mincing or strutting, or prostituting themselves with girlish voices or coy, provocative glances."[37] In fact, if you followed the old, modest way, your physique would be well proportioned (ll. 1012–19):

> BUILD, Stupendous
> COMPLEXION, Splendid
> SHOULDERS, Gigantic
> TONGUE, Petite
> BUTTOCKS, Brawny
> PECKER, Discreet

In contrast, the new Socratic teaching would ruin you:

> BUILD, Effeminate
> COMPLEXION, Ghastly
> SHOULDERS, Hunched
> TONGUE, Enormous
> BUTTOCKS, Flabby
> PECKER, Preposterous[38]

These lines say a good deal more than "Follow Socrates and you'll turn into a big prick." The new education, they say, threatens to turn homosexuals into floridly effeminate fops and queens, while the old education upholds a brand of homosexuality that makes a boy into a true man. The glorious youth of Athenian sculpture and vase painting has a most modest and well-proportioned penis; barbarians, slaves, and satyrs have big penises. The typical bisexual equilibrium maintained by Athenian aristocrats may have been somewhat precarious, and the new education was clearly perceived as a threat to that equilibrium. Both libido and aggression between father and son were contained by homosexuality, and that homosexuality was embedded in the old education. Other fantasies that find expression in this play are of madness, masturbation, and brother-sister incest.[39] It is as if Socrates had opened a Pandora's box of forbidden impulses.

Similarly Socrates' "Socratic dialogue" with Strepsiades is replete with imagery of unbridled buggery and feminization. The teacher humiliates and takes advantage of his student, induces distress, pain, castration anxiety (suggested at l. 734), and causes a marked infantile regression.[40] The education may be newfangled, but the game is old and familiar: who can screw whom and manage to get away with it. This, it seems, is Aristophanes' reading of Socrates' underlying intention.

Thus Plato's *Symposium* (in which Aristophanes is one of the participants) and Aristophanes' *Clouds* delineate, in very different ways, the central problem in education. The *Symposium* presents an educational and philosophical ideal, the progressive movement away from the concrete, from the pleasures of the body zones and the love of particular bodies. Teaching and learning must somehow have the spark of *eros* but not the overt acts of *eros*. For the comic poet, the old education, while not perfect, strikes a better balance and is more "temperate" than the new, which threatens to destroy manhood (and education) by its sexual and exploitive gratifications.

The new modes of education were reflections of changing conditions in Greek society and were also a means of coping with those changes. Dodds and others have discussed the changes in social, economic, and political organization that were associated with changes in the family. In brief, obligations to kinsmen were gradually weakened as obligations to the polis and to new political units increased.[41] The absolute authority of the father diminished, so that, for example, fathers no longer had rights of life and death over their children. By the end of the fifth century, sons could even bring their fathers to court on various charges.

The themes of the authority of fathers over sons and reversals of that authority are almost commonplace in Plato. One of the earliest dialogues, the *Euthyphro,* on the nature of holiness, opens with a father's being brought to court by his son for abusing a slave. In incidental, offhand comments one often finds mention of patricide (*Sophist,* 241D). The *Republic,* too, is replete with references to this crime, either incidentally or to illustrate a moral point. Democracy, as described by Plato in Book 8 of the *Republic,* is marked by a decline in paternal authority and the disgraceful kowtowing of fathers to their sons. In short, the traditional ways of regulating father-son rivalry seem to have been proving inadequate, or at least they were perceived as inadequate by Plato and others in fifth- and fourth-century Greece. To Aristophanes, Socrates and the Sophists appeared to be causing, or at least contributing to, this serious state of affairs. Socrates' accusers also seem to have perceived something of this sort.

Yet it is misleading to speak only of the "revolution" in which Plato was involved, for by his own lights he was a deeply conservative man. Dodds has written eloquently of Plato's attempt to stabilize and bring order to the "inherited conglomerate" of Greek tradition.[42] Plato's system of education, as outlined in the *Republic,* is at once radical and traditional. Thus we can consider Plato's ideas on education, both in the *Republic* and especially in the *Laws,* as attempts to strike a balance between a push for change based on certain intellectual principles and a need to prevent the anarchy that could follow the weakening of traditional morality. At another level, we can note reverberations of the Platonic problem of striking a balance between reason and emotion, between dialectic and appetite.

The program of training in mathematics and dialectic suggested in the *Republic* found concrete expression in the Academy. While we lack adequate information about the early years of the Academy, we can say it was the first institution of higher learning and research in the Western world, the first university. Training in dialectic, and with it instruction in the content of Plato's philosophy, may well have been the central feature of the Academy. While we find allusions to lectures, private reading must have been important. Tradition has it that a number of young men trained there went out to help in the governing of one or another Greek city.

The educational approach that found expression in the Academy served both to innovate and to stabilize. When literacy and book learning are introduced, they may divide the generations for a time; the existence of books that are authorities independent of parental authority doubtless emboldens young people to disagree with their parents. Books become not only an independent source of information but a new kind of superego, as it were. Further, literacy and the availability of texts allow one to see quickly a great diversity of opinions in the world on virtually any subject, and thus deal a further blow to parental authority. But once a generational tradition of learning and reading becomes established, fathers begin to share some of their sons' values. Now the awareness of the relativity of thought and opinion becomes a major value, and the child must grow up to realize the childishness of a black-and-white absolute morality.

I believe that Plato hoped to establish a new tradition, in which philosophy and academic learning would become accepted. I do not know whether or not Plato suspected that generational conflict is inevitable, and that if the differences between fathers and sons cannot be expressed in terms of educational values, they will be expressed in some other way. He certainly must have been aware that his own institution could not long remain immune to destructive rivalries. Indeed, soon after his death Aristotle and others split off from the Academy, and eventually Aristotle founded his own school, the Lyceum.

We can also say that the philosophic model of mind describes a person going to school, passing through the stages from elementary to secondary to university and professional education. It is a model of a person who must gradually learn to use reason and abstract discourse and to deal with the impulses that interfere with that kind of learning. The child must learn in school to sit still, to concentrate. He must gradually leave the world of his mother and be inducted into the world of men. As a young child he will be allowed to play in school, but as time goes on, he must gradually restrict his play to play in the service of learning. He must move from learning for love to loving to learn.[43] He must learn to master his material, and in the process sublimate and displace his rivalrous feelings toward peers and toward his masters. He must strive to win a victory that is fairer than the Olympic victory and to gather prizes more precious than those awarded to the Olympic victors.[44]

We should not be surprised, then, if this model of mind seems to give short shrift to appetites and passions. In important respects it gives short shrift to children, slighting their natural curiosity and emphasizing instinctual renunciation. We should now be prepared to understand how Plato could equate anything less than the full use of reason with madness and sickness of the soul. Plato articulated and ratified the split between reason and impulse, between thought and action, between thought and feeling. It is to his credit, though, that he struggled with the problem of piecing back together what he himself had done so much to tear asunder.

10

Plato and Freud

And as for the "stretching" of the concept of sexuality which has
been necessitated by the analysis of children and what are called
perverts, anyone who looks down with contempt upon psychoanalysis from a superior vantage-point should remember how
closely the enlarged sexuality of psycho-analysis coincides with the
Eros of the divine Plato.

—Sigmund Freud, *Three Essays on
the Theory of Sexuality*[1]

The purpose of this chapter is to make explicit an assumption that
has shaped the discussion of Plato in this book: that it is both useful
and possible to view Plato in relation to Freud. In the second half of
the twentieth century it is difficult to read Plato without some
awareness of Freud. From the other side, as Dodds has suggested,
Plato would undoubtedly have been very much interested in modern
depth psychology, the psychology of inner conflict.[2]

I believe that the Platonic model of mind and mental disturbance
holds an important place in Freud's thought. Outlining this one
component of Freud's thought can allow us to see more clearly its
other components. Even more important, this type of examination
highlights certain problems entailed in the notion that the mind is
divided. These problems were not satisfactorily solved in Plato's
thinking, and similarly, an examination of Freud's changing thought
over the years suggests that he too struggled with a variety of possible solutions. To anticipate the later discussion, a few of the issues
are: the place of affect, the problems subsumed under the term "sublimation," the question of whether or not a conflict psychology can
speak in process terms that are not ultimately anthropomorphic, and
the issue of the kind of verbal process, be it psychotherapy or dialogue, that is needed to change an individual.

Consider Freud's point of departure in his discussion of the ego
and the id, the so-called structural model of the mind: "The ego
represents what may be called reason and common sense, in contrast
to the id, which contains the passions. All this falls into line with
popular distinctions which we are all familiar with."[3] The "popular

distinctions" to which Freud refers are, I believe, those that first entered and became articulated in Western thought with Plato's philosophy. This fundamental distinction in Plato's thought is a most important one in Freud's.

Freud himself compared his thought to Plato's in a few scattered remarks in his early writings, particularly in *The Interpretation of Dreams* (see above, p. 169, for Plato's comments on forbidden wishes in dreams, alluded to approvingly by Freud). A more explicit comparison was made in an essay from which Freud quoted in 1920:

And as for the "stretching" of the concept of sexuality which has been necessitated by the analysis of children and what are called perverts, anyone who looks down with contempt upon psycho-analysis from a superior vantage-point should remember how closely the enlarged sexuality of psycho-analysis coincides with the Eros of the divine Plato (cf. Nachmansohn, 1915).[4]

Indeed, the majority of the references to Plato in Freud pertain to some aspect of the similarity between Eros and libido.[5] The history of studies comparing Freud and Plato has been reviewed elsewhere.[6] Suffice it to say that all of those studies suffer from some degree of failure to ascertain whether the overall configurations of the theories of these two men are sufficiently congruent to warrant a "compare and contrast" approach. If we consider that the two thinkers share a central underlying notion or structure, then the comparison is justified. That underlying notion is that man is a creature of inner conflict, split into a higher, rational part and a lower, desiring part.

How much of Plato Freud knew and the way he used that knowledge in his own thinking are of no great importance to this argument. In fact, Freud was not particularly steeped in Plato.[7] Our task is to outline certain similar structures or forms in the theories of the two men, bracketing the historical issues. It must be kept in mind that Freud did not begin by studying man in conflict or the motives of behavior. He started by treating people with "sicknesses," hysteria, neurasthenia, and the like, and came to believe (building upon the work of Jean-Martin Charcot, Hippolyte Bernheim, and others) that these sicknesses were to be understood as expressions of inner conflict. Dreams and other products of mental life similarly could be understood as products of an inner battle between wishes and prohibitions. Freud, then, placed at the center of his theories of psychiatric illness the "popular distinctions" referred to above, the split between reason and impulse, though he believed that impulse often acted outside conscious awareness. In brief, both Plato and Freud, by different routes, eventually became concerned with the issues entailed in the assumption that man could act against himself and against his own best interests.

Let us, then, consider some ramifications of the model of mind as split between a higher and a lower part. These parts are typically in conflict, and each part has its own interests, wishes, and characteristic mode of functioning. The line of cleavage is between a rational, organizing, and organized structure and a wild, undifferentiated, and unbridled part. In Plato we see the rational (*logistikon*) versus the appetitive (*epithumetikon*), psyche versus soma, and other variants of the same theme.[8] This theme persists throughout all the variations and vicissitudes in Freud's conceptions of the mental apparatus. The split can be seen in the successive formulations of the mental apparatus: conscious versus unconscious (in the topographic model), ego instincts versus sexual instincts, and ego versus id (in the structural model, where the distinction conscious–unconscious now has a different connotation).[9] Both Plato and Freud consider the impulsive, irrational part to be the more bodily, the primitive, the earlier in development, the childish, and the animal. And both Plato and Freud (until the structural theory) group moral functions with the rational, structured part, and equate rational truth with moral goodness and self-control. In Freud's topographical model, for example, consciousness and the censor represent the claims of reality, rationality, morality, and society. Even in his ego-id-superego model, Freud takes pains to point out that the division of functions between ego and superego cannot be precisely delineated.

Integral to the model is the notion of two different ways of thinking, each characteristic of one of the split parts of the psyche. In Plato, the lower parts of the psyche "think" as if asleep or in a dream. They function with shadow and illusion, shifting meanings, contradictions, and oscillations in identification and identity (see, for example, *Republic*, 380D). For Freud, the operations of the mind in dreaming show the way to the difference between conscious and unconscious and lead to the construction of the framework of primary process thinking (and discharge) versus secondary process. Such terms as "condensation" and "displacement" more formally label and specify the processes described by Plato as belonging to the modus operandi of the baser parts of the psyche. Striking, too, is the presence in Plato of the metaphor of "binding" thoughts so that they do not run amuck (*Meno*, 97D–98B), a metaphor that Freud uses to distinguish the operation of energies in the two systems (that is, primary process operates with unbound energies).

Both thinkers are concerned about the use of anthropomorphic language in descriptions of mental life. Plato freely uses the language of persons within a person, as does Freud. Both, however, seek some sort of *process* language: Plato, something leaning upon geometry and arithmetic; Freud, models seemingly physical and quantitative. Both, though warning against taking the anthropomorphic language of conflict too literally, cannot dispense with it. This observation suggests another reason for some of the congruence between the views of Plato and Freud: the model of the mind in conflict is a model in large part derived from the introspectively available experience of conflict within the person (for example, *Republic,* 439D–441C). The inner voices experienced by the person in conflict find representation in the anthropomorphic language of the theory.[10]

These considerations point to another crucial feature of the model shared by Plato and Freud: it is a model of conflict and also of *control.* Who shall rule, the higher or the lower, reason or instincts? The metaphor is political, in both Plato and Freud, but also, for both, more than metaphor.[11] The issues of inner control are in complex ways embedded in issues of control of one part of society by another, or of the individual by society. When Freud invokes Plato's Eros as a parallel to his own view of sexuality, he concludes:

> Human civilization rests upon two pillars, of which one is the control of natural forces and the other the restriction of our instincts. The ruler's throne rests upon fettered slaves. Among the instinctual components which are thus brought into service, the sexual instincts, in the narrower sense of the word, are conspicuous for their strength and savagery. Woe, if they should be set loose! The throne would be overturned and the ruler trampled under foot.[12]

Another metaphor of control common to Plato and Freud (noted by many, though not by Freud) is a man in control of a horse: a horse and rider (*The Ego and the Id*) and a charioteer and two horses (*Phaedrus*).

The other side of the problem of control is the way in which the two parts of the psyche cooperate. Freud posits a process of *sublimation* of libido (or of aggression) in the course of development, and points to infantile sexual curiosity as a major source of later curiosity and desire to learn. In the common clinical situation of inhibition of a previously well-functioning activity, a *breakdown* of sublimation is posited. A middle-aged photographer, previously successful in his work, finds himself losing interest in that work. Dreams and daydreams reveal that he is preoccupied with voyeuristic and exhibitionistic sexual wishes. We learn that his daughter's budding adolescent sexuality and his menopausal wife's fading charms have proved most unsettling. He withdraws from activities that involve looking and being looked at, including photography. Looking has become excessively sexualized and conflicted; inhibition is the defense. In fact, it is just this kind of clinical situation that calls our attention to the likelihood that in development, libidinal and aggressive drives become interwoven with skills, talents, and interests.[13] The term "sublimation," and the related terms "neutralization," "primary autonomy," and "secondary autonomy," derived from psychoanalytic ego psychology, are attempts to address the issue of how the divisions of the psyche cooperate at times, and at other times seem to have a kind of falling out. Plato's formulations on *eros* in the *Symposium* (see above, p. 195) are attempts to deal with the same problem. Theories that split the mind into higher and lower parts must posit either one source of psychic energy that can be used by either or both parts or two different kinds of energy, one characteristic of higher mental functioning and one characteristic of the lower. Even then, these two energies must bear some relation to each other.[14]

Theories that split the psyche essentially categorize the different motivations that seem to drive human behavior. The higher part has loftier motives, thinks more clearly, and has a greater capacity for delay. The lower part has baser motives, thinks in more muddled, emotional ways, and acts impulsively. As a result, the theorist who posits a division of the mind ultimately uses an anthropomorphic language that speaks of better and worse sorts of persons within the person. Needless to say, such schemas tend to be developed by people who value the intellect, and one should not be surprised to find that while their theories posit the superiority of the rational part, they are marked by a note of envy for those whose lives are governed by the lower portions of the psyche.

For both Plato and Freud this split is a basic configuration that shapes and places constraints on the particulars of the theories that emerge from it. In both Freud and Plato we find variations over time in the nuances of the split, variations in the boundaries drawn. In Freud's earliest writings (especially the *Project for a Scientific Psychology,* 1895), the ego is characterized as an organization that binds, delays, filters, and transmutes the impulses that are associated with relatively unstable neuronal systems.[15] This ego makes memory possible, among other tasks, by converting perceptions into fixed memories. This view of ego in the *Project,* and the discussion of the development of thought by way of the hallucinated absent object in *The Interpretation of Dreams,* addresses the issue of how bodily impulse and desire become transmuted into thought, judgment, and other higher mental activities. One can show that Freud's distinction between ego instincts and sexual instincts, as well as the later distinction between ego and id, conforms to the same pattern. In effect, then, we find numerous variations on the theme of the mind-body problem, for all of these schemas in the works of Freud (and of Plato) attempt to allocate some of the functions of the person to a more mindlike agency and some to a more body-like agency. Subsequent psychoanalytic theories have ascribed some degree of organized thinking to the id and/or posited more idlike characteristics of the ego. I believe these theories have merely multiplied entities within the mind, with each entity still characteristically split into rational and appetitive.

A word about the term "instincts" is in order. I have spoken as if we could equate Plato's use of such a term as "appetites" (*epithumiai*) with Freud's term "instincts" or "instinctual drives" (*Triebe*). On the whole, despite variations in usage and definition of these terms in the writings of both Plato and Freud, this equation is justified. "Instinct" as used by Freud bridges mind and body; the instinct is the *mental representative* of the bodily demand.[16] Another way of describing this relationship is to say that the instinct is the desire, the wish (that is, a mental construct), that is built upon a biological need. More peremptory and urgent desires are instinctual drives.

For Plato, on the whole, appetites are strong desires that are not easily ignored. It is true that he speaks of two different classes of appetites (*epithumiai*), necessary and nonnecessary ones (*Republic,* 558D–59D). There are those "from which we cannot turn away . . . and . . . whose satisfaction is beneficial to us" (the necessary ones) and those that we could train ourselves to be free of and whose satisfaction is harmful to us (the unnecessary ones).[17] Plato would thus divide the sexual appetites (*aphrodisiai*) into necessary and unnecessary ones. The relevant issue, however, is that all these desires are a compound, as it were, of the somatic and the psychic, though some are distinctly more psychic than others. Thus, in both Plato and Freud, peremptory desires can be arranged along a spectrum. At one end are the desires that arise from basic bodily needs and urges, while at the other are those that we might term cultivated desires. Freud would probably locate the drive to amass money somewhere in the middle of the spectrum, labeling that desire as a derivative of anal instinctual wishes but having a rational, adaptive component. Thus Freud's "instinctual drives" differ from Plato's "appetites" more in emphasis than in essential qualities.

When we turn to the notions of sickness and madness, we find another striking parallel, which is already entailed in the notion of a split of the psyche into rational and irrational parts. For Plato, sickness of the psyche is the manifestation of the wild, primitive part of the mind expressing its claims, and expressing them loudly. In Freud we find more complex formulations about sickness, formulations generally not so antagonistic to the instinctual side. The notion is clearly present that sickness is the result and an indication of a struggle between rational (and/or moral) aims and instinctual, appetitive aims. Related is the notion that the sickness of the psyche represents a form of ignorance. Removal of the ignorance requires the freeing of the parts of the mind that ordinarily should be able to know and seek out the truth. Thus Plato and Freud came upon the importance of ignorance in their working setting: Freud in the analytic dialogue, Plato in the philosophical dialogue. But this notion seems to follow inevitably when the psyche or the person is seen as split. One party within the person will deal with the other by using any device to keep the upper hand—threats, persuasion, bribery, and, finally, out-and-out deception appearing in the guise of ignorance.

"Sickness of the psyche," "therapy," "mental illness"—these are medical metaphors. "Treatment" was Socrates' metaphor for his philosophical activity. Freud, who started out as a physician, was of course explicitly treating disease. Though he never completely dispensed with the physician–patient–illness model, he clearly moved further and further away from the model into a realm of discourse that spoke of universal wishes, impulses, defenses, and prohibitions. In 1921, for example, he wrote of physicians and patients; in 1937, of analysts and analysands.[18]

Both Plato and Freud appreciate the need for a proper balance among the parts of the psyche. Freud, of course, places much greater emphasis on the dangers of instinctual suppression than does Plato, though Plato is always careful to give the appetites their due. Plato's model is a hierarchy of command and control, or a master–slave relationship. Freud's model is something like an uneasy alliance among the parts of the psyche, a shaky parliamentary democracy. Nonetheless, the struggle between instinct and reason, and this struggle in association with the notion of sickness and malaise, reverberates throughout Freud's writings. "Where id was, there shall ego be" is one version of the goals of therapy.[19] Analogously, in discussing the malaise of civilization and its discontents (in *The Future of an Illusion* and in the first chapters of *Civilization and Its Discontents*), Freud uses the same model: culture demands that people renounce instinctual gratifications, and people are resentful and ever ready to throw off the yoke of civilization. Culture must offer something to coat the bitter pill. (The second part of *Civilization and Its Discontents*, however, introduces a radically new version of the problem involving the disguised operations of guilt.)[20] Again, we must note that neither Plato nor Freud is entirely consistent in his choice of political model for the relationships between parts of the divided psyche. Freud, for instance, can view the instincts as "fettered slaves," while in some instances Plato speaks as though the parts were on friendly terms.

The problem of the nature of treatment is inextricably involved with the issue of control of the lower parts by the higher. How is this control to be achieved and maintained? Plato entertained several solutions, certainly not original in either his day or ours, entailing society's control over the individual, or that part of the individual which is wild and irrational, "sick." In the *Republic* and the *Laws* he proposed coercion, promises of reward, suggestion, benign fictions, exhortations to instinctual renunciation, and hints of rewards in the next world. He also knew how to seduce and overwhelm the other person in a dialogue. Freud too recognized a gamut of means of control, and saw the history of civilization as a succession of experiments in methods of controlling instinctual forces. From the perspective of the physician treating the patient, he recognized an array of "cures" or ways to make the patient act more rationally. Suggestion, hypnosis, reassurance, and prohibition clearly have their curative effects.[21] Both Plato and Freud, however, argued that another way is possible, a way that allows for a more complete integration of the rational with the irrational. Both knew well how much effort is needed to develop such a method and for any man to apply it.

Plato's unique contribution is the *ideal* that man can achieve control over the irrational by a special kind of training and education, emphasizing the student's abstractive, intellectual powers. This training would be aimed at cultivating the power of dialectic as an instrument for reaching truth. Analogously, Freud's unique contribution was the development of a way leading to permanent, internal reorganization. The ideal for Freud is a method of understanding, leading to self-understanding, which permits a more benign form of self-control than the patient has previously experienced.

"What do they do? They dialogue" is Freud's epitome of treatment.[22] Yet dialogue is only the surface appearance, capturing only one aspect of the analytic situation. The analyst and analysand "dialogue" in order to analyze. For Plato the dialogue leads to dialectic, a more "objective" form of discourse. Both Platonic and analytic dialogues seek to bring the conflicting parts into harmony. For Plato this means taming the wild part and strengthening reason, and in *some* of Freud's thinking the "cure" similarly results in a strengthening of the rational part. For both Plato and Freud the dialogue involves a struggle between reason and emotion. Clearly Plato's interest in suppressing and abolishing affect flows from his desire to eliminate anything that interferes with philosophy, but he realizes emotions cannot be eliminated altogether because they are needed to give motive steam to the inquiry, to join in establishing a sense of *conviction* about the truth.

A split between the two members of the dyad also appears to be a part of the conception of both the dialectical and the analytic situation. This split between patient and doctor or between student and philosopher is conceptualized along the lines of the splits within the psyche. For Plato the philosopher is to the rest of humanity as the rational part of the psyche is to the irrational. Freud also tends to equate the doctor with the rational (the ego) and the patient with the irrational (the id). For example, in discussing the transference Freud writes of a "struggle between the doctor and the patient, between intellect and instinctual life, between understanding and seeking to act. . . ."[23] Both analysis and dialectic appear to aim at reducing the split and bridging the gulf. The student or the patient should be able to do for himself and with himself what at first he is able to do only with the aid of the philosopher or the doctor.

Thus the experience of the participants in the dialogue, whether the philosophical or the analytic, is intimately related to the theoretical framework of the splits within the mind. The working setting provides the most vivid and immediate instances of the problem of reason versus emotion, rational versus irrational, and thought versus action. In the very process of dialogue, both dialectic and analytic, impediments and resistance arise to the seeking of truth. Plato speaks of *aporia,* an impasse. Participants in the dialogue become dismayed, confused; they are embarrassed and they blush. Though Freud's conceptualization of the origin and meaning of these blocks is quite different from Plato's, the observation that they exist and must be dealt with is common to both.

To sum up, my thesis is that the similarity in the models of Plato and Freud involves the following interrelated factors:

1. Each comes to see the study of man in conflict, and especially in self-destructive conflict, as central to his working task.

2. The nature of the working situation, a form of dialogue seeking to establish truth, confronts the participants with the facts of man in conflict with himself and with another.

3. Both draw upon introspective data, the data of internal dialogue, which seem to confirm the existence of conflicting parts within the mind.

4. Each develops his theory from the perspective of the leader in the dialogue, and tends to conceive of the split within the dialogue along the lines of the split within the mind.

5. Plato's theories of mind are accounts of the mind as an instrument that can engage in dialectic; Freud's are accounts of the mind that can engage in psychoanalysis, either as patient or as doctor.

Everywhere these two thinkers see conflict and a struggle for dominance: within the mind, among people, in the political world. Where should we begin to look for the source of this outlook? What is the model for the model? One interesting answer, more obvious for Plato than for Freud, is that the prevailing forms of political organization provide the basis of the divisions of the mind. This view would lead us to suspect that the divisions in Greek society, especially those between master and slave (or among the social classes), provide the model. One could argue that the *Republic* presents an idealized picture of the social structure of a Greek state, especially Sparta.[24]

Where is the political or social framework for Freud? In fact, it is ubiquitous in Freud's works and appears in a variety of forms. *The Interpretation of Dreams,* most famous for its mechanical and physical models of the dreaming process, is replete with political, social, and economic analogies.[25] For instance, the dream censor operates like the postal censor. Psychic agency (*Instanz*) is an agency in the same sense as a government bureau. Throughout his career Freud devoted much attention to the question of the relationships between mind and human society, mind and human history.

This line of argument is interesting and might deserve further investigation, particularly in the case of Freud; but it is misleading to think of the political structure as the basic model for the structure of the mind primarily because the political structure is itself a product of the mind—of minds that structure and construe the facts of social life in terms of a particular schema.

Another possible source of this model of mind is the relation between parent and child; the parent is the rational and the child the appetitive. At times they are in conflict and at times they cooperate. But obviously this is only one version of parent–child relationships and undoubtedly it is a reflection of, or a product of, a particular cultural attitude toward children, albeit a widespread attitude.

We are forced into a Scottish verdict: not proven. All we can say is that a dialectic takes place among three kinds of structures: (*a*) the structure or model that exists in the mind of the theory maker and which he imposes upon the phenomena he studies; (*b*) structures or models that are widely held within a culture, and by means of which that culture construes and constructs the world around it; (*c*) structures that in some way may actually exist (that is, it is possible that some models of the phenomenal world do correspond to structures inherent in the phenomena).[26]

At this point one can consider what may be common to the personal psychology of men who are sensitive to the existence of conflict and are prone to see it everywhere in their world. I shall venture a speculative hypothesis, based in part on Freud's own account of how, in his self-analysis, he came to discover the importance of the oedipal conflicts.

There was an unusual configuration in Freud's own family: a father who was old enough to be his grandfather, two much older half brothers (the children of his father's previous marriage), and a nephew his own age. We also now know from the extensive researches of Max Schur that in fact Freud's father had had another wife, between his first wife and Freud's mother.[27] This fact had apparently been kept from Freud, or he may have known and repressed it. We also know that Freud, the man who discovered the importance of primal scene trauma, before age four lived in one crowded room with his whole family. Undoubtedly he was repeatedly exposed to parental nudity and parental intercourse. In Freud's account of his self-analysis of his own Oedipus complex, his family configuration had presented him with a certain kind of puzzle about family life, analogous to the puzzle confronting Oedipus in Sophocles' play. We can surmise from Schur's information about Freud's early life and his father's life that Freud knew both too much and too little about the facts of birth, copulation, and the question who is the parent of whom.

For Plato we have precious little reliable biographical and autobiographical material, but it is generally accepted that his father died sometime in his youth, that his mother then married her mother's brother, and that from that union came a younger half brother, Antiphon. Plato's stepfather, Pyrilampus, had an older son by a previous marriage. Plato's own parents had three other children: two sons, Glaucon and Adeimantus, and a daughter; the birth order of the children is not known. Plato, of course, did not explicitly know of and label the oedipal conflicts, but his dialogues contain repeated references to parricidal and incestuous wishes.

We may speculate further that Plato struggled with oedipal impulses and may have felt a certain Hamlet-like outrage at his mother's remarriage and subsequent childbearing. My hypothesis about the prominence of primal scene imagery in the dialogues suggests that Plato himself struggled to master some primal scene trauma, or at the least was very much caught up with a primal scene fantasy. I would surmise that he was unusually sensitive to whatever limited exposure to adult sexuality he may have had.[28]

I suggest, then, that the atypical features of the family constellations of both Plato and Freud somehow made the mastery of (interrelated) oedipal and primal scene conflicts more problematic than it otherwise might have been. These conflicts served to make them unusually aware of conflicts of wishes and desires as a ubiquitous feature of human life. The need to master their own inner conflicts impelled them to develop theories emphasizing the ubiquity of conflict. Freud wrote *The Interpretation of Dreams* as part of his struggle to resolve conflicts about his father's death. Plato, I believe, began writing the dialogues as part of an attempt to master conflicts stirred by the death of Socrates.

Another feature of both men's style of thinking and viewing the world is the thinking in schemata, or rather searching for similar schemata in diverse phenomena. One manifestation of the style is argument by analogy, or search or discovery by analogy. Plato compares the soul to the state; Freud compares the history of the Jewish people to the developmental sequence of the human child.[29] In Freud we see the notion that contemporary patterns in the life of the adult have a history, and that history consists of childhood versions of the adult pattern. If behavior in the adult seems inexplicable, seek out an infantile configuration that will illuminate it: seek out the oedipal triangle that explicates the current adult triangle. For both Freud and Plato, the method of deducing the structure of the unknown from a structure of the known, and then moving back and forth between the two, is fundamental and far-reaching. Is there some intrinsic connection between their readiness to see a schema of conflict and their readiness to seek out schemata? Did the experience of a somewhat atypical family constellation catalyze for each not only an awareness of conflict but also an awareness of configuration? I can only offer these points as interesting speculations that might turn into suggestive leads to an understanding of the creative process in such men as Plato and Freud.

To this point I have emphasized the core of commonality between Plato and Freud: their use of a certain model of mind with its attendant definition of conflict. Further, each of these men came upon a core of similar problems, namely, those issues arising from the split between instinct and reason. Though similar problems have to be dealt with, however, the proposed solutions and resolutions may be quite disparate.

To reiterate the obvious: Freud is first and foremost a clinician, and his most original and enduring contributions are not to be found in his philosophical statements. The methods of free association and interpretation stand at the heart of Freud's work. The concepts of the unconscious and the vicissitudes of instincts, as well as the central role of interpretation of transference, go far beyond what any of his clinical, philosophical, or poetic forebears had devised.

The most profound difference between the two is in their attitudes toward conflict. As mentioned before, both thinkers are unusually sensitive to the existence of conflict, contradiction, paradox, and irony. For Freud, this is the basic given of our existence. One can do better or worse in the handling of one's conflicts, but conflict and unhappiness are probably inevitable. One of his early statements about the "cure" of hysteria is that psychiatrists must assist their neurotic patients to surrender their exotic sufferings and prepare themselves for the commonplace unhappinesses of life.[30]

Plato recognizes the ubiquity of conflict but he is not prepared to accept it. He not only yearns to eliminate conflict, he has a plan for doing so. For Plato, the solutions of many kinds of difficulties lie in the elimination of contradiction, ambiguity, and conflict. For justice to be achieved, each person must do one thing, not several; each class of the city must perform only one function. Harmony in Plato sometimes suggests a harmonious arrangement of conflicting forces, but more typically it conveys a sense of separation of elements, each kept distinct from the others, with one element dominating (for example, *Symposium,* 187A–E). In the ideal city-state of the *Republic,* rivalry, contest, and all the emotions that attend them must be minimized or eliminated. Men and women should be equalized; biological differences must be played down. Though the notion is not spelled out explicitly in Plato, implicitly the family is the seat of trouble.

From these considerations about two antithetical attitudes toward conflict we may take a look at what I consider a conspicuous absence in Plato. I refer to some notion of a superego, a moral agency that can be in conflict with the ego as well as with the id. A person can suffer from irrational guilt, and a moral agency within him can act as a fifth column. Plato, I believe, probably would not have accepted this idea very easily even if he could have read Freud. Freud's idea of the inevitability of conflict derives from the conception of the indestructibility of the infantile wishes and the objects of those wishes. This idea already carries with it the sense of internalization of the objects as experienced by the child in the course of development. As the moral, controlling, frustrating, and approving aspects of these objects are represented internally, the representations are attended by the mixture of love and hate, aggression and libido, and fear and longing that the child experiences in relation to the parents.

Plato seems to recognize that early moral upbringing can be riddled with every kind of ambivalence, but he is horrified by this fact and has a tremendous need to circumvent it, or to do away with its consequences. Freud's ideas about the superego require an agency within the mind that can harbor both love and hate toward the person himself. Plato sees the ultimate sources of moral values as exterior to man, as the forms of the true and the good. The good cannot be too good. The forms are untainted by hatred and aggression. Such negative affects are relegated to the body and its demands; the ambivalence is split.

This discussion is only a step toward a thorough comparative study of these two thinkers. Much in the complexity of Plato has been ignored, and much in Freud has to be understood within a framework of philosophies that go far beyond the Platonic.[31] But perhaps this search for similar forms can stimulate others to a more extended and richer understanding of Plato and Freud.

IV

THE MEDICAL
MODEL

11

The Hippocratic Corpus

You may be an undigested bit of beef, a blot of mustard, a crumb
of cheese, a fragment of an underdone potato.
        —Charles Dickens, *A Christmas Carol*

Of the various models we are considering, the medical is remarkable
for two perhaps related features, its simplicity and its durability. Its
simplicity lies in the assumption that all diseases of the mind are
diseases of the body, and in its corollary, that a healthy mental state
accompanies a healthy body. The organs or systems whose defects
are implicated in mental illness vary widely in the theories of ancient
Greek physicians and in those of the many physicians who have
addressed the problem since their day. But from the Hippocratic
statement that the brain is the source of all mental distress to such
modern slogans as "Behind every twisted thought lies a twisted
molecule," there is an impressive continuity in this article of faith.[1]
We noted in Chapter 3 that a body of thought, theory, and details of
practice crystallized in the Greco-Roman medicine of late antiquity
and was transmitted with astounding literalness well into the nineteenth century.

The simple model of "body acting on mind" is accompanied by
the assumption that the professional best fitted to treat mental disorders is the doctor, the man trained to understand bodies. And with
a compelling simplicity and economy of thought, it follows that the
appropriate treatments are the tools of the doctor—drugs, regimen,
and the knife. The person of the doctor, his words, exhortations,
philosophy of life, resolution of his personal conflicts, are relevant
only insofar as they are directed toward helping the patient take his
medicine, so to speak. The doctor has professional responsibilities
and a code of ethics, more or less well defined, though varying in
specifics from one historical period to another. The patient's obligations are simple enough: he must be obedient and cooperative. If
possible, he should also be intelligent and educable, the physician's
ally in the cause of fighting his illness.[2]

Further, no guilt or shame attaches to having a disease, or even to
succumbing to it—only to failure of patient or doctor in their respec-

tive obligations. Medical practice and the medical model of illness, even mental illness, offer a framework of social support for detached, nonpunitive study and treatment: illnesses of the body or mind are to be analyzed and understood with the attitudes appropriate to any natural phenomena. No spirits or bogeymen are involved, only recognizable physical agents, such as air and water, bacteria and toxins, viruses and hormones. The gods, or God, stand respectfully aside, not necessarily denied an existence by the doctor, but tending to be invoked either as a ubiquitous, nonspecific factor in all human affairs or, in some oblique way, as the final consultant to be called in on the case.

This congeries of ideas and attitudes which we call the medical model first became more or less explicit, as far as we can tell, with the rise of Hippocratic medicine in the fifth and fourth centuries B.C.

My discussion of the medical model will be based primarily on that diffuse and confusing group of writings known as the Hippocratic corpus. A host of methodological difficulties must be noted. Ludwig Edelstein's brief article on Hippocrates in the *Oxford Classical Dictionary* contains a laconic summary of all we know of Hippocrates' life:

The Asclepiad of Cos, a contemporary of Socrates (469–399), though the most famous Greek physician, is yet the one least of all known to posterity. That he was of small stature, that he travelled much, that he died at Larissa is probable; more about his life and his personality cannot be ascertained. And as for the body of works under his name: . . . the so-called Hippocratic books . . . show the most widely different attitudes toward medicine. . . . There is not a single book the authenticity of which was not disputed already in antiquity. . . . It seems likely that none of the books preserved under the name of Hippocrates is genuine.

All, however, is not lost. As distinguished a student of Greek medicine as Edelstein was, his views on the dubious authenticity of all the works in the corpus are not accepted unanimously. My own approach to the Hippocratic question focuses on the similarities of spirit that shine through the diversity of content and theory in those books, and I believe we must put some trust in the intuition of the ancient doctors and editors who saw a unity in these works.[3]

The sources of Greek medicine go back many centuries before classical times. It is difficult to ascertain what contributions came from Egyptian and Babylonian medicine.[4] The healers mentioned by Homer also functioned as warriors.[5] The doctor, as he emerges in the fifth and fourth centuries, is a craftsman rather than a professional in our sense. Undoubtedly a few physicians achieved fame in their own day and in the next few centuries—a fame that might convey the false impression that most doctors were accorded great respect. The picture reconstructed by scholars (especially Edelstein) from the tone and tenor of surviving medical works is rather of a group of craftsmen and practitioners struggling to establish their worth and reputations.[6] Many doctors were probably itinerant, and institutional medicine did not exist in the fifth and fourth centuries; that is, there were no medical schools (*pace* the modern terms "school of Kos" and "school of Knidos"). Training was by apprenticeship, and even the existence of something like guilds is doubtful. There were no hospitals, and it is unlikely that any systematic, long-term case records were kept. The Hippocratic corpus reflects the great extent to which teaching must have been oral; the corpus contains no systematic treatise or even a textbook. It does include a number of collations of clinical experience, often with vivid case descriptions, and polemical works directed to a lay audience and intended to enhance the credibility of the doctor as well as to disseminate information about diet, exercise, and drugs.

The modern reader coming to these works has an Alice-in-Wonderland experience. We encounter brilliant clinical portraits mixed with fantastic misobservations. We find theories that seem a cross between inspired guesses about physiological processes and theories that seem scarcely removed from archaic and primitive fantasies. We encounter extraordinary arrogance (or naiveté) as the author of one treatise denounces all the mistakes of his competitors and then outlines his view of things, making almost all the same sorts of errors. And we find some classical Hippocratic aphorisms and ideals that have legitimately guided and inspired clinicians over the centuries. We find fledgling attempts to create a science, or at least a scientific ambience. There are obvious similarities to modern medicine, obvious discrepancies, and a confusing borderland of information and theory with which historians of medicine have struggled for the past two millennia.[7]

What can one say, then, about the notions of madness, of normal and abnormal mental activity in this heterogeneous group of writings? First, they are scattered, and in only a few of the books can one find sustained discussion or description of mental life. Certainly they include no textbook of psychiatry from which one could extract a "system." Yet they have certain unity, and with little difficulty one can outline the few basic premises about mental functioning. The unity is all the more striking because these premises underlie several theories about which organs or humors are involved in mental activity and its disturbances.[8] In one view represented in the corpus, the brain is the seat of mental activity, especially in *On the Sacred Disease*. Elsewhere, the heart and the blood are variously the seat of intelligence.[9]

As the first step in constructing our medical model, let us consider

218   *The Medical Model*

an example of the doctor at work, describing and prescribing for a disturbance involving serious mental derangement:

Another disease due to thickening. It arises from bile, whenever the bile flows to the liver, and settles in the head. These are, then, what the patient suffers. The liver swells, and because of the swelling it enlarges toward the diaphragm, and at once pain besets the head, especially at the temples. And he does not hear acutely with his ears and often does not see with his eyes. And shivering and fever seize him. These things happen to him at the onset of the illness, but they also occur intermittently, sometimes very severely and sometimes less so. As the illness extends, in time the suffering of the body becomes greater, and the pupils of the eyes dilate [? literally "scatter"], and he sees dimly, and if you bring your finger to his eyes, he does not perceive it because he cannot see. This is the sign by which you may know he cannot see, that he does not blink as the finger approaches. He plucks at the threads of his garment (if he does see) imagining that they are lice. And whenever the liver expands toward the diaphragm, he is delirious. He thinks he sees before his eyes creeping things and other animals of various sorts, and armed men fighting, and he himself thinks he is fighting in their midst. And he speaks of such things as seeing battles and wars, and he gets up and threatens anyone who does not allow him to do so. And if he stands up, he cannot raise his legs, and falls down. And his feet are always cold. And when he is asleep, he may start up out of his sleep, and he is terrified, seeing frightening dreams. This is the way we know that he is startled and terrified by his dreams. For when he is restored to his senses, he recounts the dreams, which conform to what he did with his body and what he said with his tongue. These are, then, what he suffers. Sometimes he may lie speechless the whole day and night, breathing rapidly and heavily. And when he stops being delirious, he is at once restored to his full senses. And if one were to question him, he will reply appropriately and understand what is said. Or, a little while later, he may again lie in the same distress.

This disease befalls one especially in a foreign country, or when perchance one goes along a deserted route and fear seizes him, arising out of some frightening apparition. And it may seize him in various ways.

[Treatment:] When he has this condition, one should give him to drink five obols of black hellebore, and administer it in sweet wine, or purge him with the following:

Egyptian nitre, a quantity the size of a sheep's vertebra, grind it well, and mix in a mortar a hemicotyl of cooked honey, a hemicotyl of olive oil, and four cotyls of water from boiled beets that have been exposed to the sun. Or, if you wish, instead of the beets, mix in boiled ass's milk. Purge him with this mixture, whether he has fever or not.

For soups, let him use a mixture of well-boiled barley, with honey added. Let him drink a mixture of honey, water, and vinegar, until the outcome of the illness is decided. In fourteen days or more, it will be clear if the outcome is fatal or not.

Often this sickness, having remitted, will recur. If it does so recur, there is mortal danger. Then the outcome will be decided in seven days, as to whether or not it is fatal. If he escapes from the recurrence, he will not die, and, for the majority [the most part?], the treatment succeeds in healing. When the illness is over, he should follow a good regimen, gently adding to what the stomach receives, and not heating it, lest diarrhea supervene. For both these [heating and diarrhea] are dangerous. And let him wash daily, and take short walks after meals. Let him dress in a light and soft garment. And at the appropriate time [the right season?] let him drink milk and whey for forty-five days. If he follows this regimen, he will soon be healthy. But the illness is a severe one and demands much concern.[10]

This remarkable clinical description is written by a physician for the benefit of other physicians. It is from a collection of descriptions of various "internal diseases," a kind of clinician's notebook or lecture notes rather than a systematic text. It is an account of a delirium, an acute brain syndrome with fluctuation in level of disorientation, accompanied by visual hallucinations.[11] In our day, a common cause of such a state would be withdrawal from alcohol, delirium tremens. Impairment of hearing and vision occur along with the mental changes. The doctor has made careful observations and some shrewd deductions, as when he correlates the patient's later description of his delirious dreams with the observed delirious behavior.

We cannot readily identify the particular disease constellation that the physician has in mind. We do not know for certain whether he theorizes that the disease is ascribable to bile or if he means that in fact it involves enlargement of the liver and perhaps jaundice. It is a serious disease and can be fatal. Treatment consists of hellebore, a powerful cathartic usually prescribed for mental derangement. But a purge with another mixture plus a certain diet may also be adequate treatment.

This passage is representative of the accounts of disturbed mental life in the Hippocratic corpus, except that it is both more detailed and more vivid than most. There is no question of any "emotional" etiology to this condition: it arises from a life-threatening illness. The account is part of a catalog of diseases, most of which have no mental accompaniments, though others do. We have here the typical setting, an obvious physical disturbance, in which the doctor encounters, treats, and thinks about a mental disturbance. The doctor is interested in the details of the mental disturbance, but only insofar as they are part and parcel of a clinically useful description of the disease as a whole. Thus we have a vivid impression of the mind of the clinician at work, diagnosing, classifying, carefully observing and recording, and thoughtfully prescribing. Though the basis for the prescribed treatment cannot be deduced from this piece alone, it is a mixture of experience, trial and error, a theory of the pathogenic effects of bile, and the alleged utility of hellebore as a cholegogue (a drug for purging bile).

On the Sacred Disease

Of all the works in the Hippocratic corpus, *On the Sacred Disease* contains the most extensive discussion of mental functioning, both in health and in disease, and, by virtue of its consideration of the relationship between brain activity and thinking, feeling, and behavior, comes closest to being a systematic exposition of the medical model of normal functioning. The fact that the treatise is ostensibly about epilepsy does not diminish its relevance for our purposes, since the discussion of epilepsy is in fact typical of the way Greek physicians considered severe mental disturbances.

This work, in contrast to the passage cited earlier, is addressed primarily to laymen and explains the doctor's belief about the causes and treatments of illnesses in general and epilepsy in particular. It differs from the first selection in its lack of specific prescriptions for treatment, which would be expected in a work for practicing physicians. It is also polemical, asserting simultaneously the unique professional competence of the physician and the unique importance of the brain and its diseases.[12]

The author of the treatise asserts that the so-called sacred disease is no more or less sacred than any other, and that the epithet was first applied by charlatans who desired to conceal their ignorance and shirk responsibility for their failure to cure the disease. The sacred disease is to be understood in terms of physiology, not religion; its awesomeness gives it no special claim on divinity.

The disease, like all other diseases, has a nature and causes, and is in principle curable: it belongs in the province of doctors. It is hereditary and originates *in utero*. Disturbances of the brain cause most serious diseases, and this is no exception. When the veins that carry air to the brain become blocked—by excess phlegm, for example—disease results.[13] Among the author's many astute clinical observations is the fact, confirmed by modern medicine, that the disease rarely appears *de novo* after the age of twenty. He describes the symptoms (for example, speechlessness and frothing at the mouth) and the behavior of the patient (for example, withdrawal from company because of shame). But for us his description of the role of the brain is most important:

Men ought to know that from the brain, and from the brain only, arise our pleasures, joys, laughter and jests, as well as our sorrows, pains, griefs and tears. Through it, in particular, we think [*phroneomen*], see, hear, and distinguish [*diaginoskomen*] the ugly from the beautiful, the bad from the good, the pleasant from the unpleasant, in some cases using custom as a test, in others perceiving them from their utility. It is the same thing which makes us mad [*mainometha*] or delirious [*paraphroneomen*], inspires us with dread and fear, whether by night or by day, brings sleeplessness, inopportune mistakes, aimless anxieties, absentmindedness, and acts that are contrary to habit. These things that we suffer all come from the brain, when it is not healthy, but becomes abnormally hot, cold, moist, or dry, or suffers any other unnatural affection to which it was not accustomed. Madness comes from moistness.[14]

In short, the brain is the source of mental and emotional activity. And because it extracts from its intake of air those parts that contain intelligence and opinion, it is also the interpreter of consciousness (*ton hermēneuonta tēn sunesin*).

What is this disease called sacred? What did it mean to the contemporary readers of this work? What does it mean in terms of our contemporary medical knowledge? What is the relevance of epilepsy to larger issues about the nature and treatment of mental disorder?

Several scholars, most notably Oswei Temkin, have provided evidence that "the sacred disease" is the popular name for epilepsy. Though the term *epilēpsis* is used only once in the treatise (section XIII), and then only in the general sense of a seizure (its literal translation), it is clear that in the Hippocratic corpus and other more or less contemporary literature the term refers to epileptic seizures.[15]

The seizure or capture implicit in the condition's name does indeed come on as an attack, seemingly out of the blue, and the afflicted were perceived and perceived themselves as being seized. Thus what is being described is dramatic and episodic and, because it comes as if from outside, seems to have little to do with the person's sense of himself.

Its sufferers may fall, become speechless, make thrashing motions of the limbs, foam at the mouth, and pass excrement, and the eyes may roll.[16] Only one side may be afflicted. Nocturnal attacks of unexplained fear and madness (or delirium) are mentioned as a variant of the disease (though strange behaviors and nocturnal attacks different from those of the disease are also described).

These symptoms coincide fairly well with what is now termed grand mal epilepsy, though such features as sudden night terrors may overlap with what is called psychomotor epilepsy or may not be true epileptic attacks. In all, in view of the immense problems entailed in identifying ancient diseases, we are dealing with a reasonably well-defined entity recognizable in modern terms.

What further associations did this disease have for the Greeks? Its dramatic and occasionally catastrophic nature made it apt to be considered god-sent. The madness of Heracles was considered by some to be a case of epilepsy.[17] Thus the disease had connotations of the divine, and possibly even the heroic. Even more important, however, the term "sacred" suggests some of the ambivalent sense of the Latin *sacer,* both holy and accursed. The condition is dangerous; the sufferers are to be avoided.

The first task of the doctor is to move the disease from the realm of mythology to the realm of physiology.[18] The disease has a *phusis*, a nature, like all other diseases. It is not surprising, then, that the medical writer makes no allusions to mythical heroes who suffered from the illness; such an allusion might have run counter to his particular polemical and scientific position. To my knowledge, the Hippocratic corpus contains no mention of the mythical characters who went mad and who were portrayed so vividly on the Athenian stage and in vase painting. Even Galen, a man of wide and ostentatious erudition in the second century A.D., hardly ever cites a figure from drama to illustrate overt madness.[19]

A great deal is at stake here, as the author makes plain. Much of the argument in the first few chapters and in the summary at the end is aimed at establishing that these conditions belong in the province of the doctor, not of the magician. We can also discern the author's wish to combat the fear, shame, and guilt that attend the sufferers of this disease.

How, then, does the disease come about, if not by divine acts? Natural causes, or what were natural causes to fifth-century Greeks, provide the answer. Phlegm and air, veins and blood, winds and weather are the *dramatis personae*. If there is a villain, it is phlegm, which prevents precious air, with its intelligence, from reaching the brain. If there is a victim, it is the brain, deprived of its necessary nutriment. If there is conflict, it is not between two gods, but rather between phlegm, which cools and obstructs, and blood, which warms and helps bring air. If there are irrational and unexplained behaviors, nameless terrors in the night, they occur because the brain is temporarily deprived of the stuff that makes it rational and coherent. If the disease runs in families, it does so because phlegmatics beget phlegmatics, bilious beget bilious, not because of inherited pollution or guilt. In sum, we have substituted the impersonal for the personal, the physiological for the mythological.

We may next take note of the transition from the role of the brain and of phlegm in generating this illness to the discourse on the central importance of the brain in all mental phenomena (XVI, XIX). The author, never having paused to prove that epilepsy involves the brain, goes on to assert the crucial role of the brain in the whole of human life. What is the source and origin of the notion that the brain is of unique importance? It is not intuitively obvious that the brain is the seat of thinking.

In the early fifth century, Alcmaeon of Croton pointed to the connections between the brain and the major sense organs. If the later traditions from which we derive this information are true, he may well have asserted the hegemony of the brain (a Stoic notion) or something like it, and may have done some brain dissection. One could also point to Diogenes of Apollonia, who seems to have argued for the central importance of air in mental processes, and also may have considered the brain an organ of intelligence. Thus, by the end of the fifth century, the notion that the brain is the seat of thinking had been formulated, though we do not know how widely it had spread.[20]

Is there no clinical evidence connecting the brain with thinking? The Hippocratic physician must have had a chance to *observe* some connection between brain disorder and deranged behavior. I would argue, however, that such observations were in fact not at all easy to make, and that for inferences to be drawn about the connection between brain and thinking or brain and behavior, it was necessary for the physician to have already assumed the connection. In the case of epilepsy, for example, there is little obvious connection between brain and disease, except for an occasional epileptic who might grasp his head or complain of funny feelings in his head. But then again, epileptics might experience odd sensations in many parts of the body, such as some precordial anxiety, olfactory or auditory hallucinations, illusions, or coenesthetic sensations.

Did not observations of head wounds afford an opportunity to see the connection between brain damage and disordered thinking? We do find a report of head injury with brain damage, the formation of pus, delirium, and death. In the same passage we find mention of spasms, or perhaps convulsions, that can ensue when the skull in the temporal area has been trephined, and it is noted that these spasms appear on the side of the body opposite the site of trephining.[21]

What about the finding reported in this treatise that goats with seizures may be found on autospy to have dropsied and foul-smelling brains? These and other bits of suggestive evidence allowed the physician to have a plausible basis for asserting that the brain is associated with both seizures and thinking.

Strictly speaking, however, none of this evidence can be interpreted as pointing to the brain as the *chief* organ of mental life, motor control, and so on. The clinical texts report delirium and madness to be associated with many conditions that do not obviously involve the brain. Seizures occurring in the course of febrile illnesses, for example, do not obviously seem to be mediated through the brain.

Further, we know that it was entirely possible to ascribe some role to the brain in mental and emotional processes while maintaining that the heart, for example, is the main locus of such activities. This, in fact, is the view found in Aristotle: the brain plays a part in the proper cooling of the blood that goes to the heart, and such cooling is necessary to enable the heart to carry on the intellectual and emotional activities of the body.[22] The question of heart versus brain was not definitively settled in antiquity, and perhaps not even for many centuries later.

In sum, I would argue that the available clinical evidence certainly suggested the importance of the brain but by no means unequivocally pointed to it. Some act of inference or intuition by the physician must have been involved. I doubt that we can, in fact, accurately reconstruct the processes that went into this brilliant piece of insight.

I suggest, however, that the author of *On the Sacred Disease* had a *motive* for assigning great importance to the brain. First, as R. Onians has pointed out, in Greek popular belief the head is an organ of life, a seat of the psyche, an organ of generation, and a symbol of the continuity of life and family.[23] The head of the body is like the head of a household. The motive of the physician can best be discerned in Plato's *Timaeus,* a dialogue that builds on popular beliefs and develops the analogy between body and psyche and, implicitly, the state.

The *Timaeus,* as Plato makes plain, is intended as a sequel to the *Republic.* In the *Timaeus,* too, the psyche is divided into three parts, but here they correspond to parts of the body rather than parts of the polis: the rational to the head and brain, the spirited-affective to the heart, and the appetitive to the area below the diaphragm (probably the liver).[24] The imagery is of great interest, for political metaphors crop up here too (70A–B). The brain (the rational part) is cast as the body's "acropolis," which sends orders to the thorax or "guard-room" (the seat of the "emotive-spirited") to put down the rebellion that the appetitive part has stirred up in the rest of the body.

Plato has thus constructed a physiology of thought, emotion, and desire, ordered it, and politicized it for his own ends. In the process he has set up the brain as the seat of the functions that he himself, *qua* philosopher, exercises. He has arrogated the brain for himself and for his professional philosophical functions (which include political ruling functions). He may have chosen the brain for all its earlier connotations as an organ vital for life and generation, but also because he needed to define a unique part of the body as exercising the unique functions he says are those of the philosopher. He has said, in effect, "The philosopher is the brains of the organization."

Something similar is to be seen in *On the Sacred Disease.* Here the brain corresponds to the physician. Having devoted the first part of the treatise to staking out the claims of the professional competence of the physician vis-à-vis other practitioners, the author devotes the second part to the claims of the brain vis-à-vis other parts of the body which had been held to represent the sites of mental activity (the diaphragm and heart). The diseases of the brain, he asserts, are the most grievous and serious of all diseases. This is imperialistic

behavior, less consciously and conspicuously so in the medical treatise than in Plato's work, but imperialistic nonetheless.[25]

Just as for Plato the activities of the brain are analogous to the
activities of the philosopher, so for Hippocrates they are analogous
to those of the doctor. But the contrast between Hippocrates and
Plato is also important. For Hippocrates the brain is not the absolute
ruler that it is for Plato. The brain is subject to influences beyond its
control—the quality of phlegm in the body, the season of the year,
the prevailing winds.

The Hippocratic physician sees his power as distinctly limited. He
is subject to the constraints of nature and of the illness. He cannot
radically alter the condition of the patient, but must hope at best to
tip the balance in favor of recovery. The words of the Renaissance
surgeon Ambroise Paré, "God heals the wounds, I dress them,"
capture the spirit of the Hippocratic view of the physician's limitations. There is no medical utopia where the doctor cures all ills of the
body as there is a philosophical utopia where the philosopher king
cures all ills of the state.

A second point of comparison between the brain and the doctor
may be found in their roles as interpreters. The brain, for Hippocrates,
interprets sensory phenomena, provided by air, the stuff of intelligence. It is a messenger (*ho diangellōn*) to consciousness (*sunesis*).

The physician, in his relationship to the patient and to his illness,
does not command but explains. He reconstructs with the patient the
history of the illness, interpreting the relationship among his symptoms, his regimen of life, and the prevailing pathogenic forces (such
as the winds). He also ventures a prognosis and formulates treatment
and explains them to the patient.[26]

The Doctor-Patient Relationship

Some of the surviving works of the Hippocratic corpus are clearly
designed for the general educated public, others for physicians. This
alone is an important index of the degree to which the Hippocratic
physician saw himself as an educator. In many works, especially
those dealing with proper regimen, one senses the physician explaining these matters to the patient, and at times the author explicitly
advises the physician to make all this perfectly clear to the patient.
While the term *hermeneutēs,* translator, is not specifically applied to
the physician, it captures the flavor of what the doctor is doing. He
is, in effect, translating his knowledge of theories and clinical experience into terms useful to the patient. The physician has made a
practical interpretation of philosophically based theories about nature
and about the body, useful to himself, to other physicians, and
thence to his patients and the public at large. If Socrates was the man

who, according to Cicero, brought philosophy down from the heavens to the marketplace, Hippocrates was the one who brought philosophy down from the level of theoretical discourse to the practice of caring for and curing the body.[27]

Obviously, there must have been tremendous variation, depending on the physician and patient, in the extent to which the physician would trouble to explain to and educate his patient. Something of this variation is reflected in Plato's comments about the differences between the "scientific" physician, who treats freemen, and the slave physician, or the physician's assistant, who treats slaves.

The slave [doctor] . . . never talk[s] to [his] patients individually, or let[s] them talk about their own individual complaints: [he merely] prescribes what mere experience suggests, as if he had exact knowledge. . . . But the other doctor, who is a freeman, . . . carries his enquiries far back, and goes into the nature of the disorder; he enters into discourse with the patient and with his friends, and is at once getting information from the sick and also instructing him as far as he is able, and he will not prescribe for him until he has first convinced him; at last, when he has brought the patient more and more under his persuasive influences and set him on the road to health, he attempts to effect a cure. [*Laws*, 720]

If one of those empirical physicians [i.e., slaves] . . . were to come upon the gentleman physician talking to his gentleman patient, and using the language almost of philosophy, . . . he would say, . . . "Foolish fellow, . . . you are not healing the sick man, you are educating him; and he does not want to be made a doctor, but to get well." [*Laws*, 857][28]

Even if Plato exaggerates somewhat in order to make his points clearer, he does convey some of the ideals of the doctor-patient relationship. Plato's portrait of the scientific physician with his patient is certainly consonant with much of the Hippocratic corpus.

One also senses that the physician sees himself and his patient as part of the natural scheme of things. As such, he can help rectify a disturbed balance of humors and qualities, but has only a limited ability to cure.

What does the physician explain to the patient? The author of the treatise on epilepsy describes the task of the physician all too briefly. On the basis of the patient's condition, an examination of his diet, his place of living, and the season of the year, he must decide, for instance, which humor might be present in excess. Appropriate foods can reduce the amount of bile or phlegm in the body. The proper medicines can also affect the balance of humors by causing an increased expulsion of phlegm or bile. (We find no mention of a drug considered specific or helpful for epilepsy.) The drugs considered most appropriate for the treatment of the various mental disturbances in this and other treatises are the group of hellebores, powerful cathartics and emetics that were believed to eliminate excess yellow and black bile. We shall return to these drugs and to consideration of their use in mental disturbances.[29]

Now, if the doctor spends all this time and effort talking with the patient, explaining, eliciting information, and educating, obviously a relationship is established between the two. Does the Hippocratic doctor ever discuss with his patient what we might call personal problems, whether immediately relevant to the presenting problem or not? In instances of blatant mental disorder, did the doctor ever attempt to understand the patient's emotional difficulties? These questions lead to the issue raised by Laín Entralgo: can we speak of verbal psychotherapy in the context of the Greek doctor-patient relationship?[30]

First, it is abundantly clear that the Hippocratic doctor had no professional interest in the patient's personal emotional difficulties, whether the illness was conspicuously physical or mental. Such a concern was simply not part of the physician's conception of his professional activity. We do hear of discussions of dreams, but only to help the physician diagnose physical illness. (The underlying assumption here was that occult bodily disturbances might be registered first in dream content, before the patient was consciously aware of them.)[31] It is highly likely, however, that the sympathetic physician, or one with a talent for understanding emotional difficulties, would talk over such matters with the patient. It is also likely that the physician, even in his role as clinical detective, might try to ferret out some information about the inner feelings of his patient. We have definite indications from later antiquity that the shrewd physician kept an ear open for indications of "lovesickness," to avoid mistaking it for an ailment of the body. An anecdote from Galen tells how he discovered that a female patient was pining away with unrequited love for the actor Pylades: her pulse would quicken at the mention of his name.[32] Later authors also wrote of the need to handle madmen with firmness or kindness, or to distract them with discussion of neutral topics, or even to shake a man out of his delusional state with tricks.[33]

But, overall, ancient medicine did not develop a concept of the healing power of words and dialogue, just as it did not develop a concept of disturbances of the mind apart from disturbances of the body. On the contrary, one gets from the Hippocratic authors the sense that anything not couched in physiological and physical terms already touched on magic and charlatanism.

Undoubtedly some nonspecific psychotherapy took place, partly through the constant presence of the kindly physician. Even more the physician's statement that the patient has an intelligible physical problem, treatable by physical means, must have gone a long way toward alleviating guilt and shame and providing a restorative mechanism of defense.[34]

12

Aristotle on Melancholy

> I have neither the scholar's melancholy, which is emulation; nor the
> musician's, which is fantastical; nor the courtier's, which is proud;
> nor the soldier's, which is ambitious; nor the lawyer's, which is
> politic; nor the lady's, which is nice; nor the lover's, which is all of
> these: but it is a melancholy of mine own, compounded of many
> simples, extracted from many objects.
>
> —Shakespeare, *As You Like It*

The Hippocratic writings contain many brief references to melancholy but no single extended discussion. We learn more about melancholy from the medical writers of later antiquity, who in their
commentaries and encyclopedias tell us much about the conceptions
held in the fifth and fourth centuries B.C.[1] In the Hippocratic corpus,
melancholy is unusually mentioned in lists of diseases caused by a
surplus of black bile, and this linkage is evidence of a close connection between melancholy and epilepsy, which is also attributed to an
excess of black bile.[2]

Thus we are dealing with a condition that, like epilepsy, was
thought to have a clear physical cause and a definite relationship with
other diseases of black bile. Hemorrhoids, dysentery, stomachache,
and skin eruptions round out the group of black bile diseases. Like
others in the group, melancholy may increase in the fall of the year—
or, alternatively, in the spring (each humor was thought to increase
in a different season).[3] Melancholy, or melancholia, may have presented difficult problems of treatment for the Hippocratic physician,
but, as this list of rather prosaic conditions attributed to black bile
suggests, they approached it with a clinical matter-of-factness.

Melancholic illnesses were occasionally associated with *mania* (raving madness), but no intrinsic or cyclic connection between the two
is implied. Although the Hippocratic corpus contains no extended
description of the experience of melancholia, scattered comments
allow us to understand what the Hippocratic author means when he
says, "When fear and sadness last a long time, this is a melancholic
condition." A vivid account of "anxiousness" very likely describes
one form of melancholia:

Anxiousness—a difficult disease. The patient thinks he has something like a thorn, something pricking him in his viscera, and anxiety [perhaps loathing or nausea] tortures him. He flees from light and from people, loves the dark, and is attacked by fear. His diaphragm swells, and he feels pain at the touch. He worries and sees frightening visions, fearful dream images, and occasionally dead people. The disease attacks mostly in the spring.[4]

Treatments include hellebore, ass's milk, and cleansing of the head. If the treatment succeeds, the disease will remit in time; if not, the patient will suffer from it for the rest of his days.

If we combine evidence from the Hippocratic corpus with bits and hints from later Greek medical literature, melancholic diseases seem to be characterized by anxious concern, nameless fears, blackness of mood, suicidal impulses, and sullen suspiciousness. Again, the entire flavor is of a somatic condition, with both mental and physical disturbances treated by physical means; no possible cause is sought in emotional disturbances.

We find the same assumptions of organic and somatic causes in Aristotle's *Problemata,* but we also find more elaborate discussion of the mechanisms by which black bile relates to character, temperament, and melancholic illnesses. The treatise in section 30 of the *Problemata,* beginning "Why are men of genius melancholics?" and usually attributed to Theophrastus or some other disciple of Aristotle, gained great popularity during the Renaissance.[5] Its interest lay less in its physiological content than in its discussion of the issue that so engaged many Renaissance thinkers (especially the NeoPlatonists) about the connections among genius, inspiration, and madness.[6]

The piece begins with the assumption that all men of talent are melancholics, and asks why. Here, as we shall see, "melancholic" does not necessarily imply disease; it may simply denote a melancholic temperament.

Why is it that all those who have become eminent in philosophy or politics or poetry or the arts are clearly melancholics, and some of them to such an extent as to be affected by diseases caused by black bile? An example from heroic mythology is Heracles. For he apparently had this constitution, and therefore epileptic afflictions were called after him "the sacred disease" by the ancients. His mad fit in the incident with the children points to this, as well as the eruption of sores which happened before his disappearance on Mount Oeta; for this is with many people a symptom of black bile. Lysander the Lacedaemonian too suffered from such sores before his death. There are also the stories of Ajax and Bellerophon: the one went completely out of his mind, while the other sought out desert places for his habitation. . . . Among the heroes many others evidently suffered in the same way, and among men of recent times Empedocles, Plato, and Socrates, and numerous other well-known men, and also most of the poets. For many such people have bodily disease as the result of this kind of temperament (*krasis*); some of them have only a clear constitutional (*phusis*) tendency toward such affliction, but, to put it briefly, all of them are, as has been said before, melancholics by constitution.[7]

We are now in the realm of a fairly well-formulated theory of humors and their relation to "constitution." We are speaking of the melancholic in contrast to the phlegmatic, the sanguine, and the choleric. In a person with this temperament, with the balance of humors dominated by black bile, frank melancholic diseases may erupt. On the other hand, one can also be melancholic by temperament without suffering from the associated diseases.

The author compares the effects of black bile and the effects of wine. By providing an example of a known substance that produces a variety of effects on the mind and temperament, he lends plausibility to the notion that an internally occurring substance can produce similar mental effects. Wine makes some men angry, some kindly and merciful, and some impulsive. Further, one can observe that wine produces these changes gradually. When a man who is sober and "cold" (without much natural heat) begins drinking wine, he becomes a bit more talkative; with increasing amounts of wine he may become a "speechmaker" and be more bold, then impulsive, then maniacal and raving, then foolish ("morons"), like some of those who have suffered from epilepsy since childhood.

The variety of traits induced or elicited by wine is naturally distributed among men; that is, variations in the amount and quality of black bile are responsible for the incidence of these naturally occurring traits. Wine produces them for only a short time, while black bile produces long-term and permanent effects.

Both wine and black bile are "pneumatic," full of air and frothy, and both can vary in the qualities of heat and cold. Wine makes men lustful, and lust is related to air; air causes erection and ejaculation. A clinical observation is introduced: melancholics' veins are hard and distended by air. (Note that the brain is not mentioned; this hypothesis does not say that these chemical agents act on the brain, which then causes the mental states.)

The author seeks to build a theory that will invoke only one simple substance as the cause of a variety of phenomena in melancholics. Thus he argues that the qualities of black bile may vary, particularly its temperature, and that the variations in qualities can explain why a variety of effects may be produced by only one substance. Cold black bile leads to apoplexy, numbness, fearfulness, and being disheartened (*athumia*). Hot black bile produces "cheerfulness, bursting into song, and ecstasies, and the eruption of sores."

Now, the ordinary amounts of black bile arising from food ingested do not affect the characters of most people, though in sufficient quantity bile may lead to some physical melancholic disease (presumably transitory). But in those with the basic melancholic constitution one finds characteristic illnesses, the nature of which depends on the proportions of hot and cold black bile. Coldness and a moderate amount of bile make men sluggish and stupid, while excessive quantity and heat lead to euphoric, erotic, impulsive, and garrulous behavior. If hot black bile is too near the seat of intellect (probably the heart here), the individual is affected by a "manic" and "enthusiastic" state. Such people may become Sibyls, Bacchants, or "god-struck."[8] But when the amount of black bile is more moderate (and presumably of the right temperature), melancholics become more intelligent than most other people and tend to demonstrate talent in education, the arts, or politics. Cold bile makes one cowardly, while warm bile allows one to deal with fear and remain steadfast.

Daily fluctuations in mood, from sad to cheerful, are also explicable in terms of variations in the mixture of hot and cold bile. These everyday fluctuations, however, must not be confused with deep, long-lasting mood states. If cooling is too sudden or excessive, extreme despondency leading to suicide can result, especially in the young.

Finally, the author summarizes his position: not all melancholics are alike, because black bile varies in its qualities and effects. All melancholics are exceptional, but it is not the melancholic diseases that make them so, though they may be predisposed to such diseases.

Who are these exceptional men, the *perittoi?* Heracles is one. His melancholic diseases include outright madness (which led him to kill his children), epilepsy (perhaps synonymous with the attack of madness), and sores. Another is Lysander (died 395 B.C.), a famous Spartan commander who defeated the Athenians on several occasions and attempted to help establish the Oligarchy of the Thirty in Athens.

Ajax, memorialized in Homer's *Odyssey,* in post-Homeric poems, in countless vase paintings, and most powerfully in Sophocles' play, is the greatest melancholic of them all.[9] The transformation from epic hero to medical case is instructive and, for the Greeks, quite simple. Ajax is associated with rage and sulking and with images of blackness and heaviness. Perhaps we can glimpse the transition in some lines surviving from a lost post-Homeric epic, *The Sack of Troy,* which state that the two sons of Asclepius the healer became "specialists," one in surgery and the other in diseases hidden within (internal disease). The latter physician "was the first to understand the flashing eyes of Ajax raging and his mind weighted down."[10] *Barunomenon,* "weighted down," is the metaphor that appears in our term "depressed."

Bellerophon is famous from the story in Book 6 of the *Iliad* and also from numerous works of art. With his winged horse, Pegasus, he slew the Chimaera. The *Iliad* hints that he flew too high, so to speak, and so became hated by the gods. He wandered alone, staying away from the haunts of men, and was thus suited to be labeled mad by our author (though he was not called mad by Homer).

Empedocles was an early fifth-century philosopher, shaman, and physician, an enigmatic figure, undoubtedly considered strange if not a bit mad.[11]

Even Plato is included. Perhaps all philosophers (especially Socrates) are strange and a bit "touched." Plato wrote with considerable feeling about "divine madness" in his *Phaedrus*. In later antiquity we find the tradition of Platonic *tristitia*, or sadness.[12] And we have the line from middle comedy (late fourth or early third century):

> Oh Plato, all you know is how to frown,
> And solemnly raise your eyebrows like a snail.[13]

The reason such men are melancholics, of course, lies in the quantity and quality of black bile within them, not in the inner conflicts that might beset them, the tremendous competitive pressures to which they might be subject, or the extremely high standards that they might set for themselves.[14] Thus the portrait of a melancholic presented to us by Sophocles in his *Ajax,* rich in subtleties of the psychology of shame, of ego ideal, of displaced rivalries, and of aggression turned against the self, forms a striking contrast. Note, however, that the author of the *Problemata* does not refute the kind of psychodynamic detail presented by Sophocles, but seems to ignore it. Psychology is translated into physiology, but we do not get any sense of conflict between the two. This is not a polemical piece; it offers no rebuttal to the opinions of others.

I believe that two frames of reference apply to this treatise and to the singular ease with which passions and conflicts are explained in terms of the vicissitudes of black bile. I refer first to the discussions of mind and body in which Aristotle attempts to achieve clarity and methodological precision in accounting for both somatic and psychic factors. The second framework harks back in time. I refer to the multiple connections seen in fantasy, folklore, and subjective feelings among melancholy, blackness, poisonous thoughts and feelings, and the burden of anger, grief, and unrelieved emotion. This second framework is relevant to the psychoanalytic formulations on melancholia which attempt to bring a new kind of scientific ordering to such subjective and elusive data.

In the person of Aristotle we find both philosopher and biologist, and it is in Aristotle that we find the greatest depth of understanding of the problem of the split between mind and body and, at the same time, the widest variety of solutions offered.

Briefly, Aristotle's main lines of approach can be summarized as follows:

1. All life has "soul," but it varies in degree: plants and the lower animals have nutritive (or vegetative) souls; the souls of more highly developed animals give them the capacity for movement; a soul that does some reasoning inhabits men and some animals; only man has a rational soul. (*De Anima* is the main exposition of this view.)

2. In speaking of mental life in man, Aristotle, like Plato, has several schemas of subdivision, which attempt to cover the gradations from appetitive to intellective and the mixtures of intellect and desire that characterize most human activity. In his *Nicomachean Ethics* he speaks of human choice: "Choice [*proairesis*] can be described either as appetitive intellect or intellectual appetite, and such a principle [*archē*] is man" (1139b4–5).

3. The importance of "complementary" descriptions of the same phenomena is emphasized. In *De Anima* Aristotle speaks of the intimate connection between emotions and the body; emotions are of the soul but cannot exist apart from the body:

> The passions are materialized formulae [*logoi enuloi*]. . . . But the physicist and the dialectician will in every case offer different definitions in answer to the question, for example, "What is anger?" The dialectician will define anger as a craving to return hurt for hurt, or something of the sort; the physicist, as a surging of blood and heat around the heart. The one is describing the matter, the other the form or formula or the essence. [403a25–403b2][15]

4. The division into matter and form (and the divisions into four kinds of causes: material, efficient, formal, and final) is another attempt to deal with the "mind within the body" and the "body that contains mind." (Incidentally, we might take note of the "mentalistic" character of Greek biology from Aristotle to Galen. It assumes a teleology, that is, a plan in the mind of the maker. The mind of the biologist is sufficiently similar to that of the maker that the biologist-philosopher can, in fact, hope to discover the maker's plan and purpose.)

5. Aristotle's earlier theories (now largely lost) seem to have viewed the soul as external to and detachable from the body. The soul is a divine essence that interacts with the body but is not united with it.[16]

6. The humoral theory of the temperaments of mankind provided a psychophysiology. Such a theory attempts to solve the mind-body problem by positing a combined mind-body factor, in this case a humor.

We have reason to believe that Aristotle's successors tended to hypostatize this last solution to the mind-body problem. The author of the treatise on melancholy might have said that he was presenting a theory of the *material cause* of melancholic disturbance (analogous to the material definition of anger as a "surging of blood and heat around the heart"). The *logos,* the formula, of melancholy (analogous to "anger as a craving to return hurt for hurt") might be some such statement as "Melancholia is the disposition to react to injured pride and loss of face with brooding, sulkiness, and despair." The author of this treatise made no such formulation, nor did any other ancient writer. He limited his interest to one set of causes for melancholy and did not broaden it even within the framework of Aristotle's thinking on the mind-body problem.

From the perspective of the theory of temperaments, however, he did his job admirably. It is tempting to say that he outlined for us the equivalent of one of the modern biochemical theories of the etiology of affective disorders. His arguments about black bile constitute a respectable precursor of the catecholamine hypothesis of depressive and manic disorders of the brain.[17] Briefly, this theory states that excesses of norepinephrine and related substances, acting in certain parts of the brain, lead to mania, while deficiencies and depletions of these substances lead to depression. I think it more significant, however, that he explicitly and implicitly raised some of the important issues to which contemporary hypotheses must be addressed: the relationship between normal mood variations and pathological mood states and the search for a few simple substances that act at a particular brain site to produce specific disturbances. Where do such substances originate? Do they occur naturally in the body, or are they derived from foodstuffs or from some other external source? If our author has neither attempted nor achieved a comprehensive synthesis of the psychological and the physical, we cannot easily fault him. Aristotle himself fell short of such a synthesis in his discussion of the soul, and we are just beginning to get a glimpse of the requirements for such a synthesis, even in the narrowly focused area of depressive disorders.

As for the second framework, I can clarify what I have in mind by posing a question raised by F. Kudlien: Where in the world does this notion of black bile come from, let alone the idea that it is related to mental depressions and agonies?[18] Is black bile a substance that Greek physicians thought they could see, as they could see yellow bile, blood, and phlegm, or is it a hypothesized (or imagined) form of bile? Medical historians have tended to search for clinical situations in which dark or black substances might appear to be coming out of the body and be associated with diseases that seem to be accompanied by depression. Kudlien argues persuasively that no one has seen black bile and that probably the Greek physicians did not really think they were seeing it either. There is really no good evidence that, for example, the black stools of patients with gastrointestinal bleeding or the coffee-ground vomitus of gastric hemorrhage were associated with black bile. One would be hard pressed to demonstrate that anyone saw the bile of man or animal as black under any conditions where one might observe bile (though one could see *dark* bile— brownish rather than yellowish). Even if one could argue that black bile might designate dark or brownish bile, we find remarkably little evidence that Hippocratic physicians even claimed that they saw black bile in abundance in cases diagnosed as melancholia. Book 3 of Hippocrates' *Epidemics,* it is true, tells of a woman who passed black urine and who was said to have "melancholics."[19] But even here the connection is not explicitly made between black bile and melancholia, and, to my knowledge, this example is unique in the Hippocratic corpus.

I believe that Kudlien is basically correct when he says that we must give greater attention to the realm of magical thinking and popular belief. He brings together various quotations from Greek literature, from Homer down to classical times, which demonstrate, among other points, that (1) "melancholia" was a popular term for the condition of those considered crazy, or batty, probably before or contemporaneous with its earliest medical usage; and (2) there is a nexus of associations among anger, darkness or blackness surging up with such anger, and blackness as poisonous (for example, *Iliad,* 17.591—"a black cloud of distress"). Thus *cholos,* anger, and *cholē,* bile, often overlap in poetic and literary usage. One could extend these arguments and show that the connections extend also to the images of anger and grief as burdens, or weights, which lead to "depression" and bitterness.[20]

We begin to see that the associations of blackness, bile, and dejection arise from common (perhaps universal) subjective experiences and associations involved in becoming and feeling depressed. These subjective experiences undoubtedly have a reciprocal relationship with particular views and even patterns of experience that are presented to the individual by his culture. The way any individual experiences, reports, and explains his depressed state is influenced to a significant degree by cultural patterns.[21]

In any case, the connection between mind and body implied in the term "melancholy" is not the tortuous one posited by certain medical historians—for example, gastrointestinal disorders that produce black excrement or vomitus may also be associated with depressed, fearful states. Rather, it is a primordial, subjective, psychosomatic fantasy based on the blending of mental and somatic sensations. If, indeed, clinical observations were to be reported associating dark bile with gastric or hepatic disorders, flatulence, and melancholia (as suggested by some of the Hippocratic lists of black bile disorders), I would argue that such "observations" were built upon the more primordial and subjective connections detailed above.

But this line of argument has further implications. We may, in fact, have pinpointed a major way in which theories of mental disturbance, psychological as well as physiological, are built up. The black bile theory seems to have developed when subjective experiences led to a search for causal agents that had some sort of intrinsic connection with the quality of the experience. If there is a black mood, there must be a black substance; a bitter feeling, a bitter substance. This step from sensation to substance can, in principle, be a beginning of bona fide testable theory making, or it can prove to be a false step, a blind alley, a misleading and untestable theory. What is done next is crucial to the outcome, as is the degree to which the theory maker is aware of the tentativeness of his hypothesis. The existence of black bile might well have served as a useful initial hypothesis in a search for somatic causes of depression. In fact, in the treatise on genius and melancholia one detects a tone of intellectual curiosity, of the tackling of complex questions, of a search for some experimental or quasi-experimental verification of the hypothesis. The analogy between the effects of black bile (the hypothesized substance) and wine (the known substance) might have led to a more refined experimental model of a mental disturbance. That it did not do so, that black bile became the final rather than the first explanation—and a false explanation that lasted many centuries—should not be laid at the feet of the theory or of the substance.[22]

When Freud formulated the theory presented in "Mourning and Melancholia," he first observed the patient's excessive self-reproaches and then posited a mental agency in charge of self-reproach (the superego).[23] If the degree of self-recrimination is excessive and pathological, then the agency that regulates self-reproach and self-praise must be malfunctioning. The degree to which the theory may be regarded as scientific depends not on this reasoning but rather on the steps that are taken next, the consequences of those steps, the way data are used, and the willingness of the theory maker to revise or abandon his initial notion. Freud's original formulations of the dynamics of severe melancholia emphasized the interplay of ambivalence toward the lost or disappointing person, injured narcissism, guilt, and aggression turned against the self rather than the other. The posited superego, a self-punitive agency of the mind that behaves sadistically, as it were, is also central to the theory. In all, such formulations have stood the test of time, though in some respects they have been found incomplete. That they generated both new observations and new formulations is an indication that they are indeed scientific.

What is our current understanding of the nature, causes, and treatment of melancholia? Modern psychiatry, I believe, is at the threshold of a valid synthesis of the psychic and the somatic in relation to severe depression.[24] On the psychological side, a wealth of observational data now point to the crucial importance of such factors as losses and separations in early childhood, intense maternal ambivalence in child rearing, and difficulties in the regulation of guilt and in the expression of appropriate aggression. The appreciation of the complex interplay among these and other factors creates the possibility of increasingly effective kinds of psychotherapeutic treatment for depression. The diagnosis and classification of types of depression have also been refined. On the somatic side, several rather sophisticated biochemical models are now available, models that are amenable to proof or disproof. These models are also of great use in the development of a rational basis for the pharmacological treatment of the severe depressions, an area in which great advances have been made in the last twenty years. Important beginnings have been made in the classification of manic–depressive and depressive disorders into several distinct genetic subgroups. Both laboratory research and more naturalistic research (on primates and lower animals) are beginning to yield precise information on the physiological sequelae of mother-infant separation and other disruptions in the social nexus of the animal. Such studies are beginning to generate models that may lead to testable hypotheses in relation to human depression. An understanding of the interplay of biological, psychological, and social factors in the origin and continuation of depression may well be achieved in the next few decades. The quest begun by the Greeks for a resolution of the antinomies of nature and culture (*phusis-nomos*) and of psyche and soma has thus reached a new level of sophistication, only dimly adumbrated by those who first articulated these problems.

13

Hysteria and Social Issues

Menstruation—the sanguineous tears of the disappointed endometrium.

—Anonymous medical aphorism

Hysteria, the disease of the "wandering uterus," was given its name by the Greeks. The condition and its diagnosis and treatment must be understood in the context of the intrapsychic and social conflicts that accompanied relationships between men and women. By using the idiom of physiology to describe these conflicts, the Greeks defensively disguised their social origins and placed them in the sphere of physical illness.

In order to understand hysteria's place in the medical model, it will be necessary to examine many aspects of the disease, among them ancient and modern medical and psychoanalytic considerations, the place of women in Greek society, and the use to which group hysteria and uterine disorders were put in Greek tragedy.

Psychoanalytic and Clinical Psychiatric Considerations

"Hysteria" derives from the Greek *hustera,* womb. As is well known, the ancient Greeks believed that certain physical symptoms in women (shortness of breath, pain in the chest, lump in the throat, pain in the groin and legs, some instances of fainting and some seizures) were caused by a wandering or displacement of the uterus. Hysteria was considered more likely to affect widows and virgins than married women, and so the treatment usually involved a prescription of marriage and intercourse. This view was held, more or less firmly, by medical men and laymen alike for many centuries. Sometime in the seventeenth and eighteenth centuries physicians began to give primacy to "animal vapors" within the body, to "nerves," and, finally, to the brain, minimizing the importance of uterine movements. In the nineteenth century, particularly under the impact of Jean-Martin Charcot, the medical profession began to think of hysteria (or, properly speaking, hysterical conversion) as a neurological disease without any demonstrable neuropathology, a functional disease brought on by psychological trauma and treatable by psychological means. Even Charcot, though, in his earlier years, used "ovarian compressors" to help abort a hysterical seizure.[1]

Freud articulated a notion that was in the air in his day—that hysteria has its origins in psychological factors. Specifically, Freud said, hysteria is caused by the patient's unresolved unconscious conflicts; the symptoms themselves express those conflicts symbolically, and treatment consists in helping to make the conflicts conscious. In addition, as Freud quoted one of his medical teachers as saying, "c'est toujours la chose génitale"—it is always a sexual matter. He also made explicit the intimate connection between hysteria and sexuality. He pointed out that hysteria could occur in men, a fact recognized in late antiquity. In both the popular and the professional mind, however, hysteria is still most closely associated with women.[2]

A number of psychiatrists and psychoanalysts have expanded upon these germinal insights of Freud. Several constructive attempts have been made to classify and clarify different sorts of hysterical phenomena. The communicative and interpersonal setting of hysteria has been increasingly emphasized, as in Szasz's *Myth of Mental Illness*.[3] And psychoanalysts have argued that hysteria involves important intrapsychic issues other than the resolution of the Oedipus complex. These issues pertain to the earlier phases of the mother-child relationship, and have been variously characterized as oral, schizoid, and narcissistic.[4]

We have also learned a great deal about hysteria from the work of medical and social historians who have explored the social and economic setting in which hysteria in nineteenth-century England and America must be viewed.[5]

Let us look at the terminology of hysteria.[6]

Hysterical conversion is a state in which the patient complains of a bodily disorder for which no clear organic cause can be found. Among the classic symptoms are paralysis of a limb, blindness, and anaesthesia of one side of the body, as well as such less exotic complaints as the sensation of a lump in the throat (*globus hystericus*) and certain forms of headache. Hysterical seizures mimicking epilepsy are typically condensations of the acts of childbirth and intercourse. When the term "hysteria" appears in medical literature from antiquity down to the early twentieth century, it refers to these symptoms.[7]

Hysterical character (or hysterical personality) is a term applied to patterns of behavior and of social presentation rather than to formed symptoms. The hysterical character, usually a woman, tends to be histrionic and represses and ignores much important social interaction, particularly in the sphere of sexuality. This kind of patient does not frequently consult medical doctors about specific somatic complaints. If she seeks psychiatric help, she most often complains of inability to get along with people or to be successful in love. The frequency of minor hysterical conversion symptoms is probably higher than normal in such patients, though the data are not altogether clear. In recent years it has been pointed out that the "hysterical character" may well be a man's version of what women are like in general. Clinical experience suggests that female therapists tend to diagnose hysterical character far less often than do male therapists. Hysterical character may be ascribed to men but seldom is.

Hysteria and massive dissociative phenomena are rather exotic conditions that have great appeal to the popular imagination. Patients who experience massive amnesias with loss of personal identity have been the subjects of numerous plays and novels. Multiple personalities, such as the famous case presented in *The Three Faces of Eve,* are relatively uncommon now, or at least less prominent than they seem to have been in Freud's day. In the nineteenth and early twentieth centuries they were intensively studied by psychologists, hypnotists, and some psychiatrists. Such patients are usually quite seriously ill, often barely warding off massive disruption of the personality. Some have been, or later become, frankly psychotic; others may be seriously impaired in their overall life functioning. This group merges with others: (a) persons exhibiting *pseudologia phantastica,* a kind of habitual and fantastic lying, which serves to allay anxiety; (b) patients who deliberately consult doctors about fictitious medical problems and are willing to undergo painful or dangerous operations and diagnostic procedures; (c) the classic impostors, people who *must* live with a false identity.[8]

The interrelationship among these three main categories is not at all clear. Overall, those so diagnosed behave as though certain of their impulses and behaviors were disavowed and not recognized as belonging to the self. Repression and "ignorance" are also important. The psychosexual issues characterizing hysteria cluster around oedipal themes—for example, the vicissitudes of triangular relationships among parents and child, involving rivalry, jealousy, aggressive wishes, and expressions of wishes for sexual possession. Although a variety of dyadic themes—that is, themes involving early mother-child ties—have emerged from the study of hysterical patients, the oedipal triangular themes seem to be most characteristic of hysteria. Such terms as "bad hysteric" and "primitive hysteric" reflect the clinical fact that for some patients, early unresolved mother-child issues seem more prominent than oedipal conflicts. It seems to me that for this group of patients the later oedipal rivalry between mother and daughter has brought to light, or aggravated, earlier disturbances in their relationship.

Hysterical conversions, the somatic representations of conflicts, are interpersonal communications. They can be fruitfully viewed as a sign language, a secret code designed to communicate in circumstances in which the patient cannot openly say what he means. Similarly, hysterical ignorance is a communication. At an unconscious level, these symptoms are intended to influence people around the sufferer and to influence his own inner objects.[9] The "audience" for hysteria is a fusion (and usually a confusion) of internalized object representations and people actually present in the person's life.

The hysterical conversion symptom is an enactment of a fantasy, including a fantasy map of the human body, particularly the sexual and generative organs. The contents of such a fantasy are similar to typical normal infantile sexual theories, a child's misunderstanding of the reproductive process. The fantasy, an unconscious one, also represents a story or a scene, usually of some sexual activity observed and/or fantasized by the patient in childhood.[10]

Dramatic and exhibitionistic elements are important in hysteria. A successful hysterical performance engages and influences the audience. Exotic hysterical conversion symptoms often signify that the patient has identified with (and unconsciously acted the part of) a person close to him who has had a bona fide physical illness. The hysteric is a good mime, though not a deliberate one.

Circumstances in the life of an individual (and perhaps of a culture) that seem to foster the use of hysterical symptoms involve a certain climate of "motivated ignorance" in the family. Major conversion symptoms in middle-class patients may occur when a parent is carrying on an extramarital affair "in secret," but somehow everyone knows.[11] Important too (in both family and cultural style) is an official suppression of sexuality (and repression of the knowledge of sexuality), particularly in the female, coupled with a good deal of overexposure and overstimulation. The paradigm is the Victorian lady who fainted in the parlor while her husband made love to the maid on the back stairs.

Hysteria also seems to be related to the status ascribed to male and female in the family and in the culture. When the male is considered superior and the female second-rate, deformed, male and female social roles and sexual mores tend to differ sharply, and female sexuality is considered either nonexistent or an inferior form of male sexuality. Childbearing is the only raison-d'être of female sexuality. The male is permitted sexual outlets outside of marriage, while the female must be chaste before marriage and faithful afterward. Hysterical conversion, in particular, is more likely to be seen in social groups whose members are encouraged to express open dependency and helplessness. In most cultures, these groups would consist of women and children, but each culture has its own subgroups (the poor, for example) to which this observation is applicable.[12]

It should be kept in mind that these statements, particularly those linking social factors to individual cases of hysteria, now have the status of suggestive hypotheses, with some empirical confirmation, but require much more extensive and detailed evidence before they can be accepted as facts. Such formulations, however, are useful in orienting ourselves as we explore the significance of hysteria in classical Greek culture.

Hysteria in Greek Medicine

The attention given hysteria by Greek writers is a good indication of important strains and conflicts in Greek society, in particular those involving male-female relationships and the status assigned to male and female sexuality. A hysterical symptom, for a Greek woman, permitted a safe expression of certain unmet needs, and the relationship with the doctor allowed a form of gratification that would otherwise be forbidden. The doctor who treated such a woman was permitted certain muted sexual gratifications while simultaneously preserving culturally held beliefs that ignored female sexuality, unless it was aimed at producing heirs. Thus the hysterical symptom and the doctor's treatment might serve a social-regulatory function.

Hippocrates' *Diseases of Women* illustrates an explicitly hysterical disease:[13]

If a woman suddenly becomes voiceless you will find her legs cold, as well as the knees and the hands. And if you then palpate the uterus, it is not in its proper place; her heart palpitates, she gnashes her teeth, there is copious sweat, and all the other features characteristic of those who suffer from the "sacred disease" [epilepsy], and they do all sorts of unheard-of things.[14]

The uterus, traveling far and wide, caused trouble wherever it lodged, either by pressure or by blocking a passage. Respiratory difficulty, *globus hystericus,* pressure in the loin, headache, and drowsiness could all be caused by the wandering uterus. Such illnesses were to be found primarily in women who did not engage in intercourse, and one theory stated that the uterus so deprived would dry up, lose weight, and rise in search of moisture. Retained menses somehow could cause similar effects and had a similar cause. The condition described—loss of voice, coldness, sweating, palpitations, gnashing of teeth—resembled but differed from epilepsy. The anatomical difficulties of the theory of uterine migration were ignored, doubtless partly because of ignorance of human anatomy. At least as important was a *need to be ignorant* of the insides of the female body, particularly the details of the generative system.[15]

Treatments varied with symptoms, but commonly involved bandaging (to prevent further ascension of the uterus), orally administered medicaments (wine, for example), fetid fumigations to the nose (to repel the ascended uterus), and aromatic fumigations inserted in the vagina (to attract the wandering uterus back to its proper place). Marriage (or remarriage), intercourse, and procreation were prescribed for victims who were virgins or widows.

Mental derangements related to these physical symptoms are most vividly described in the case of virgins. From our perspective, they lie on the border between hysteria and melancholia.[16] The treatise *The Sickness of Virgins* describes a group of conditions caused by the retention of menstrual blood.[17] In these cases retained menstrual blood presses on heart and diaphragm, thereby causing mental symptoms. (Here the heart is considered the seat of mental activity.) Such women are susceptible to delusional thinking (*paraphrosunē*) and raving madness (*mania*), have suicidal thoughts, and may actually hang or drown themselves. If they recover, they falsely ascribe the recovery to Artemis and dedicate their finest clothes to her. The physician, however, asserts that the true cause of the cure is the removal of any hindrance to menstruation. He advises such women to marry and become pregnant to ensure against relapse. Married women afflicted by the disease are likely to have been hitherto barren.

Can we rule out the possibility that a potpourri of organic conditions is being described rather than a psychogenic condition? We simply cannot be certain. Are these conditions the same ones we call hysterical conversion? It seems likely. From the time of Hippocrates to the present, physicians have recognized a condition more frequently found in women than in men, particularly in women who are sexually deprived which mimics every variety of known physical illness, and which the society and the doctor and the patient consider an illness. The remedies explicitly or symbolically entail sexual gratification. Hysteria, as a culturally sanctioned dumb show in which patient, doctor, and family all participate, has a continuous history from antiquity to the present.

Along with the persistence of hysterical conversion, we can find certain rather durable beliefs about male and female sexuality, about copulation and birth. These myths can appear as popular beliefs, as biological and medical theories stated in the scientific vocabulary of each age, and as conscious and unconscious fantasies in hysterical men and women. They enshrine the conviction that women are inferior to men, and that female sexuality is an inferior or derivative form of male sexuality (the belief that women are castrated men, for example, or that the clitoris is a *forme fruste* of the penis).[18] Hysterical symptoms are, in effect, mimetic enactments of such fantasies, with the woman herself taking simultaneously or alternately both male and female roles.

The Status of Women in Greek Society

A psychodynamic understanding of hysteria allows us to pick out certain themes in Greek culture that show that Greek hysterical afflictions, with their supposed etiologies and treatments, were well suited to reflect conflicts and tensions within Greek culture. The Greek myths, especially as embodied in Homer, at first seem to express a free acceptance of human sexuality. Lust, conjugal affection, and sexual intercourse are freely acknowledged and deemed important. The poets tell of the sexual lives of both gods and heroes without prurience or puritanism. If anything, a certain amount of awe attends the power of the sexual urge, as exemplified by the attitudes toward Helen in both the *Iliad* and the *Odyssey*. Her attraction to Paris, and his to her, are the work of the gods. The aged Priam (whose city is endangered and whose sons are being killed because of the passion of Helen and Paris) can still admire Helen's beauty and remark calmly that it is no wonder that mortal men should fight over her (*Iliad,* 3.156–60). Demodocus' song (*Odyssey,* 8.266–366) tells of the adulterous relationship of Aphrodite and Ares. When they are caught by Hephaestus, Aphrodite's husband, great mirth breaks out among the gods as they see the pair caught naked in Hephaestus' net. There is embarrassment and recompense, to be sure, but also laughter. Yet even in the Homeric epics, where no anxiety accompanies sexuality, a double standard clearly prevails. Zeus can have his dalliances, but not Hera. Agamemnon may have concubines, but Clytemnestra is supposed to await chastely the return of her husband over ten long years. Odysseus may sleep with any number of goddesses (a year with Circe and seven with Calypso), but Penelope cannot spend a night with one of her suitors.

When we examine what we know of Greek life in the fifth century B.C., we find that public sexuality tends to mean male sexuality.[19] Some of its expressions in vase paintings and literature are quite striking. In the Dionysiac processions that preceded dramatic festivals, the participants carried giant phalluses, much like the floats in Macy's Thanksgiving Day parade. Quite common, perhaps in the courtyard of every household, was the "herm," a head of Hermes on a rectangular column with a huge erection (only head and genitals are represented). The leather phallus was a stock item in Greek comedy.

However much an individual Greek husband, father, brother, or son may have loved and respected a woman, men were clearly accorded superior legal status.[20] Only sons inherited (they were obligated to provide dowries for their sisters); if a man left only female

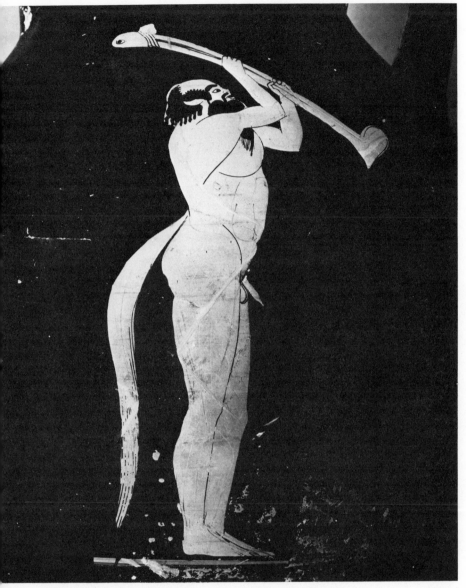

Phallic exuberance in Greek art. The eye on the head of the phallus, quite common in erotic art, suggests a view of the penis as a living creature.

Detail of red-figured amphora by the Flying Angel Painter, fifth century B.C. Courtesy Museum of Fine Arts, Boston.

heirs, some male relative had to marry one of the daughters and supervise the inheritance. In the upper classes, sons were better educated and perhaps even better fed than daughters. A married couple was more likely to live with the husband's family than with the wife's. Single men had sexual freedom, and they lost little of it when they married; women, married or not, had none. Women, especially of the upper class, were often confined to the house and were not permitted to appear unchaperoned in public.

Though the evidence is not clear for the fifth century, we know that in the fourth century female infanticide was practiced, usually by exposure.[21] Female infanticide may well have provided a means of population control. Daughters were not valued and were expensive to rear because they required dowries at marriage. Jokes were made about brothels' being staffed by the daughters of even the best households—that is, the prostitutes included girls who had been exposed and rescued as infants. Incidentally, female prostitution was well established in Athens, and prostitutes were readily available to those who could pay.

There are subtle indications of male disdain and fear of mature female sexuality. Representations of heterosexual intercourse, though frequent in vase paintings, are usually included in scenes of banquets and orgies. Or one sees a man having intercourse from the rear with a boyish-looking woman, and it is difficult to be sure whether the penis is in the rectum or the vagina.[22] Greek women depilated their axillary and pubic hair to please their men, probably an indication of male dislike for indications of adult female sexuality. More striking is the age discrepancy between male and female at marriage—typically girls were in early adolescence, fourteen or so, while the men were thirty. Thus the man had a bride who was sexually mature but in other ways barely out of childhood. The usual pattern was for the young couple to establish their marriage within the groom's family, and thus the bride was placed in an uncomfortable situation, without the daily support of her mother and female relatives.

Philip Slater has developed the most detailed argument to date about the Greek male's fear of the female and of female sexuality.[23] He noted, as have others, that for the Greeks, bogeywomen were more prominent than bogeymen. The loveliness of the Muses was counterpoised by the murderousness of the Harpies, Sirens, Sphinxes, and snake-haired Furies. Psychoanalytic understanding of such monsters suggests that they embody one of the small child's views of the mother—powerful, dangerous, and equipped with both breasts and penis; in short, the phallic mother.

Mythology suggests that men considered the female sexual drive more powerful and more dangerous than the male.[24] This awe, if my

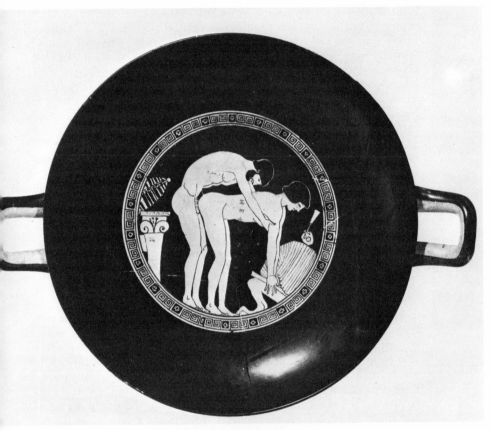

Love scene. The captions say: "The girl is beautiful" and "Hold still!"
Interior of Attic red-figured kylix, fifth century B.C. Courtesy Museum of
Fine Arts, Boston.

construction is correct, was dealt with by social restrictions and, to a certain extent, by the splitting of women into two classes, those who were wives and those who were sexual objects.[25]

Needless to say, vocational possibilities for women were distinctly limited. Management of the household was the task of upper-class women, and lower-class women, as everywhere, had to participate actively in the tasks necessary to eke out a living. The seclusion of women was an upper-class luxury: lower-class women, lacking slaves and servants, had to go out to buy and sell, to barter their labor, and to run the family errands. Even in myth and fantasy the growing girl had no available model of a woman who could function independently of men. Medea complains about the difficult role of the woman but offers no constructive solution, even for herself (such as making her own living as an independent witch doctor).[26] We know of few, if any, women philosophers or artists in the fifth and fourth centuries.[27]

Of course, this may be a somewhat skewed view of the overall status of women. It would take many more data than we now have to get a balanced picture of the way women managed, survived, and perhaps at times flourished. In some ways Athenian society accorded more legal rights to women than did other cultures. Women had rights of divorce seemingly equal to those of men. Athenian women of all classes probably attended the great tragic performances, so that though their lives were more restricted than men's, they had some access to the great art and literature around them.

The other sort of information we lack about the life of women relates to the support and intimacy they received from other women. It is of course extremely difficult to understand such a crucial aspect of a culture's life as male-female relations without having the opportunity to live in and with the members of that culture. Anthropological perspectives gained in cross-cultural studies of sex-role differentiation are helpful and suggestive. Analyses of themes in literature and myth which reveal major points of stress and strain in the culture are also of use. But in the absence of knowledge of the roles played by love and affection in the day-to-day life of the members of the culture, we cannot be sure we have a balanced picture of the situation. It might have been far worse or far better than we imagine, though I am inclined to speculate that our current modes of analysis highlight the stresses and conflicts and slight the sources of pleasure and gratification that may be more difficult to observe. Discord tends to be noisy, while the forces that bind men and women together may well operate silently.[28]

It is not possible to discuss the position of women in classical Greece without considering the question of Greek male homosexuality. (We have virtually no reliable information on female homosexuality in classical times, other than that it existed and was acknowledged to exist.) A number of scholars have written on the social and educational contexts of male homosexuality in some detail.[29] Again, we must keep in mind that the composite picture that emerges from the writings of these authors (particularly Slater) tends to emphasize points of strain in the culture and may well minimize stabilizing and even positive features of functioning between the sexes and between the generations.

Nevertheless, we must recognize that the Greek male was far more valued than the female. Since descent was recognized only through males, the immortality of the parents, as it were, depended on having sons to continue the family line. The female, both feared and devalued by the male, had several options in the rearing of her male children. Her son was an object for displacement of rage against her husband and father, and he was her great hope, a surrogate phallus that alone could give her pride and prestige. At the same time, relations between men were characterized by marked competitive, agonistic, and phallic-narcissistic attitudes. This competitiveness could extend to the relations between father and son if they were to become intensely involved with each other. Fathers played a relatively minor role in the rearing of young children. (Male slaves did play an important part in the later rearing of boys, possibly during the latency age.) Father-son relations presumably were characterized by idealization of the father, with a de facto distance and perhaps formality, and, given the intense phallic-competitive atmosphere, a large measure of castration anxiety. Greek boys must have found little opportunity to experience casual, tension-free encounters with girls, particularly after puberty.

The initiation into sexuality and manhood often came about through a homosexual relationship with an older man, which might serve multiple purposes: the educational function of indoctrinating the youth into the roles and duties of an adult male; provision of a form of male intimacy perhaps lacking in the father-son relationship; and deflection of aggression from the father. The Spartan aristocratic culture of the fifth and fourth centuries institutionalized homosexuality as a formal part of the education and rearing of the adolescent boy. In Athens the homosexual relationship was not a formal institution. Indeed, Athens had laws against homosexual relations between older men and adolescent boys which were not sanctioned by the boy's family. But a sensual and erotic homosexuality was not only common in Athens but quite public.

Several points must be made here: (1) Homosexuality as practiced in Sparta and Athens was not incompatible with heterosexuality and marriage. On the contrary, in a very real sense homosexual behavior was a preparation for manhood, including marriage and the procreation of children. Both cities imposed social and financial penalties on men who did not marry.[30] (2) "Educational" homosexuality was built around the belief and the fantasy that the virtue and strength of the older man was passed on through his semen into the anus of the young boy. The *arete* of the man was in the semen.[31] (3) As in all things Greek, modesty and moderation were expected in homosexual behavior. There were rules for courting and for being courted. Homosexual relationships that were too obvious or too promiscuous were ridiculed.[32] (4) In the upper classes (where most of the literature was written) male homosexuality was tied to civic education and the exclusion of women from public and educational life. The practice was associated with fear and disdain of women.

The male sexual function, then, was considered a prop of the culture as a whole and not just a source of pleasure or procreation, though procreation (especially of sons) was accorded immense importance.

Several factors seem to have combined, then, to make hysterical conversion a "sensible" and plausible condition for women, and particularly for virgins and widows: (1) an overevaluation of male sexuality associated with male fear of mature female sexuality; (2) public expression of phallic sexuality associated with a great deal of stimulation (or overstimulation) of sexual desire; (3) official suppression of female sexual activity outside of marriage (or prostitution), perhaps associated for individual women with their own repression of sexual knowledge and desire; (4) the fact that a woman's social position and self-esteem depended very heavily on having a husband; (5) the need for a socially acceptable means of expressing suppressed desire and protest against social oppression: when these needs were expressed through a physical condition, especially in the form of an illness, doctor, patient, and family alike could deny its unconscious meanings.

What can we say, however speculatively, about the intrapsychic life of the woman in Athenian society? Undoubtedly she internalized the cultural split between female as legitimate wife and female as sexual object. Similarly, she must have internalized the male attitudes about the dangers of female sexuality, as well as the overvaluation of the phallus. Thus she suffered from an internal conflict based on several contradictory fantasy representations of what it is to be a woman. The woman who fell ill with hysteria was one who temporarily failed to integrate these conflicting self-images and who expressed the conflict in a physical symptom. All of these factors, of course, impinge on the growing girl as well as the grown woman. The degree to which her parents, particularly her mother, had comfortably integrated these inner contradictions would undoubtedly influence the degree to which the girl could master them. While such a hypothesis does not pretend to be a comprehensive explanation of conversion hysteria, it does provide a framework that may help to explain the choice of neurosis and symptoms.[33]

Hysterical conversion may well be a kind of illness that includes its own cure. That is, the illness is only half of a drama designed to say something about the plight of the woman and her feelings toward men. The doctor may well have played an important transference role. Unconsciously he may have represented the wished-for good father who understood and recognized the daughter's sexual and social needs. We know well that in modern cases when treatment does not work and the doctor's efforts are frustrated (these are not written up as readily as the successes), an unconscious element of revenge against men, and in particular against male relatives, plays a role.[34] When the treatment succeeded, the Greek doctor not only may have provided some release from a strict superego and from social disapproval but may also have influenced male relatives to facilitate marriage or remarriage for the afflicted woman. The doctor, for a variety of reasons, was well placed to be seen as a caring and loving father. For one thing, as we can glean from the medical literature on problems of women, he was interested in helping barren women conceive, and even offered suggestions on how to increase the chance of having a male child.[35] In all, the doctor may well have been the individual best suited to mediate the social and intrapsychic conflicts of the afflicted woman.

For the moment, we shall leave the disease of the wandering uterus and turn to the disease of the wandering woman—the group orgiastic rites described in Euripides' *Bacchae*—to explore the connection between hysteria in the individual woman and the kind of group hysteria involved in women's ritual worship of Dionysus.

Group Hysteria: Ecstatic Possession and Bacchic Frenzy

Much has been written about the relationships between the social status of women in various cultures, including the Greek, and ritualized forms of possession, especially group possession. Indeed, the group and the individual phenomena seem so obviously cut from the same cloth that we must exert some effort to pinpoint the nature of their interrelationships.

First, the bodily behavior of an individual woman having a hysterical seizure is remarkably similar to that of women involved in some group ecstatic or semiorgiastic experience. The disheveled hair, the head tossed back, the eyes rolling, the body arched and tense or writhing, the sudden cessation and quiet—these can be found in the graphic accounts of Charcot's ward at the Salpetrière, in Attic vase paintings of Maenads, and in descriptions of contemporary Haitian voodoo rituals. It is indeed likely that these body movements express a similiar meaning in each case: sexual excitement and ecstasy, childbirth, yearning for liberation from restraint, and striving toward fusion with powerful fantasy figures.

The inner experience of an individual having a seizure is also remarkably similar to that of a member of an ecstatic group—the feeling that what is taking place is out of one's control. In states of ecstatic possession, tension gradually builds to the point where the god takes over and the person seems under his control; in the individual's seizure, the onset is usually more sudden, with varying degrees of amnesia for the experience and its antecedents. The term that best applies to both experiences is "dissociation." The woman in this special state is dissociated from her usual self, as if under the control of someone else. From a psychodynamic viewpoint, the behavior is disowned by the person. A demonstrable continuum exists from the small-scale motivated ignorance of the hysterical character, or the person with a minor hysterical conversion syndrome, to the dissociated state of a person in a fugue, a massive amnesia, or a state of possession.

Students of the phenomena of group ecstatic possession and the associated ritual healing rites, notably I. M. Lewis, have outlined some of the social functions of these states. E. R. Dodds, citing several cases of dancing mania, has pointed to the impressive similarities between the Dionysiac rituals described in the *Bacchae* and other group ecstatic experiences around the world.[36] These group experiences seem to serve as expressions of protest and of wishes for liberation by oppressed groups. Around the world, the most commonly oppressed group is women, and ecstatic phenomena are likely to be found in cultures in which sex roles are strictly differentiated, with men clearly dominant. Group rites can involve men as well as women, particularly groups of men who are in marginal and subservient positions in the culture. There is no doubt that these experiences not only provide release but give importance and dignity to otherwise disenfranchised groups. In many rituals the oppressed groups take on (in symbolic or more literal form) some of the attributes of the dominant group. The women portrayed in the *Bacchae* take on male functions and male powers, in particular those of warriors. They leave their looms and their children, take up arms, and defeat men. Pentheus threatens to capture all the Asiatic Bacchantes and put them to work at domestic tasks. They carry the thyrsus, which symbolizes the disembodied phallus.

Anthropologists and students of cross-cultural psychiatry are fa-

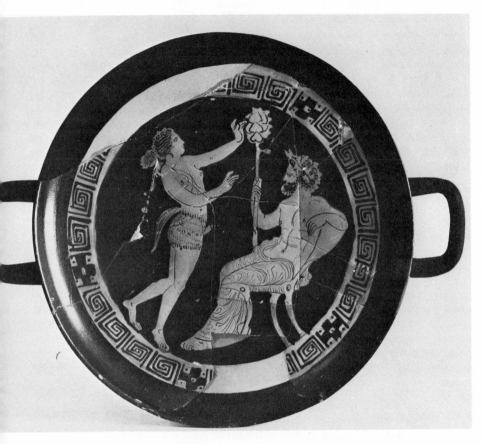

A maenad with tail and penis, wearing a skin. This unique scene seems to be a concrete representation of the fantasy of the maenad as phallic woman. Interior of Attic red–figured kylix, early fourth century B.C. American School of Classical Studies at Athens, Corinth Excavation.

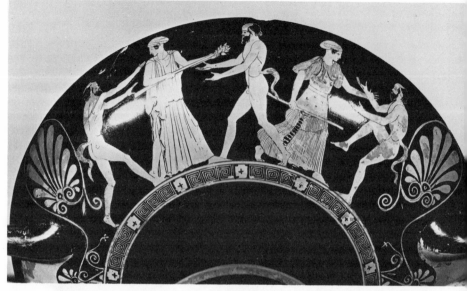

Maenads fending off satyrs with their thyrsi. The thyrsus is the female counterpart of the phallus.

Exterior of Attic red-figured kylix, fifth century B.C. Courtesy Museum of Fine Arts, Boston.

miliar with hysterical illnesses that occur only in specific cultures and which are culturally defined as possession by a god or spirit. The healing of this culture-specific illness takes place in a group setting, either a cult group or a group of friends and relatives, while the healer (or shaman) performs the dramatic ritual. The ritual is intended either to exorcise the spirit or to persuade him to dwell peacefully and responsibly within the person. The ritual often involves a wedding between the afflicted woman and the spirit, who then agrees, as it were, to provide protection and good fortune for her. In fact, the marriage between the woman and her spirit husband is sometimes formalized in a document, and the woman agrees to stay away from her human husband on certain days of the week when her spirit husband will consort with her.[37]

A particularly vivid example of this kind of attack and the associated ritual healing is supplied by Grace Harris in her description of *saka*, a possession hysteria in women in an East African tribe.[38] These women at first show signs of a general restlessness or anxiety, and then suddenly begin the characteristic convulsive movements. The shoulders shake rapidly while the head moves rhythmically from side to side. Often the eyes are closed and the face is expressionless, and the woman seemingly loses consciousness. Some women perform monotonous repetitive acts, while others repeat strange sounds that mimic foreign words. The people of the tribe consider this a disease of "the heart" which involves abnormal urges and cravings as well as fears. One disease related to *saka* is a form of kleptomania. *Saka* is an illness of "wanting and wanting." The attacks are frequently triggered by a desire for something belonging to the victim's husband or something (usually requiring cash) that he has been unwilling or unable to procure for her. The healing takes place at a public or semipublic ritual, with other women present, and involves dance and drums. The spirit that allegedly possesses the woman demands that she be given the objects she craves, often items associated with the activities of men. During the ritual the woman wears male garb and carries a man's walking stick. The items that the husband must provide seem unexotic but are important to her: cigarettes, bananas (from the foreign-owned plantations where the men work), manufactured cloth. Recovery from the illness is usually rapid if the husband provides these items, and harmony seems to be restored. In this culture, boundaries between the roles of men and women are sharply demarcated. Men work outside the village and have cash to spend. Women have very limited rights and limited scope in dealing with land and cattle, the mainstays of the tribal life. They cannot inherit or dispose of land or cattle without their husbands' consent.

The sickness and its cure belong to the realm of complex social rituals that serve several functions, though they do not always serve all of them equally well.[39] The ritual states a problem, provides a pathway of solution, and holds up a model of resolution that will be of benefit to the community at large.

In sum, we have good reason to believe that both the hysteria described in Greek literature and the group ecstasy of the Dionysiac rituals served to express and potentially to redress a certain imbalance in the relationships between men and women. Both served as a socially contained (more or less) and socially acceptable way of presenting, negotiating, and readjusting serious disturbances in intrapsychic equilibrium.

We have no evidence that at the time Euripides' *Bacchae* was first performed (406 B.C.) Athenian women performed Dionysiac rituals—that is, acted as Maenads—at Athens. A Dionysiac ritual was performed elsewhere in Greece, and delegations of women from the various Greek cities held a biennial festival at Delphi. It is unlikely that that festival included the more gory aspects of Maenadism, the *sparagmos* and *omophagia* (tearing apart and eating raw) of an animal or human. (Dionysus was worshiped in Athenian dramatic festivals and at various rustic Dionysia, but these rituals did not involve Maenad-

ism.) There are suggestions that the Bacchic rituals involving Maenads in other parts of the Greek world—notably Macedonia, where
Euripides wrote the *Bacchae*—were more orgiastic and primitive, and
that animals were indeed torn apart and eaten raw. Tradition has it
that Olympias, the mother of Alexander the Great, was very much
involved in the sort of rituals described in the *Bacchae*.[40]

Vase paintings from the second half of the fifth century and later
show Maenads tearing animals apart or carrying their torn members.
We do not know to what extent these paintings were intended to
illustrate either the myth of Dionysus or recent enactment of the
ritual. Thus, while the raw ritual was not to be found at Athens,
awareness of it was not far from the consciousness of Athenians who
witnessed the *Bacchae*.

In the last decade of the fifth century, several gods associated with
orgiastic worship were imported to Athens. We do not know details
of their rituals as practiced at Athens, or for which sex they were
intended, but such rituals clearly represented a push toward more
orgiastic forms of worship. We hear of ritual ecstatic groups called
Corybantes, who seemed to have played a role in healing emotional
distress, including psychosis.[41] These rituals involved dancing accompanied by flute (for the Greeks, an orgiastic instrument) and kettle-
drum. Men particpated. Other kinds of cult worship, centering
around various gods and goddesses (Rhea, Hecate, Pan), served as
forms of healing for particular afflictions. Again, details are few. Plato
suggests a connection between Corybantic and Bacchic rhythms and
the rocking and singing by which mothers put crying children to sleep
(*Laws*, 790B–90C). The ritual may have served as a fantasy reparation
of an early mother-child disruption.

In Aristophanes' *Wasps*, Philocleon, the old man who suffered
from jury mania, was taken to the Corybantes in an attempt to cure
his madness. I. M. Lewis has suggested that ecstatic possession rituals (peripheral possession) are important for disenfranchised groups,
groups peripheral to the center of power. Philocleon seems to have
belonged to a group (older men of a class that did not have considerable wealth) that relied on jury service as a means of access to
power as well as money (ll. 548–58 and 578). Aristophanes portrays
the jury service as a form of peripheral possession. One avenue of
cure for this "disease" is a more formalized ecstatic possession
group, the Corybantes.

There certainly is reason to believe that Dionysus was an egalitarian god, more accessible to all groups and all social classes than was,
for instance, Apollo. Women, as a disenfranchised class, would certainly be attracted to the worship of Dionysus.[42] Aristophanes' ridicule of Dionysus in *The Frogs* was motivated in part by a wish to

attack such feminist murmurings as are portrayed in some of his other plays (*Ecclesiazusae, Lysistrata,* and others) and in part by a wish to counter the relatively sympathetic portrayal of women found in Euripides' work.[43]

Dionysiac ritual and myth served some of the same purposes as hysterical illness and its treatment: both offered a way of expressing and redressing serious social and psychological imbalance between the sexes. Dionysus, a male god, understands the feelings and needs of women. In this sense, the god (in myth) and the cult leader (in reality) correspond to the physician in the treatment of the hysterical woman. The doctor who sympathetically listens, carefully examines abdomen and genitalia, inserts suppositories, and recommends intercourse is attuned to the inner needs and social dilemmas of his patient. The drama of Dionysiac ritual is paralleled by the quieter ritual of the doctor-patient relationship.

It is likely that as a means of expressing conflict and attempting to resolve it, hysteria served the needs of the sexually deprived woman while cultic ecstasy served the needs of the married woman with children. The Dionysiac rituals and myths seem to be capable of expressing rage and ambivalence toward children more directly than hysteria can express them. These last statements must of necessity remain conjectural. We simply have no information on the frequency of hysteria or the extent of women's participation in ecstatic ritual or the extent to which a woman might be subject to hysteria *and* participate in an ecstatic ritual.

Diseases of the Uterus in Greek Tragedy

Greek tragedy contains no women who are called hysterics, but the problems of two of its female characters, Phaedra and Hermione, are strikingly rendered in the quasi-physiological language of "women's troubles."[44]

In Euripides' *Hippolytus,* Phaedra suffers from a thwarted passion for a man forbidden to her—Hippolytus, her husband's son. Theseus, her husband, is absent, gone to consult an oracle. Theseus, of course, is a notorious womanizer, and Hippolytus is the offspring of one of his many dalliances. Phaedra has been agitated and has not eaten for three days; she wishes to die. The Chorus, trying to make sense of her illness (ll. 120–50), asks if she is possessed by one of the gods associated with madness and frenetic behavior. The question is in part diagnostic, for before an appropriate healing ritual can be chosen, one must know which god is the cause of the problem.

The Chorus continues to speculate on the causes of Phaedra's condition and focuses directly on the kinds of difficulties a woman might have: Has she heard that her husband is in another woman's bed? Or has some sailor brought bad news from Crete about her husband? The language of the whole passage is sexual, so that the "bad news" (usually taken to mean that Theseus has been killed) might even mean that he is coming home with another woman. Then follows a passage describing women's temperament. The meaning seems to be generally clear, but it is difficult to understand and translate precisely: "There loves to cohabit with an awkward temperament an ill and wretched helplessness involving pains and loss of good sense."[45]

Such lines ambiguously describe a blend of "women's troubles," pregnancy, and delivery. The Chorus sings of "a breeze through the womb," seemingly suggesting the notion of hysteria. Perhaps it is referring to a compound of hysteria and the melancholia described in the Hippocratic treatise *The Sickness of Virgins,* an illness caused by a uterine disturbance leading to madness and suicide.[46] Thus the poet connects madness, adultery, and diseases and distress of the female reproductive system. I believe he has also intuitively sensed something important about the role of mothers and mothering figures in the life of the hysterical woman, for the play is rich with nuances in its portrayal of the relationship between Phaedra and the nurse. The poet appears to have seen a connection between the disturbances of the woman's insides and the behavior of the man she loves. The wandering uterus is a response to the wandering husband.

In Euripides' *Andromache,* Hermione is the legitimate wife of Neoptolemus; Andromache is his concubine. Note the cast of characters: Hermione is the daughter of Helen of Troy; Neoptolemus is the son of Achilles, who was slain by Paris at the gates of Troy. Andromache is the enemy incarnate: she is the wife of Hector, the Trojan hero. At the capture of Troy, Neoptolemus killed Astyanax, the infant son of Hector and Andromache. The action of the play revolves around Hermione's insane jealously of Andromache, for Andromache has borne a son to Neoptolemus and Hermione is sterile. Neoptolemus is away (like Theseus) and Hermione intends to kill Andromache. Hermione accuses Andromache of using witchcraft and malignant drugs to seal her womb and make her sterile, thereby stealing her husband's affection. Andromache protests (ll. 31–37):

I'm persecuted cruelly. She is behind it, charging I've made her unable to conceive with secret drugs and dosings, made him hate her. Charging I want this house all to myself and mean to crowd her out of it, bed and all—a bed that from the first I never wanted and now reject for good.[47]

Both Andromache and the Chorus make it clear to Hermione that she has fallen out of favor with her husband not because of malignant drugs but because of malignant jealousy. Her husband does not love her, and, by implication, she is sterile because she is a bitch, not because she is bewitched.

The Chorus sings (ll. 181–82): "There is something very jealous in women by their nature, and it becomes especially ugly in the case of women who share a husband." And Andromache gives Hermione a stern lecture on the proper behavior of a good Greek wife (ll. 207– 228):

> It's not beauty but
> Fine qualities, my girl, that keep a husband. . . .
> A woman, even when married to a cad,
> Ought to be deferential, not a squabbler. . . .
> Well, we women are infected
> With a worse disease than men [jealousy],
> But try to conceal it.
> O dearest Hector, for your sake I even
> Welcomed your loves, when Cyprus sent you fumbling.
> I was wet nurse to your bastards many a time
> Only to make your life a little easier.
> And for such conduct he approved and loved me.
> But you!—you hardly dare to let your husband
> Out in the rain. He might get wet!

Hermione, then, claims to be afflicted with a uterine disorder. Her position is more paranoid than melancholic—her uterus is being poisoned from without. Thus the poet makes most explicit the intimate connection and interchangeability of somatic and interpersonal terms. To claim that something is wrong with your uterus (even that somebody else is causing the trouble) is to evade your real problem. It's your foul character and your failure to understand how a woman is supposed to play the game with a man, especially a man who goes off at a whim to another woman.

The rivalry between Andromache and Hermione illustrates the competition between women that is implicit in the inferior position of women in Greek culture. Given the fact that men are supposed to have the qualities and abilities that women are presumed to lack, the competition among women for what men have and can offer becomes correspondingly intense.

Plato's Account of the Wandering Uterus

These two examples from tragedy suggest that the equation of the unhappy uterus with the unhappy woman was available to the Greek consciousness, or at least to the intuition of Euripides. Plato makes far more explicit the link between hysteria and the desires and frustrations of women.

Plato's interpretation of hysteria is contained in his account of the creation of woman and of sexual desire (*Timaeus,* 90E–91E). The souls of wicked and cowardly men were reincarnated as the first women. The creation of woman necessitated sexual desire for procreation. The male organ is compared to a wild animal stung with lust. The uterus is likewise an animal that desires procreation.

When remaining unfruitful long beyond its proper time, [the uterus] gets discontented and angry, and wandering in every direction through the body, closes up the passages of the breath, and, by obstructing respiration, drives them to extremity, causing all variety of disease, until at length the desire and love of the man and the woman, bringing them together and as it were plucking the fruit from the tree, sow in the womb, as in a field, animals unseen by reason of their smallness and without form.[48]

Plato's account of hysteria begins to decode two messages in the Hippocratic theory. The first is that the frustrated uterus is really the frustrated woman. The second is that female sexual desire does not exist; it is procreation that women desire. The account is couched in more interpersonal language than we find in the medical discourse. Plato attributes desire and motivation to the womb, which obstructs the air passages if it does not get what it wants.

In the sixteenth century, Rabelais, praising Plato, invoked this passage in his caricature of women, describing the uterus as a dangerous place, wherein arise "humors, brackish, nitrous, boracious, acrid, mordant, shooting and bitterly tickling. . . . "[49] Rabelais seems more fearful than Plato of the woman's insides, though the fear is latent in Plato. Such a view of female sexuality becomes self-fulfilling as the hysterical woman arouses more immediate male fears by her strange behavior. Plato's rendering of the Hippocratic theories suggests that they were more valid as statements of psychology and sociology than of medicine and physiology.

Motivated Ignorance

Repression is a universal, readily available mechanism of defense in all human beings, both normal and disturbed. The term refers to a set of operations, by no means completely understood, whereby one can shut out, disregard, and be genuinely ignorant of things that are too uncomfortable or too painful to know. Freud used an aphorism of Nietzsche to illustrate the motivation for repression: " 'I did this,' says my Memory. 'I cannot have done this,' says my Pride and remains inexorable. In the end—Memory yields."[50] Hysteria is the condition par excellence of large-scale and continuous repression. It can properly be called the disease of motivated ignorance. The operation of repression in a woman with a hysterical character structure is seen in the following clinical report:

A married woman in her thirties, mother of three, was referred for psychiatric evaluation of an anxiety state, accompanied by diffuse somatic complaints for which no clear medical explanation could be found. In an initial interview the psychiatrist thought he discerned features of a hysterical character structure but could not make any clear sense of the presenting symptoms. Accordingly he arranged a second interview a week later, hoping to clarify the situation. A few days later, however, the patient, rather agitated, called from a phone booth to cancel the second interview "because I'm bleeding from down below and have to go to the hospital." The psychiatrist asked if she was bleeding from the vagina, rectum, or urinary tract. The woman said she didn't really know, but was on her way to the hospital. The psychiatrist later saw her in the hospital, on the gynecology ward. She had been pregnant, had not known it, and had had a spontaneous abortion. When asked about her seeming ignorance of the source of the bleeding, she explained, "You see, I really don't know much about these things. We never knew much about them as kids, since I was brought up on a farm in upstate New York." Further inquiry revealed that in fact, as one might expect, the farm was a place where knowledge of the sexual life of animals was readily available—hardly avoidable, in fact—and the human community was far from wanting in every variety of sexual activity. In short, there emerged a clear picture of a person who did not know and did not see because she did not want to know or see. She had been exposed to too much too soon and had dealt with the problem by defensive ignorance. She handled her current conflicts over motherhood and marriage by being "ignorant" of her pregnancy. In families and cultures that provide a good deal of overt sexual stimulation but forbid women to engage in sexual activity, conversion symptoms and hysterical ignorance are likely to flourish.

Fifth- and fourth-century Greek literature and tragedy frequently contain themes of ignorance and misidentification. *Oedipus Rex* is the play par excellence about unconsciously motivated ignorance and is a brilliant portrayal of the step-by-step process by which repression and ignorance are lifted. Recognition (*anagnorisis*) is prominent in many other plays, such as Euripides' *Iphigenia in Tauris*. For Socrates, "Know thyself" and "No man knowingly errs" are the cornerstones of the philosopher's mission. For Plato, knowledge is power, ignorance is despicable, and madness is a species of ignorance.

Surprisingly, Plato, the philosopher of truth, argues for certain socially useful forms of ignorance and lying. The most famous is the "noble lie" in the *Republic* (382A). That lie is clearly analogous to the motivated ignorance of hysteria, for it specifically attempts to conceal the basic facts of the relation between sexual intercourse and birth. Further, Plato's plan for his Republic (perhaps only for the guardians) insists that each person must be ignorant of the identity of his true biological parents. In the *Statesman* (271A) we find a myth that eliminates the place of women and intercourse in birth. The myth of Cadmus and the sown men who rising out of the earth, as well as the wish of Euripides' Hippolytus (ll. 616–39) that women were not needed for reproduction, also attest that such fantasies were widespread in Greek culture. What are we to make of Plato's lie? I alluded in Chapter 9 to an important aspect of the lie: its connection with Plato's analysis of the political turmoil of his day. Plato tried to find a way to reduce and finally eliminate all rivalry, possessiveness, and jealousy as a way of ensuring loyalty to the state. He located the origins of competitiveness and jealousy in the family constellation and in the sense of exclusive possession that attends marital sexuality. He then proposed to eliminate the family for the good of the state. Many other utopian schemes (as well as totalitarian states) have posited the need for radical rearrangement of conventional sexual mores.

Anthropology provides a relevant footnote. A few societies have allowed their members, at certain periods in their lives or under other carefully defined conditions, relatively promiscuous sexuality. The result in one group, the Muria of India, seems to be a great reduction of intense jealousy and of the deleterious social effects of excessive competition and possessiveness. The Muria have devised a common dormitory, the *ghotul,* which boys and girls enter between the ages of three and four and where they stay until they marry late in puberty. There they engage in open sexual activity and cultivate the art of sexual pleasure, but pairings are prohibited. According to the ethnographic report on this group, the Muria have been remarkably successful in maintaining a culture with a high level of individual happiness, strong marital fidelity, little competitiveness, great pleasure in sexuality, and a disciplined sense of social cooperation.[51] This culture seems to use the institution of the *ghotul* as a way of minimizing tensions between parents and children, and also between the sexes. (The Muria themselves see the institution as necessary to prevent children from witnessing the primal scene.)

Now Plato's scheme appears to play down not just sexuality but the importance of gender differences. Gender is no more important for guardians than for watchdogs; that is to say, it is relevant to breeding but to nothing else. It would seem that Plato, in his own way, was addressing the issues of conflict between men and women that were so important in Greek society. His scheme appears to have been an attempt to stabilize relations between the sexes, but his method relied heavily on a denial of sexuality. If this is true, to consider Plato merely a misogynist is to miss something important.[52] He may well have understood something central in the life of the Greeks, something that impinged on political life, and that something is the relatively degraded position of women. It is as if he had decided to put repression to good use for the suppression of rivalry in the body politic. His solution is, in a rather literal sense, perverse, since we know from psychodynamic studies that the clinical perversions (exhibitionism, fetishism, and so on) are enactments of fantasies that disclaim any differences between the sexes. In the unconscious fantasy of male perverts, women usually have penises; since there are no castrated creatures, there is no danger of castration. The man who seemed to divine (in the *Timaeus*) that hysteria has to do with the psycholgoy of women as well as with their physiology is also the man who proposed a radical social solution to the problem of inequality between men and women. If he seems to have thrown out the baby with the bath water and proposed a cure worse than the disease, we must still give him credit for his attempt to address a major source of friction in Greek culture.

We must take note of a certain paradox here. Though motivated ignorance is not hard to find in Greek literature, Greek society produced many individuals who did, in fact, dare to look.[53] The doctors who described hysteria and prescribed for it did look at female genitalia and whatever other parts of the sexual anatomy they could observe. In short, the prominence of the theme of knowledge versus ignorance in the products of Greek culture may also be a reflection of a relatively *successful* struggle to look and to see. *Oedipus Rex* ends in blinding, but the audience and playwright looked at incest, murder, and tragic horror, and came away the better for it. Hysteria in Greece might be considered only an index of significant social stresses. But Greek efforts to understand hysteria were part of a great creative ferment that led to a release from ignorance, thereby enriching the entire human race.

Greek Medical and Biological Theories of Conception

Fantasies about the nature of the male and female generative processes appear in Greek culture both as popular beliefs and as seemingly rational scientific theories.[54] The theories are embedded in a biological hierarchy, the "scale of nature," in which male is generally superior to female, and the male human occupies the highest place of all. Such a schema clearly mirrors the actual structure of Greek society.

Implicit in early Greek thought is the notion that brain, marrow, spinal cord, and semen are all one substance, the essence of life.[55] Because men have semen and women do not, they have a greater supply of brain. This view, held even before the brain was accorded primacy as the seat of thought, is implicit in the Homeric epics and seems to underlie the theories of Alcmaeon, the pre-Socratic philosopher. It finds explicit expression in Plato's *Timaeus,* where brain, marrow, and semen are all "seed," and "psyche" is seed or is in the seed. It underlies several passages in the Hippocratic corpus, including the curious discussion of the effeminacy of the Scythians (*Airs, Waters, Places*), which, according to Hippocrates, was caused by pressure on the testicles from excessive riding and the wearing of tight pants. The treatment was to bleed the veins behind the ears, as if a blood vessel ran between the head and the genitals. The herms, because they show only head and genitalia, similarly exemplify the fantasy that head and genitals together are the important life-giving organs.

Naturally, a man would not want to lose or waste this valuable substance. A hint of this concern is seen in Aristotle's discussion of semen as a nutritive substance that the body may need to draw upon, and his emphasis on exhaustion as the result of intercourse (*The Generation of Animals*, 725b).[56] One is reminded of Stanley Kubrick's film *Dr. Strangelove*, in which the paranoid colonel is obsessed with the fear that the Russians are trying to destroy his "precious bodily fluids."

It was widely held that when a child was conceived, the man contributed the vital life principle, psyche; the mother was merely a vessel.[57] This belief can be seen in Aeschylus' *Eumenides*. Apollo, in his debate with the Furies, argues for the primacy of male rights and of male power (ll. 658–66):

She who is called the child's mother is not its begetter, but the nurse of the newly sown conception. The begetter is the male, and she as a stranger for a stranger preserves the offspring, if no god blights its birth; and I shall offer you a proof of what I say. There can be a father without a mother; near at hand is the witness, the child of Olympian Zeus.[58]

The same view is enshrined in more sophisticated and more carefully argued form in Aristotle's theory of human reproduction. As elaborated in his great work *The Generation of Animals*, the male *sperma* (seminal ejaculate) contains the *gonē* (the begetting principle) and mingles with the female's menstrual residues. The male contributes sentient psyche and the female contributes matter. Aristotle did not subscribe to the right-left theory of male-female differentiation (that is, males are conceived and carried on the right side of the uterus, females on the left—the inferior—side), but held that the male is "hotter" and the female "colder." Heat causes more elaborate concoction and tends to yield males, while lack of heat tends to produce females. The determination of sex takes place after the embryo has begun to form and is associated with the formation of the heart, the source of heat. Aristotle is famous (nowadays infamous) for saying such things as "The female is as it were a deformed male" (*Generation of Animals*, 737a27–28) and "We should look upon the female state as being as it were a deformity, though one which occurs in the ordinary course of nature" (ibid., 775a16–17). Aristotle's observation is curiously deficient in regard to the female. Noteworthy is his view that the menstrual periods do not occur according to a rhythm peculiar to each woman but tend to occur when the moon is waning. Clearly Aristotle did not exercise here the same care he brought to bear in other observations of the natural world. We may be seeing a degree of male hysteria, a defensively motivated ignorance about female sexuality.

When we examine the writings on conception and reproduction in the Hippocratic corpus, we encounter a diversity of views. Predominant is the "pangenesis" view, a view that does not explicitly assert the superiority of the male's contribution to conception.[59] But, even in a work that argues that the stuff of the fetus is drawn equally from all parts of both mother and father (*On Generation*), the author emphasizes the special importance of brain and marrow—which of course were thought to be made of the same stuff as semen.[60] Moreover, the right-left theory is found scattered throughout the Hippocratic writings.[61] Thus, while the Hippocratic views seem to be more egalitarian than Aristotle's, they still show signs of a belief that the male's contribution to the embryo is greater than the female's.

Galen's views embody many older ones.[62] His work, produced in the second century A.D., was influential well into the eighteenth and early nineteenth centuries. Galen also believed hysteria to be a disease of the uterus, but he made some interesting modifications of the Hippocratic view.

Galen disagreed with Aristotle on the issue of female sperm. There *is* female semen, he stated, though it is inferior to the male's, and the male's contribution has more of the reproductive principle. Females are seen as imperfect males: the female sexual and generative organs are the inverse of the male, because they have less innate heat. Galen identified the ovaries, but considered them female testes, which manufactured female semen. He also held to the right-left theory. The right spermatic artery, which supplies blood to the right (male) side of the uterus, he observed, originates from the aorta and brings blood of fine quality. The left spermatic artery, however, he incorrectly asserts, arises near the kidney, and the blood it brings to the left (female) side of the uterus is more watery—that is, urinary.

Galen also talks of male hysteria, and posits retention of sperm (due to lack of intercourse) as the common cause of hysteria in both sexes. Thus the ascription of a major female contribution in reproduction—women have semen too—goes hand in hand with a more egalitarian distribution of hysteria.

Here is an example of Galen at work, as he tells of a widow's hysteria:

Following the warmth of the remedies and arising from the touch of the genital organs required by the treatment there followed twitching accompanied at the same time by pain and pleasure after which she emitted turbid and abundant sperm. From that time on she was freed of all the evil she felt. From all this it seems to me that the retention of sperm impregnated with evil essences had—in causing damage throughout the body—a much greater power than that of the retention of menses.[63]

Note the suggestion of an ejaculation-like phenomenon in the female, which was to be a recurrent theme in Victorian pornographic literature.[64] In psychoanaltyic terms, such a notion suggests an unconscious fantasy that the female has a hidden phallus. This fantasy serves as reassurance against male castration anxiety, by implying that there are really no penisless people.

Doctors of the Body, Doctors of the Soul

For the ancient Greeks, then, hysteria, like melancholia and other emotional disturbances, was a medical disorder, and it remained so for many centuries. What can we say of the assets and debits of the medical approach to mental disorders? The assets include simplicity, the potential for experimental and clinical confirmation or refutation, and a framework in which mental disturbances can be viewed by patient and doctor as natural phenomena not to be encumbered by guilt and shame. A medical model allows one to approach the patient who exhibits puzzling and frightening thinking and behavior, spend time with him, and learn more about him. The doctor need not take personally things the patient says or does, for it is "his sickness talking, not himself." Lastly, the model may recognize the fact that emotions obviously partake of both mind and body, and that to understand disturbances involving passions and strong feelings one must pay attention to both psyche and soma.

Among the debits are the converses of these propositions: the medical model can prove not merely simple but simpleminded; it may serve as a way of avoiding paying attention to important but upsetting psychological material emanating from the patient. Psychoanalysts have discovered that the doctor should, in a sense, take personally what the patient says and does, for if the doctor understands the nature of the patient's productions as transference, he may be able to illuminate dark corners of the patient's past and present behavior. Overemphasis on the role of the body may lead to premature closure on the task of understanding important and complex phenomena in the mental life and psychological makeup of the patient.

I believe, however, that many of the good features of the medical model can be borrowed and applied by therapists who are not physicians.[65] To a great extent, psychoanalysis has shown how a psychotherapist may adapt the clinical detachment of the physician for psychotherapeutic purposes. The good physician is not uninterested but disinterested. Clinical medical practice also provides an example of responsible caring for the patient, a kind of caring that is the sine qua non of a genuine psychotherapeutic relationship. It is possible to be scientific in one's approach to problems of the human heart without necessarily being a scientist. The physician of the soul need not literally be a physician. The Hippocratic oath laid down a set of ideals for physicianly responsibility which placed the welfare of the patient above all else. Those ideals are available as a model for all who would undertake to alleviate the suffering of another human being.

One gets little sense of a rivalry, let alone an incompatibility, between medical and psychological or philosophical frameworks in Greek classical antiquity. They seemed to coexist peaceably, albeit often in separate spheres. Rivalry clearly existed between groups of physicians and between physicians and others who claimed to be healers. We do not, however, hear of tragedians denouncing the views of the doctors on hysteria or vice versa. As far as we can tell, no one protested when Phaedra was said to have suffered from a drafty womb rather than an illicit desire for the son of her wandering husband.

A few aspects of this apparent lack of competition are worth consideration. First, in later antiquity—that is, in late Hellenistic times and the early centuries of our era—doctors and philosophers do in fact seem to have felt themselves to be rivals in prescribing the way a person should live.[66] When the doctors began to make claims of promoting happiness rather than merely curing illness, they entered the moral marketplace of the philosophers.

Second, with the rise of Christianity, with its ideals of healing through faith and its denigration of the claims of the body, a new rivalry emerged between doctors of the body and doctors of the soul. Christ's healing of the possessed madman and expulsion of the demon (Mark 5:9) became an appealing model for the healers of both mind and body. How and why Christianity became associated with a greater degree of separation of mind and body are important questions, but consideration of them would take us too far afield. The role of new concepts of guilt and sin, the renunciation of sexual desire, belief in an afterlife, and questions about the place of Christians in the social order of the ancient world are among the factors that would have to be taken into account.

Third, we must consider the possible role played by the limitations in detailed knowledge of both mind and body in early classical antiquity. The fund of knowledge about anatomy and physiology was much larger and more secure in the first two centuries A.D. than it had been in the fifth or even the fourth century B.C. By the second century B.C. the nerves, both peripheral and cranial, had been discovered and their functions defined. Earlier theories about the transmission of information from brain or heart to body were totally inadequate.[67] Similarly, philosophy of mind had increased in complexity and detail and had become a more specialized field. Though the ideal of a broadly educated man, including a broadly educated physician, persisted until the end of antiquity, it does seem that the physician was pressed to master more and more specialized knowledge about both mind and body. In this regard, however, we still see relatively little competition, though the philosophers often borrowed and leaned upon current medical theories to supplement and illustrate their positions.

Perhaps we can best understand the relative lack of mind-body competition by referring to the notion of teleology, which was so important in ancient biology and medicine. From Plato through Aristotle to Galen, the notion that the body and its parts were created with a certain end (*telos*) in mind was axiomatic; that is, the creator, whether gods or God or some other intelligent agency, created according to a plan.[68] The ancients posited a mind (or purpose) in the body, saw a mind at work in the body, and so asserted the link between mind and body.

Perhaps even more fundamental was a certain sense of awe and reverence for the order of nature. A sense of beauty and worship of the beautiful pervaded Greek antiquity, and beauty encompassed bodies, minds, geometric shapes, and arrangements of the parts of animals. We are heirs to a greater split between mind and body than our Greek forebears. As we struggle to reconcile and synthesize the two in many areas of life, including our approach to mental illness, we have tended to place our hopes for the reunion of mind and body in the credo of science and scientific inquiry. Science may well succeed for us in this task. Perhaps, however, we might pause from time to time to recall what the Greeks called *to kalon,* the beautiful, and try to recapture something of the quiet ease and charm with which the Greeks experienced an indissoluble unity of the beauty of the mind and the beauty of the body.

V

MODELS OF
THERAPY

14

The Psychoanalytic and
Social Psychiatric Models

1st Gent: Our deeds are fetters that we forge ourselves.
2d Gent: Ay, truly: but I think it is the world that brings the iron.
——Shakespeare, *Two Gentlemen of Verona*

With hysteria, my analysis of ancient models of mental illness is complete. My formulations regarding hysteria, however, have left one important question unasked: How does one go about treating this condition? What is proper therapy for a condition that involves a complex of individual psychological and social psychological factors? If medical treatment does not directly address the underlying issues, what form of therapy does? Should every hysterical woman be psychoanalyzed? Is society itself in need of "treatment"? Would legal, political, and economic action that altered the formal relationships between men and women eliminate hysteria? How does a person achieve enough distance from his own culture to diagnose a widespread cultural malaise and devise a method to treat it? All of these issues bring us back to the initial problem posed in this book: What is a psychiatrist? What does he do that cures?

The Psychoanalytic Model

Let us begin by defining psychotherapy, a generic term for verbal therapies, and then proceed to characterize psychoanalysis and psychoanalytic therapy.[1] Psychotherapy is a socially defined helping relationship between two people, one of whom is designated as the psychotherapist and the other as the person seeking help for emotional distress. The explicit means by which this process is carried on is dialogue, in which it is agreed that emotions and thoughts relevant to the patient's distress will be discussed. The psychotherapist is a professional, or at least has societal sanction for his work, and usually receives some form of recompense. He has received specialized training in his craft and enjoys the prestige such training brings him. He is supposed to work primarily for the good of the patient. He is bound by ethical rules of conduct to avoid all exploitation of the patient. The patient, for his part, expects a sympathetic and informed listener and some sort of guidance as to how he is to behave while with the therapist. The dialogue takes place over a period of time, in the course of which a relationship develops between patient and therapist. The patient is responsible for carrying on his part of the dialogue and must cooperate in the tasks of the treatment.

The therapist's chief contribution to the dialogue takes the form of comments that help to clarify and organize the patient's problems. It is assumed that, while the major form of communication is verbal, important messages may be communicated by nonverbal means, such as gestures and intonations of voice.

Schools and versions of psychotherapy differ, often quite dramatically, in what they assert to be the proper content and nature of the dialogue. They also differ in respect to the theory that informs and shapes the therapeutic procedure (or that at least is consonant with the procedure). Psychoanalytic therapy (and psychoanalysis) of the variety associated closely with the work of Freud emphasizes that the content of the dialogue should be the patient's honest reports of all thoughts, feelings, memories, images, dreams, and bodily sensations. He is to report them as he experiences them, whether they relate to past, present, or future; those that pertain to the relationship between patient and therapist are especially important. Jungian, Adlerian, Sullivanian, existential, and other modes of psychotherapy have their own conceptions of what is central, what is relevant, what must be reported, and what the therapist must interpret.[2]

The Assumptions of Psychoanalysis

Psychoanalysis and psychoanalytic therapy are guided by a number of theoretical assumptions. I am using the term "psychoanalytic model" to refer to this set of assumptions and the associated therapeutic methods.

It is assumed that an unconscious level of mental functioning exists (in both patient and analyst) and that the nature and content of that thinking must be elucidated. As a corollary, it is also assumed that the major sources of emotional difficulty stem from unconscious wishes and motives that appear in disguised and distorted forms. It is the task of the therapist to help the patient to remove the disguise, to learn about the motives for disguise, and to understand the modes of disguise and self-deception he habitually uses (some of these modes are called mechanisms of defense). One analyst has in fact defined psychoanalysis as "the systematic study of self-deception."

Another important assumption is that the childhood of the adult patient has played a powerful role in the shaping of his current behavior and often exerts its influence in ways that are outside his awareness. Figuratively the adult patient views the world through a set of lenses that systematically color and distort personal and social reality. He is not aware that he has these lenses. Nor is he aware that if reality does not conform to his expectations, he goes to considerable lengths to find people who will confirm them and conform to them. Other people are often unwitting actors in a repetitive drama staged by the patient. These lenses are, as it were, the internalized representations of early childhood relationships.

The nature of these internalized relationships is gradually revealed through a conjoint scrutiny of the person's life history, including his current relationships. The effect of these internal representations on the patient's interaction with the therapist is what is meant by "transference." The patient, in the intensity of the therapeutic relationship, will reexperience earlier relationships, with the therapist playing the parts of the principal figures in the patient's past. If therapy is to succeed, the transference must be understood and interpreted, not merely developed and experienced.

It is a commonplace that the goal of psychoanalytic therapy is change by means of understanding or insight. Insight is often mistakenly assumed to be a purely intellectual or cognitive awareness of the sources of one's difficulties. This notion is not more true, however, than the converse, that the goal of therapy is an exclusively emotional release, catharsis, or abreaction. Either a purely intellectual or a purely emotional response is a caricature of insight and represents a resistance to true understanding and permanent change.

I have argued that the Socratic imperative "Know thyself" is a root of the notion of understanding as part of the process of healing. Further, I have argued that Plato's attack on poetry and drama was in part motivated by a need to move beyond myth and ritual as ways of understanding.[3] It is as if he saw that myth does not allow one to free oneself from endless repetition and reenactment of old problems and conflicts. From a psychoanalytic perspective, the knowledge that a mythical monster dwells inside each of us is important but not sufficient. We must understand the monster's resourceful and protean nature. We must understand that we have played our parts in the creation of our monsters, that we may have chosen to handle our fears of the bogeyman by becoming bogeymen to others.[4] It is not enough for a patient to know that he acts immaturely and impulsively; he must also know when, how, and why he does so.

The task of analysis is to help the patient to understand the variety of solutions he has attempted and to assess the degree to which they have been successful. Psychoanalytic exploration and interpretation of dreams, for example, demonstrate to the patient that he has, in effect, been matching conflictual situations from the past with ones in the present.[5] He may come to see his misinterpretations of the present and understand his maladaptive attempts to handle the same old conflicts. Freud's dream, quoted in the first chapter, shows situations from the relatively recent past matched with a situation from the previous day. His interpretations of the dream revealed how prone he was to react to criticism and disclosed the variety of devices he used to protect himself from it, most notably criticism of his critics.

Thus the notion of insight refers to a personal kind of understanding of the relationship between past and present, sufficiently detailed in both intellectual and emotional terms to represent a form of knowledge that carries genuine conviction. It is this kind of self-understanding, not a formulaic recitation of "I know I hate my father," that is associated with change in behavior, thought, and feeling.

Throughout this work I have used the term "working through," particularly in relation to the tragic conception of knowledge through suffering. The term, in this sense, connotes a willingness to suffer the consequences of one's choice, and not to short-circuit the process of grief and anguish by seeking palliatives.

The technical sense of "working through" is defined in Freud's "Remembering, Repeating, and Working Through" as the fundamental processes of psychoanalysis.[6] George Santayana's dictum that those who do not remember history are doomed to repeat it conveys a similar point. Unless one can reconstruct and recollect one's emotional past history and assimilate it to the present by the process of working through, one is doomed to endless symbolic repetition of the past by acting out. Insight cannot be acquired just once; it must be applied and reapplied in many different situations.

It is not insight alone that allows for change and growth; the process of gaining the insight is probably at least as important as the insight itself. Psychoanalytic theory attempts to explain something of this process, which is the crux of the interaction between patient and therapist, but I do not believe we yet have a complete or sufficient knowledge of all that is entailed in this process. Certainly, the attainment of an insight implies a good deal of emotional involvement and arousal on the part of the patient. The extent and nature of the therapist's emotional involvement are also only partially understood.[7] Such terms as "countertransference" and "listening with the third ear" hardly begin to encompass the intricacies of the therapist's engagement with the patient.

Psychoanalytic theory and practice posit a large measure of detachment on the part of the therapist, yet he cannot be too detached. Schools of psychotherapy differ considerably in their estimate of the optimal stance and optimal degree of involvement of the therapist.

Existential psychotherapies, for instance, emphasize the need to break down the distance between therapist and patient so that the therapist can totally experience the patient's situation. Classical psychoanalysis speaks of the need for empathy but warns of the dangers of overidentification with the patient.

Psychoanalysis and the Freedom of the Individual

One of the major goals of psychoanalysis is to help the individual to achieve a great degree of freedom and of freedom of choice. Such a statement is deceptively simple. For one thing, it posits an individual who is potentially distinct from and differentiated from his "group," which includes the society at large and the crucial family figures of his childhood. While psychoanalysts assume that each person must come to terms with his group and that "no man is an island," they also consider a large degree of individuation to be desirable.

From the perspective of psychoanalysis, individuality is impaired not by group allegiances per se but by unrecognized and unacknowledged allegiances, particularly to the early family figures who are now represented internally. The importance of elucidating the transference lies in the need to demonstrate to the patient the extent to which he is bound to his primordial group and the constraints these allegiances place on his adult interpersonal relationships. Freedom lies in releasing some of the energy invested in these internalized representations so that it may be directed into richer and more varied relationships in the present. The guarantor of freedom is in part the insight acquired in analysis and self-analysis. Insight requires the use of the rational faculties, but the rational faculties themselves must be freed from their bondage to the service of rationalization. The instinctual drives and the intense passions that attend them are other guarantors of freedom.[8] The natural forces of growth and development must also be given their due. Reason and instinct, if stripped of disguise, protect the autonomy of the person.

The relationship between psychoanalysis and a particular conception of the individual has been most eloquently discussed by the sociologist Philip Rieff. In *The Triumph of the Therapeutic,*[9] Rieff argues that a particular type of individual, which he calls "psychological man," emerged in the late nineteenth century—in contrast to "corporate man" (my own antonym), the man who hitherto sought security and salvation in corporate institutions. According to Rieff, the traditional institutions—religion, the extended family, and the state—no longer have the moral weight they carried for centuries, and therefore no longer provide the psychological security they once did. Modern man cannot find comfort, solace, and moral direction in cultural conglomerates as he did in the past. Psychoanalysis is the therapy par excellence for this new psychological man for whom traditional institutions no longer afford meaning and continuity in life. "Psychoanalysis," Rieff says, "is yet another method of learning how to endure the loneliness produced by culture. Psychoanalysis is its representative therapy—in contrast to classical therapies of commitment."

The systems of control and consolation that Western man has had available in religion or in the worship of the authority of the state are "therapeutic," as opposed to "analytic."

All such systems of therapeutic control, limiting as they do the area of spontaneity, are anti-instinctual; what we mean ordinarily by cultures are just these systems. We call these systems "therapeutic" because these controls are intended to preserve a certain established level of adequacy in the social functioning of the individual, as well as forestall the danger of his psychological collapse. Needless to say, such systems of control—whether Christian, Buddhist, or any other—are authoritarian. The classic modes of anti-authoritarianism revolve around therapeutic respites from control; anti-authoritarianism, therefore, has always been vulnerable to the charge of being culturally (i.e., morally) subversive.

In Freud's conception, therapy [psychoanalysis] is indeed a mechanism for establishing self-control. But therapy is morally neutral. Faith, however, even one that accents the remission of control, is never neutral. The analytic attitude is an alternative to all religious ones.

In Rieff's analysis of our culture, psychological man, the man who lives in the analytic rather than the therapeutic mode, is a fragile creature, and he may already be on his way to extinction less than a century after his birth. Rieff argues that the isolation of the analytic mode is too great for most individuals to bear and that modern man has sought to devise new therapeutic modes that have subtly reinstated faith and commitment to the conglomerate.

I agree that psychoanalysis is related to a certain ideal of individuality that became prominent in the first half of the twentieth century. It is not clear, however, whether a new character type has emerged, or only a new ideal. While it is unlikely that new ideals arise without accompanying changes in behavior, it is also unlikely that new ideals per se radically alter the behavior of the majority of people. This difficulty renders such formulations as Rieff's problematic, though not necessarily incorrect. If interpretation of the record of the present and recent past is difficult, prediction of future trends in character types and corresponding forms of pathology and therapy is even more perilous.

Does ancient Greece provide a parallel to the emergence of new ideals of individuality in the twentieth century and their connection with new forms of therapy, such as psychoanalysis? Consensus exists among students of classical Greek antiquity that new ideals and ideas about individual freedom and autonomy arose in the fifth and fourth centuries B.C., particularly in Athens.[10] In a very general way, the emergence of Platonic dialogue and dialectic and, with Aristotle, the crystallization of the ideal of philosophy as a way of life were intimately related to these new ideals of individuality. We can see evidence in Greek culture, from the time of Homer to the time of Aristotle, of both subjective and objective changes in the relationship between the individual and the group. Civic and political institutions developed in ways that affected the relationship between the individual and his blood group. Law, economics, and voting rights reflected and confirmed these changes. I have also suggested that the advent of literacy opened up new possibilities for individual autonomy. The ability to use reading and writing creatively implies a certain freedom from received authority, particularly when that authority is embedded in the oral tradition.

In literature, drama, and philosophy we find a new sense of man as an autonomous, self-activating agent, capable of defining and making moral choices. Protagoras' famous dicta "About the gods, I am not able to know whether they exist or do not exist" and "Man is the measure of all things" suggest something of the boldness of man's assertion of his new sense of his own importance.[11]

In the Platonic dialogues, particularly the early ones, the language is strained as Socrates gropes for words to describe the individual, the self, uniqueness, and related concepts. The notion that the few, the philosophers, can be right and the many wrong is central to Plato's philosophy. For Plato the first guarantor of the freedom and autonomy of the individual is use of the rational part of his psyche. Philosophy and dialectic make men free, even if to us the freedom appears distinctly limited when translated into the political design of the *Republic* or the *Laws*.

When all is said and done, the figure of Socrates debating, cajoling, persuading, disconcerting all around him with his irony, yet a man alone, represents an ideal of radical independence. He has the stubbornness of the epic hero, he is a new Achilles.[12] At the same time, his ethos overturns many of the epic ideals of life and verges on the starkly antiheroic.

Greek tragedies, especially those of Sophocles, demonstrate another aspect of what it is to be an individual. The hero is not a radical, but rather someone who, like Antigone, may proclaim allegiance to a more profound and authentic set of societal values than those held by her antagonists. Similarly, the hero's individuality is expressed by a stubborn defiance of conventional wisdom and a relentless drive to carry out what he knows must be done, as exemplified by Oedipus in *Oedipus Rex* and *Oedipus at Colonus*. The gulf between Sophocles' hero and the group is different from the gulf between, say, Achilles and the rest of the Achaeans in the *Iliad*. While Achilles in some way adumbrates the Sophoclean hero, he is *not* a man holding out for a more authentic set of values than those of his group. Rather he is holding out for his fair share of *timē*, honor, recognition, and material restitution. The Oedipus of *Oedipus Rex*, in contrast, holds out for the truth, no matter where its pursuit may lead. While the heroes of Greek tragedy cannot be equated with modern existential heroes, let alone antiheroes, they do assert a notion of autonomy and separateness from the group. If nothing else, they assert that the time-honored group methods of consolation and restitution are not enough; a more radical recognition of their inner needs and drives is required.

I believe, then, that what Rieff calls the analytic attitude parallels in some significant measure the attitudes that emerged in the tragedies and in the Platonic dialogues. I further contend that historically the analytic attitude begins with the Socratic quest for self-knowledge and the tragic definition of heroism. Many of the conclusions to which Plato's philosophy led him seem to be antithetical to the analytic attitude, but his attempts to devise a method of inquiry are not. While Rieff lists Plato as the archetype of therapeutic control (that is, control through conformity and a basic authoritarianism), there is more tension around this issue in Plato's works than Rieff would allow.[13] Insofar as Plato emphasized the importance of detached inquiry, no matter where it might lead, and insofar as he established the notion that knowledge should derive from underlying principles rather than from tradition and authority, he was a precursor of the analytic attitude. Insofar as he conformed to the picture that Rieff paints (deriving largely from the *Laws* and to a lesser extent from the *Republic*), Plato was anti-individualist, and his doctrines conform to Rieff's definition of therapeutic control.

The Social Psychiatric Model

Social psychiatry, by our definition, seeks to determine the significant facts in family and society which affect adaptation (or which can be clearly defined as of etiological importance) as revealed through the studies of individuals or groups functioning in their natural setting. It concerns itself not only with the mentally ill but with the problems of adjustment of all persons in society toward a better understanding of how people adapt and what forces tend to damage or enhance their adaptive capacities.[14]

This is an early definition of social psychiatry, proposed by one of the pioneers in the field, which encompasses, in principle, almost any aspect of man living in society. Global as it is, the definition omits one aspect of social psychiatry—the study of ways to correct mal-adaptation and promote individual and communal health. As the field has developed from the early 1950s to the present, the interest in therapy has grown dramatically, at times threatening to overshadow the more modest effort to diagnose and understand.

In an earlier chapter I mentioned some aspects of modern psychiatry that pertain to social psychiatry. A. B. Hollingshead and F. C. Redlich's *Social Class and Mental Illness*[15] typifies both the subject matter and the methods of social psychiatry. Family studies link family interaction with individual psychopathology. Social labeling theory provides a model for the social processes by which one enters a "career" as a mental patient. Thomas Szasz and R. D. Laing assert that the social milieu can drive a person mad, and proclaim that pathological needs of families and of entire cultures are gratified by the "creation" of madmen.

While one can adduce precursors and prototypes of the idea of social psychiatry—Plato's *Republic* is certainly one—the psychiatric theory that underpins modern social psychiatry was developed in the 1930s and 1940s.[16] The name most prominently associated with this theory is Harry Stack Sullivan, who coined the term "interpersonal psychiatry." In fact, for him psychiatry is

the study of processes that involve or go on between people. The field of psychiatry is the field of interpersonal relations, under any and all circumstances in which these relations exist. It was seen that a *personality* can never be isolated from the complex of interpersonal relations in which the person lives and has his being.[17]

To Sullivan and his followers, the relationship between therapist and patient requires the psychiatrist's careful scrutiny. The therapist is not a detached observer of the patient's psychic processes but a "participant observer." As such, he constantly influences the field he is studying, a conception analogous to the indeterminacy principle in modern physics (which states that the act of measuring the behavior of a particle always influences that behavior). For Sullivan, the person is the sum of his history of interpersonal involvements, starting with the earliest mother-child interactions. In his most extreme statements, the "person" is regarded as a mythic conception, formulated in an attempt to impose a static view of complex and changeable processes. Processes in dyads—whether mother-child, patient-therapist, or any other—are, then, only limiting cases of group processes in general. (This view is the converse of the psychoanalytic perspective, which tends to see groups as conglomerates of persons and group interactions as the result of interactions of individual minds.) Sullivan's view, then, makes for an easy transition between the study of "individuals" or dyads and the study of larger groups, ranging from the family to the larger social environment of the growing child to the entire society, and finally even to interactions among societies.

Sullivan's conception of the role of the psychiatrist, whether of an individual or of a group, is epitomized in the following quotations:

> The people in, and in a sense constituting, the interpersonal field are more or less aware of the tensions and energy transformations which occur. They have all the primary data there is. If you are one of them and if you are skillful enough, you may be able to observe the progress of events, tensions and energy transformations well enough to have something to analyze, and on which to base inference. As your skill increases, you will be able to validate inferences, your provisional hypothesis about events, by influencing the interpersonal field.

The ideal of the psychoanalytic model of treatment is the therapist as interpreter. Sullivan's ideal therapist is one who understands and influences the interpersonal field in which he is a participant.

> You will have grasped the fact that we . . . subscribe to the dictum of "know thyself" in the very particular sense of "Learn to recognize the interpersonal fields in which you find yourself, and how to influence the field forces in the direction of more certain definition of the fields and their more adequate and appropriate integration."[18]

(Obviously Socrates wins the prize for brevity.)

Such, then, is the task of social psychiatry, be it the psychiatry of the patient, the family, or the society: understand by interacting and observing; form a hypothesis about the ongoing stream of relationships; test your hypothesis by specific interventions and behavior that influence others; observe the effects; and then begin the cycle again. Indeed a Sisyphean task!

Ritual Healing: The Prototype of Social Psychiatric Therapy

Just this kind of work has been done the world over, albeit without necessarily either the theory or the techniques specific to interpersonal psychiatry. Ritual healing rites, as practiced in various forms and cultures, frequently involve a healer (the shaman) who ferrets out the sources of tension within the group to which the afflicted person belongs.[19] This kind of "diagnosis" of the social field is done very much in symbolic terms. The shaman divines which ghost or spirit is possessing the patient or ascertains who has tried to bewitch him. He interprets signs that he alone understands, including those that appear in dreams. The healer himself has usually suffered from the illness that he is now expert in treating. He has been cured either by the ritual that he now conducts for someone else or by himself—perhaps by a fast that induced visions. The forms of both illness and cure are specific to each culture.

The ritual healing process often involves symbolic representation of these group tensions (as by a portrayal of a struggle between spirits of the mother's and father's sides of the family). In addition, the members of the social nexus are brought together and made to confess their grudges and misdeeds against the afflicted person, and vice versa. They often end by making symbolic and real restitution for evil wishes or deeds directed against the sick person. Those responsible for the illness may pay the cost, often considerable, of the healing rites.

Victor Turner has provided an instructive example of ritual healing that involves just this sort of social diagnosis and prescription.[20] The sick person, a member of the Ndembu tribe of Rhodesia, was afflicted with rapid palpitations of the heart, severe pains in the back, limbs, and chest, and fatigue after short spells of work. Feeling that people were talking against him, he withdrew from the affairs of the village—in which he had settled upon his marriage to a local woman—and shut himself in his hut for long periods of time. He complained that the villagers ignored his sufferings and had made no attempt to bring in a diviner to help diagnose and cure him. While Turner cannot attest with absolute certainty that the man had no organic illness, he saw many indications that the disturbances were primarily psychogenic.

The patient was an unassertive sort of man in a society that still valued the traits of the skillful and aggressive hunter. His wife was having a rather blatant affair with a neighbor. He had not been especially happy or well liked in his village of origin, and now he was in a particularly vulnerable social position as a newcomer in his wife's village. In addition, he was torn between loyalty to his matrilineal affiliations and obligations to paternal kin (a typical conflict in the tribe).

Divination revealed that he suffered from a disease caused by the bite of an *ihamba,* a tooth of a departed hunter ancestor. In addition, evidence of witchcraft had been discovered in the village, and the healer tactfully but pointedly suggested that the patient's wife and mother-in-law were responsible. To cure the illness, he performed a ritual designed to remove the ancestral incisor.

The ritual addressed tensions in a number of areas in the life of the patient and of the village as a whole: relationships among blacks and whites, among the patient's kin, among the villagers, and between the patient and his wife and her family. The healing ritual seems to have been successful, for the patient was cured and seemed still to be well a year later. The ritual resulted as well in a significant healing of some of the important breaches in the life of the village. As Turner concludes:

the Ndembu "doctor" sees his task less as curing an individual patient than as remedying the ills of a corporate group. The sickness of a patient is mainly a sign that "something is rotten" in the corporate body. The patient will not get better until all the tensions and aggressions in the group's interrelations have been brought to light and exposed to ritual treatment. . . . conflicts in one social dimension may reverberate through others. The doctor's task is to tap the various streams of affect associated with these conflicts and with the social and interpersonal disputes in which they are manifested—and to channel them in a socially positive direction. The raw energies of conflict are thus domesticated in the service of the traditional social order. . . . The sick individual, exposed to this process, is reintegrated into his group, as, step by step, its members are reconciled with one another in emotionally charged circumstances.[21]

This kind of healing can be said to exemplify the social psychiatric model.

Of course it is tempting to say that we could learn something from these primitive techniques and might usefully expand and revise some of our notions of psychotherapy to include similar methods. The problem is the difficulty of establishing efficacious rituals *de novo*. The power of such rituals is in many ways precarious, for it depends on the stability and relative homogeneity of the society and its cultural values. Anthropologists recognize that such rituals do change with time and with shifting social circumstances.[22] New devils and spirits are introduced; and they are often white and blue-eyed. New rituals often serve as a rear-guard action designed either to hold what is left of the culture together or to assuage the guilt of those who have moved away from it.

Undoubtedly many of the newer therapies (or new versions of ancient therapies) that have proliferated in the United States in recent years—encounter groups, marathon group sessions, primal scream therapy, and so on—are in part motivated by the wish to establish ritual forms of healing. One of the tantalizing therapeutic challenges of the day is how to develop symbols, myths, and rituals that have the power to heal.[23] One problem is the need to establish the corporate and group consciousness that seems necessary if these rituals are to be effective. My own impression is that the task is basically impossible, though individuals and groups will repeatedly strive to develop such therapies. And proponents of the notion of reestablishing ritual and myth as potent healing forces tend to forget that if symbols can heal, they must also be able to hurt. If we are to introduce (or revive) ritual healing, we must be prepared to accept ritual illnesses. Ritual healing procedures tend to be associated with the more dramatic and hysterical forms of disturbance.[24] The recent revival of interest in possession and exorcism may represent a response to the increased interest in ecstatic and cathartic therapies, such as primal scream therapy.

The bard who composes oral epic poetry is also kin to the interpersonal psychiatrist.[25] The bard's task is to produce a form of poetry that has the power to help individuals to deal with their own distress by means of symbolic identifications with characters in the story. These identifications in turn facilitate a diagnosis of the trouble: you suffer from injured pride, like Achilles, or from nostalgia, like Odysseus. At the same time, the equation of one's private troubles with those of a traditional model fosters a symbolic reintegration with the group. Undoubtedly the bard also helps with group tensions and crises that do not necessarily directly entail individual illnesses. If we had more detailed knowledge of the way the pre-Homeric bards operated, we would probably see that they were shrewd interpreters of the moods and problems of the groups before whom they peformed and that they skillfully shaped their tales around those issues. In order to make such a diagnosis, the bard himself must be in touch with the group tensions, and, as a member of the group, subject to its distress.

The bard must also experience a significant degree of identification with the characters in his poem. The identifications with both audience and characters entail a blurring of the boundaries of self. The degree to which the bard (or any other ritual healer) temporarily loses some of his own identity varies considerably. At one extreme, shamans may enter dissociative trance states during their healing rituals. Tribal peoples of Siberia believe that when the shaman is in trance his soul leaves his body to search for the lost (or robbed) soul of his patient.[26] At the other extreme, the accounts of Claude Lévi-Strauss, Victor Turner, and others suggest that some healers are in constant touch with their surroundings and are little more than skillful masters of ceremonies.[27] Modern psychotherapies can also be characterized by the degree of involvement or merging required of the therapist. Of necessity, the therapist must undergo some degree of regressive identification with his patient. To be effective, however, he must be able to help regulate the degree of regression and loss of ego boundaries experienced by the patient. The therapist, in this sense, is not only a participant observer but participant regulator.

Turner has extended his analysis of the way rituals operate to bind together and heal both individuals and communities beyond the level suggested in his discussion of Ndembu healing ritual. In brief, he considers the potential ability of ritual healing to open up new forms of integration and provide a pathway toward new solutions of both

old and new problems.[28] Societies need rituals of innovation as well
as rituals of conservation. Analogously, the model of social psychiatry need not imply only a return to a status quo ante bellum but also
an advance to a new level of integration and equilibrium that might
represent a powerful and imaginative solution to problems of the
individual and of his society. From time immemorial brilliant and
charismatic leaders have used ritual and mythic versions of their
people's history and destiny to achieve a remarkable integration of
old and new, a compelling synthesis of the time-honored tribal values with the demands of changing conditions. In sum, ritual, myth,
and ritual healing may help create and mold the future, not merely
serve to cope with the present.[29]

Social Psychiatric Models of Man

I have suggested that the psychoanalytic model of therapy is associated with a particular model of man, "psychological man." Does
an analogous model of man underlie the social psychiatric model?
Two basic models can be identified, one applicable to relatively
stable societies, the other to societies undergoing rapid or perpetual
change. The first is exemplified by the Homeric model of mind and
the attendant conception of the self.

The representations of mental life that I call the Homeric model
are closer to fantasies about the mind than to theories. They are,
however, the kinds of fantasy that constitute data for interpersonal,
or field, theories of human mental life. As such, the Homeric model
of mind is a primitive analogue of later interpersonal theories.

Recall the characterization of Homeric man offered by Herman
Fränkel: "The self is not encapsulated, but is an open field of forces."
I have argued that such a conception of the self is appropriate for and
adaptive to a society that values tradition and stability and requires a
self that is amenable to the influences of others. These influences tend
toward conservation of traditional ways of thinking, feeling, and
behaving. The person must be open to the forces that help define and
maintain his role. The Homeric conception of man is thus antithetical to Rieff's psychological man but appropriate for the ritual healing
aspect of social psychiatry. The primary goal of ritual healing is a
reinstatement of a traditional balance and reintegration of the individual into his group.

The second model of man will be familiar to students of twentieth-century art and literature. It is a model of the ego not as a stable,
recognizable entity that occasionally breaks down and must be put
back together but as what we might call a collage.[30] In much of
modern art, the individual is shown not as he appears to the human
eye but as a collection of partial views juxtaposed in such a way that

there is no single view, no unique perspective from which the person must be seen. Figures in the works of Georges Braque and Pablo Picasso are shown in many dimensions at once. Human beings, animals, and inanimate objects are dismantled and recomposed in new and strange ways. Such recompositions force us to scrutinize our usual perceptions and urge us to try new ones.

Marshall McLuhan's characterization of modern man as postliterate similarly captures the shifting sense of the self that marks twentieth-century culture.[31] Literate man is a creature of privacy, a man with a stable inner world. Postliterate man, so McLuhan argues, is nourished by the pansensory, nonlinear electronic media. The stable, inner-directed man who slowly, through books, assimilates new information and outlooks no longer exists in our society. Postliterate man becomes the sum product of an overwhelming kaleidoscopic flow of sensory stimulation. McLuhan is optimistic about the long-range effects of the loss of the anchoring and continuity associated with the culture of literacy, but that optimism is incidental to his central thesis.

I believe that an analogous theme can be seen in various psychological characterizations of twentieth-century man, some intended to sing his praises, some to condemn him. An example of the former is the term "protean man," coined by Robert J. Lifton; "narcissistic character disorder" is an example of the latter. According to Lifton, we are witnessing "the emergence of contemporary or *protean man as rebel*—the effort to remain open, while in rebellion, to the extraordinarily rich, confusing, liberating, and threatening array of contemporary historical possibilities, and to retain in the process a continuing capacity for shape-shifting."[32] He argues that the introduction of atomic destruction in World War II and the subsequent threat of nuclear holocaust constitute an unprecedented rupture in man's sense of historical continuity. Those who reached maturity after Hiroshima, in particular, must live as if there may be no future generations, and accordingly their lives are not governed by the need to pass on the values and traditions of the past. With no anchoring in past or future, modern man constantly experiments with new roles, taking on multiple identities as he concentrates on his own survival. For Lifton, protean man is a new type of hero, creating a morality *a nihilo* in full knowledge of the fact that no external source of morality exists. With the possibility of total destruction of the human race, there can be no more epic heroes, no more singers of heroic deeds, and no audience to hear the tales. Heroism, whether military or moral, is no longer a guarantee of immortality, for there may be no future generations to keep the heroes alive in memory. Lifton points to the youth movements and student rebellions of the late 1960s as the leading edge of the idea that only by constant nonideological rebellion and emphasis on immediate experience (especially pleasurable or mind-numbing) can any valid meaning be found in life. Psychological man with his stable inner core, the well-analyzed man, must yield to protean man, for a stable inner identity is no longer adaptive and perhaps no longer possible.

The first social critic of the idea of protean man, I believe, was Plato. In his attack on *polupragmosunē,* doing and being too many things at once, Plato argued the need for some stable and predictable inner identity. He was ready to ground that identity in a rigid social and occupational hierarchy. What Lifton calls protean man Plato would have seen as the end result of a culture that relies on *mimēsis,* promiscuous imitation. The man caught up in *polupragmosunē,* being a psychic busybody, is, in Plato's view, a psychic nobody.[33]

Some modern social critics, while subscribing to Lifton's characterizations of emerging ideals and behaviors, take a much dimmer view of them. They argue that we are witnessing regressions to infantile, impulse-ridden, and socially irresponsible modes of behavior. They see a threat to certain basic human values, values that transcend ideology and particular political systems. Some psychoanalysts have reported that they are seeing increasing numbers of patients who suffer from tremendous inner emptiness and inability to form strong commitments to others. The clinical term "narcissistic character" is the one most widely used to describe these disorders, but other terms have been used as well: borderline personality, character disorder, anhedonic personality, schizoid personality. These patients differ from the classical neurotics (such as hysterics and obsessives) in that instinctual expression is encouraged while superego and ego ideals are repressed. Thus sexual expression of every sort is permitted; only guilt is prohibited.[34]

In brief, one could say that the classical neuroses arise in a social setting of structured conflicts between the generations and between the sexes. When a society provides a relatively stable system of authority (and relatively stable rules for rebellion against that authority), the battle is over who controls instinctual expression and the circumstances in which it is permitted. Narcissistic disorders arise in settings where differences between the generations or the sexes are minimized or denied and authoritarian control of instinctual expression is a minor issue. Here intimacy and commitment become focuses of struggle and neurotic conflict. It has become fashionable to apply the clinical term "narcissistic character" to the social and political scene. Lifton's protean man exhibits a pathological narcissism. He is "facile at managing the impressions he gives to others, ravenous for admiration but contemptuous of those he manipulates into providing it; unappeasably hungry for emotional experiences with which to fill an inner void; terrified of aging and death."[35]

Those who praise and those who condemn this version of modern man agree that a severe crisis in social institutions has led to a severe crisis for the individual. This formulation poses a massive problem for social psychiatry. The model of ritual healing, of healing by reinstating the sick individual in his proper social nexus, cannot work when the social nexus is shifting and variable. The multifaceted self of modern art, collage man, is the counterpart of shifting institutions and shifting values.

My own opinion, which can be stated but not argued in detail, is that the notion of protean man serves a therapeutic, social psychiatric function. It provides a shared ego ideal and sense of community for a wide variety of people who feel themselves alienated from and disenchanted with existing communities (the establishment, the family, the university). In fact, this kind of ideal, far from being revolutionary, is an aspect of a healing ritual. It is, in Victor Turner's term, a ritual of "anti-structure," one that facilitates the passage (especially of the young) through difficult and tumultuous times. Whether new forms of social or psychic structure may emerge from this ritual passage is problematic. Whether stable and durable new forms of therapy will emerge (forms that are neither psychoanalytic nor ritual) is equally difficult to predict.

Can the Psychoanalytic and Social Psychiatric Models Be Integrated?

Despite some important efforts in recent years, the integration of psychoanalytic and social psychiatric models has yet to be accomplished. A certain de facto integration can be seen in the way many psychiatrists work at their craft. I believe, however, that this appearance of integration is an illusion, based on the ability of some psychiatrists to wear more than one costume and to become adept at rapid changes between the scenes. One source of the difficulty can be readily surmised. A major limitation of the social psychiatric model is its lack of a theory that explains the internalization and transformation of social forces by the mind of the individual. The individual of the social psychiatric model is a hypothetical construct—a unit, something like the infinitesimal in calculus, that allows the theory to function. The mind of that individual is a relatively passive agency that registers and responds but does not transform and innovate. In fact, the social psychiatric model cannot easily explain how social psychiatrists come to be. The fact that a person can take sufficient distance from his own social field to diagnose and understand its difficulties demands a more complex theory of the mind and person than one finds in the theories that attend the social psychiatric model. Whether or not this limitation is inevitable is not clear at this juncture.

Conversely, the psychoanalytic model lacks a theory adequate to explain social phenomena. As psychoanalytic theory approaches situations in which the number of agents multiplies, it becomes progressively less able to formulate and predict. Psychoanalytic theory, as it currently stands, makes certain simplifying assumptions about the way past and present cultural forces impinge upon the person. The assumptions are in danger of becoming simplistic rather than simplifying, especially outside the immediate clinical situation. The psychoanalytic model posits that the person has two psychic agencies responsive to social forces, the ego and the superego, and one agency that is recalcitrant, the id. It has relatively little power to account for regularities of group behavior. Further, both the psychoanalytic and the social psychiatric models offer explanations of their therapeutic power that are either inadequate or inaccurate.

We may well be forced to a position of strict complementarity: while either the psychoanalytic or the social psychiatric model can be used to describe man, they cannot be used simultaneously. Man as subject and man as object can be studied only alternately or in succession.[36]

None of these remarks is intended to slight previous attempts at integration of the two models. The efforts of those who have worked in such diverse areas as ego psychology, psychohistory (as well as psychoanthropology and psychosociology), information theory and general systems theory, object relations theory, and the relation between learning theory and psychoanalysis have furthered our insight into the nature of both individual and society.[37] They represent distinct advances over the schema typified by Plato's *Republic*, according to which psyche and society are declared to have congruent structures and therefore to be unified.

Nor are we free to desist from the work just because we cannot complete it. I see two areas where the union of social psychiatric and psychoanalytic models is of utmost importance. The first is the possibility of developing a universally applicable mode of psychotherapy, one that is culture-free, or at least culturally neutral; one that is premised on the commonality of the human psyche in all cultures, yet recognizes that every human psyche exists in a particular culture. Such a psychotherapy would indeed be a most exciting achievement. As the world grows smaller and smaller and as we learn more and more about the characteristics that unite mankind, we must strive more and more to develop a way of treating those disorders that signify that man is divided against himself and against his fellows.

The second area is the problem first delineated in Plato's *Republic*, that of establishing social, economic, and political structures in which the human psyche can thrive and reach its fullest potential. It is here that the psychoanalytic model of interior man and the social psychiatric model of man as a political animal must together define the conditions under which the psyche and the state can truly and harmoniously be joined. Whence and in what form the solutions to these problems may come I do not know now, but I do know that it is worth the effort to continue the inquiry and to use all our wits and imagination to resolve these dissonances. In so doing we must provide our own rewards: the pleasure of seeking the truth and the knowledge that we continue to strive.

Let us recall the message at the end of the *Republic,* Plato's attempt to understand the polity that is within the man and the man that is within the polity. Socrates concludes the tale told by Er, the tale of how, after death, the psyches had the opportunity to choose their lives in their next incarnations. Socrates urges us to remember the tale and hold fast to its lessons:

And so, O Glaucon, the tale was saved and not lost, and so it may save us, if we can be persuaded by it. And we shall safely cross the river of Forgetfulness and not defile our psyche. But if you will be persuaded by me, and consider the psyche as immortal and able to endure all manner of good and evil, we shall always follow the road leading upward and practice justice with wisdom in every way. And thereby we shall be loving to ourselves and to the gods, both while we remain here and then later when we shall reap the rewards as the Olympic victors who gather in the prizes. And both here and in that journey of a thousand years, through which I have led you, we shall fare well.[38]

Eu prattomen.

Abbreviations

AHD	*The American Heritage Dictionary*
AHP²	S. Arieti, ed., *American Handbook of Psychiatry*, 2d ed. (New York, 1974)
AJP	*American Journal of Philology*
Am. Im.	*American Imago*
Am. J. Psychiat.	*American Journal of Psychiatry*
Arch. Gen. Psychiat.	*Archives of General Psychiatry*
Brit. J. Psychiat.	*British Journal of Psychiatry*
Bull. Hist. Med.	*Bulletin of the History of Medicine*
Bull. Instit. Class. Stud.	*Bulletin of the Institute of Classical Studies of the University of London*
Class. Bull.	*Classical Bulletin*
CP	*Classical Philology*
CQ	*Classical Quarterly*
CR	*Classical Review*
CTP²	A. M. Freedman, H. I. Kaplan, and B. J. Sadock, *Comprehensive Textbook of Psychiatry*, 2d ed. (Baltimore, 1975)
Freud, *SE*	*Standard Edition of the Complete Psychological Works of Sigmund Freud*, ed. and trans. J. Strachey, A. Freud, A. Strachey, and A. Tyson, 24 vols. (London, 1955–74)
GRBS	*Greek, Roman, and Byzantine Studies*
HSCP	*Harvard Studies in Classical Philology*
Int. J. Psa.	*International Journal of Psycho-Analysis*
Int. J. Soc. Psychiatry	*International Journal of Social Psychiatry*
Int. Rev. Psa.	*International Review of Psycho-Analysis*
J. Am. Hist.	*Journal of American History*
J. Am. Med. A.	*Journal of the American Medical Association*
J. Am. Psa. A.	*Journal of the American Psychoanalytic Association*
J. Hist. Behavioral Sciences	*Journal of the History of the Behavioral Sciences*
J. Hist. Ideas	*Journal of the History of Ideas*
JHS	*Journal of Hellenic Studies*
J. Nerv. and Mental Diseases	*Journal of Nervous and Mental Diseases*

LCL	Loeb Classical Library
LSJ	H. G. Liddell, R. Scott, and H. S. Jones, *A Greek-English Lexicon,* 9th ed. (Oxford, 1940; reprinted 1961)
Mus. Helvet.	*Museum Helveticum*
*OCD*²	*The Oxford Classical Dictionary,* 2d ed.
OCT	Oxford Classical Text
OED	*The Oxford English Dictionary*
Proc. Brit. Acad.	*Proceedings of the British Academy*
Psa. and Contemp. Sci.	*Psychoanalysis and Contemporary Science,* ed. R. R. Holt and E. Peterfreund (New York, 1972-)
Psa. Q.	*Psychoanalytic Quarterly*
Psa. R.	*Psychoanalytic Review*
Psa. Study Child	*The Psychoanalytic Study of the Child*
Psa. Study Soc.	*The Psychoanalytic Study of Society*
RE	A. Pauly, G. Wissowa, and W. Kroll, *Realencyclopädie der klassischen Altertumswissenschaft* (Stuttgart, 1894-).
REG	*Revue des études grecques*
Rev. fr. psa.	*Revue française de psychanalyse*
Rh. M.	*Rheinisches Museum für Philologie*
TAPA	*Transactions of the American Philological Association*
TLS	*Times Literary Supplement* (London)
Trans. Am. Philos. Soc.	*Transactions of the American Philosophical Society*
YCS	*Yale Classical Studies*

Notes

1. On the Babel of Tongues in Contemporary Psychiatry

1. *Psa. and Contemp. Sci.* 1 (1972): 38–54.
2. Freud, SE 4:96–121. See Erik Erikson, "The Dream Specimen of Psychoanalysis," *J. Am. Psa. A.* 2 (1956): 5–56, and M. Schur, *Freud: Living and Dying* (New York, 1972), pp. 79–92.
3. See D. Pivnicki, "The Origins of Psychotherapy," *J. Hist. Behavioral Sciences* 5 (1969): 238–47.
4. See J. Breuer and S. Freud, *Studies on Hysteria,* SE 2. Also H. F. Ellenberger, *The Discovery of the Unconscious* (New York, 1970).
5. Plutarch, *Moralia: Lives of the Ten Orators,* trans. H. N. Fowler, LCL, vol. 10 (Cambridge, 1936), sec. 833, para. C, p. 350. See P. Laín Entralgo, *The Therapy of the Word in Classical Antiquity,* trans. L. J. Rather and J. M. Sharp (New Haven, 1970), pp. 97–107, for discussion.
6. See *OED,* s.v. Psychosis.
7. Trans. J. Zinkin (New York, 1950). The following quotations are on pp. 14–17.
8. A similar analysis may be found in R. D. Laing, *The Divided Self* (London, 1960), pp. 29–31.
9. W. Gaylin, *In the Service of Their Country: War Resisters in Prison* (New York, 1970).
10. The American Psychiatric Association was organized in 1844 with only thirteen members; it had about a thousand in 1920 and more than twenty thousand in 1973 (*Biographical Directory of the American Psychiatric Association, 1973,* p. ix).
11. See in particular R. D. Laing, *The Politics of Experience* (New York, 1967).
12. See, for example, such standard works as AHP^2 and CTP^2.
13. Psychiatrists' need to wear a variety of hats and their means of coping with contradictions in their roles are illustrated in M. J. Kahne and C. G. Schwartz, "The College as a Psychiatric Workplace," *Psychiatry* 38 (1975): 107–23.

2. The Development of Models of Mental Illness

1. M. Foucault, *Madness and Civilization,* trans. R. Howard (New York, 1965), p. 250.
2. *Laws,* 908C–909B; and see above, chap. 9.
3. T. Freeman et al., *Studies on Psychosis* (New York, 1966), esp. chaps. 5, 6, and 7.
4. E.g., D. L. Rosenhan, "On Being Sane in Insane Places," *Science* 179 (1973):250–57. For a critique, see R. Spitzer, "On Pseudoscience in Science, Logic in Remission, and Psychiatric Diagnosis," *Journal of Abnormal Psychology* 84 (1975): 442–52, articles by I. Weiner, B. T. Millon, and S. Crown, and Rosenhan's reply in the same volume.

5. See J. D. Frank, *Persuasion and Healing*, rev. ed. (New York, 1974), esp. chap. 2.

6. See the following works by G. Devereux: *Mohave Ethnopsychiatry and Suicide* (Washington, D.C., 1961), pp. 488–89; *Ethnopsychanalyse complementariste* (Paris, 1972), chap. 10; *Essais d'ethnopsychiatrie générale*, 2d ed. (Paris, 1973), chap. 10. I believe that auditory verbal hallucinations were not considered part of the stereotype of madness until the eighteenth and nineteenth centuries (on the basis of on my own survey of available case reports, as in O. Diethelm, *Medical Dissertations of Psychiatric Interest* [Basel, 1971]). That is to say, hearing voices is considered to belong not to the category of madness but to some such category as religious experience. M. Millar, "Géricault's Paintings of the Insane," *J. Warburg and Courtauld Institute* 4 (1940–42):151–163, gives a brief résumé of the stereotypical representation of the insane in art. Millar demonstrates Géricault's innovation in portraying the insane as individual, suffering people.

7. See G. Zilboorg and G. W. Henry, *A History of Medical Psychology* (New York, 1941), chap. 6. A *New Yorker* cartoon by Ed Fisher shows a scene of Salem witch burning captioned, "The time will come when we'll realize that people don't cause storms, blight crops, and spoil the village butter because they're evil but because they're sick" (cited by H. N. Boris, *The Unexamined Life: Motivation, Methodology, and Community Mental Health* [NIMH Report, June 1967]).

8. See N. E. Waxler, "Culture and Mental Illness: A Social-labelling Perspective," *J. Nerv. and Mental Diseases* 159 (1974): 379–95.

9. Zilboorg and Henry, *History of Medical Psychology*, chap. 14.

10. A famous exception is the village of Geel in Belgium, according to legend founded by St. Dymphna as a haven for the mentally ill.

11. E.g., J. S. Bockoven, *Moral Treatment in American Psychiatry* (New York, 1972).

12. B. Sicherman, "Mental Health in the Gilded Age: The Paradox of Prudence," *J. Am. Hist.* 62 (1976):890–912.

13. Zilboorg and Henry, *History of Medical Psychology*, p. 551. Probably the use of iodine supplements to treat goiter was the first specific medical treatment for a psychosis caused by nutritional deficiency.

14. Electric shock is quite effective for serious depression and is still appropriately used for that condition.

15. Maxwell Jones, *The Therapeutic Community* (New York, 1953).

16. Despite Freud's support of lay analysis: SE 20:179–258.

17. T. Szasz, *Manufacture of Madness: A Comparative Study of the Inquisition and the Mental Health Movement* (New York, 1970).

18. Fuller critiques of Szasz's work may be found in D. A. Begelman, "Misnaming, Metaphors, the Medical Model, and Some Muddles," *Psychiatry* 34 (1971):38–58; and S. Reiss, "A Critique of Thomas S. Szasz's 'Myth of Mental Illness,' " *Am. J. Psychiat.* 128 (1972):1081–85. More sympathetic is F. M. Sander, "Some Thoughts on Thomas Szasz," *Am. J. Psychiat.* 125 (1969): 1429–31, and Szasz's reply, pp. 1432–35. See also E. Becker, *The Birth and Death of Meaning*, 2d ed. (New York, 1971), and *The Revolution in Psychiatry* (New York, 1974).

19. See R. Boyers and R. Orrill, eds., *R. D. Laing and Antipsychiatry* (New York, 1971). See also E. G. Mishler, "Man, Morality, and Madness: Critical Perspectives on the Work of R. D. Laing," *Psa. and Contemp. Sci.* 2 (1973):369–94.

20. E. M. Lemert, *Human Deviance, Social Problems, and Social Control* (Englewood Cliffs, N.J., 1967), and T. Scheff, *Being Mentally Ill* (Chicago, 1966). See also Waxler, "Culture and Mental Illness." (I thank Dr. Steven Leff for discussion and bibliography in this area.) For a recent critique of social labeling theory, see J. Murphy, "Psychiatric Labelling in Cross-Cultural Perspective," *Science* 191 (1976): 1019–1028.

21. A. B. Hollingshead and F. C. Redlich, *Social Class and Mental Illness* (New York, 1958). The sociological characteristics that differentiate the "analytic-psycho-

therapeutic" from the "directive-organic" psychiatrists are discussed on pp. 155–65. A follow-up on the original patients studied is offered in J. K. Myers and L. L. Bean, *A Decade Later: A Follow-up of Social Class and Mental Illness* (New York, 1968), which tends to confirm the interpretation of the earlier work: that the higher prevalence of psychosis in the lower class is in large part a function of longer hospitalization and less likelihood of clinic treatment (pp. 206–215). R. Bastide, *The Sociology of Mental Disorder*, trans. J. McNeil (New York, 1972), is a useful survey.

22. M. Siegler and H. Osmond, "Models of Madness," *Brit. J. Psychiat.* 112 (1966):1192–1203.

23. New York, 1974. See their table on pp. 16–18.

24. See, for example, S. S. Kety, D. Rosenthal, P. H. Wender, and F. Schulsinger, "Mental Illness in the Biological and Adoptive Families of Adopted Schizophrenics," *Am. J. Psychiat.* 128 (1971):302–311. The best summaries of recent research on schizophrenia are to be found in R. Cancro, ed., *Annual Review of the Schizophrenic Syndrome* (New York, 1971–) and *Schizophrenia Bulletin* (NIMH), 1969– .

25. See Bateson's formulation of the double bind in the family of the schizophrenic: G. Bateson, D. D. Jackson, et al., "Toward a Theory of Schizophrenia," *Behavioral Science* 1 (1966):251–64. See also *Family Process* 2 (1963):154–61, and C. C. Beels and A. Ferber, "Family Therapy: A View," *Family Process* 8 (1969):280–332.

26. See D. L. Burnham, *Schizophrenia and the Need–Fear Dilemma* (New York, 1969).

27. See J. G. Gunderson and L. R. Mosher, eds., *Psychotherapy of Schizophrenia* (New York, 1975).

28. See B. Simon and H. Weiner, "Models of Mind and Mental Illness in Ancient Greece: I. The Homeric Model of Mind," *J. Hist. Behavioral Sciences* 2 (1966): 303–314.

29. E.g., A. C. Vaughn, *Madness in Greek Thought and Custom* (Baltimore, 1919); A. O'Brien-Moore, *Madness in Ancient Literature* (Weimar, 1924); and J. Mattes, *Der Wahnsinn in griechischen Mythos und in der Dichtung bis zum Drama des fünften Jahrhunderts* (Heidelberg, 1970).

3. The Greeks and the Irrational

1. *The Portable Nietzsche,* ed. and trans. W. Kaufman (New York, 1954), p. 478.

2. B. Rush, *Medical Inquiries and Observations upon the Diseases of the Mind* (1812; reprint New York, 1962), p. 29.

3. For detailed discussion of Nietzsche's classical background and influence, see W. Arrowsmith, "Nietzsche on Classics and Classicists (Part III)," *Arion* 2 (1963):5–31; also *Arion* n.s. 1 (1973–74):279–380 for Arrowsmith's translation of Nietzsche's notes for *Wir Philologen*. See too H. Lloyd-Jones, "Nietzsche and the Study of the Ancient World," *TLS,* 21 February 1975, pp. 199–201, and *The Justice of Zeus* (Berkeley, 1973), p. 157.

4. *The Birth of Tragedy,* in *The Philosophy of Nietzsche* (New York, 1927), p. 951.

5. For Freud's classical background, see H. Trosman, "Freud's Cultural Background," *Psychological Issues* 9 (1976):66–70, and R. Ransahoff, "Sigmund Freud: Collector of Antiques, Student of Antiquity," *Archaeology* 28 (1975):102–111.

6. Freud, *The Interpretation of Dreams,* SE 4:261–62.

7. For a synoptic view of the history of psychiatry in ancient Greece and Rome, consult the following with their bibliographies: C. Ducey and B. Simon, "Ancient Greece and Rome," in *World History of Psychiatry,* ed. J. G. Howells (New York, 1974), pp. 1–38; G. Mora, "Historical and Theoretical Trends in Psychiatry," in *CTP²,* pp. 1–75; G. Rosen, "Greece and Rome," in *Madness and Society* (Chicago, 1968), pp. 71–136; P. Laín Entralgo, *The Therapy of the Word in Classical Antiquity,*

trans. L. J. Rather and J. M. Sharp (New Haven, 1970). There is a need for a thorough ethnopsychiatric study of ancient Greece comparable to G. Devereux, *Mohave Ethnopsychiatry and Suicide* (Washington, D.C., 1961). Some relevant material can be found scattered throughout J. C. Lawson, *Modern Greek Folklore and Ancient Greek Religion* (New Hyde Park, N.Y., 1964), and A. C. Vaughn, *Madness in Greek Thought and Custom* (Baltimore, 1919). See also R. Blum and E. Blum, *Health and Healing in Rural Greece* (Stanford, 1965) and *The Dangerous Hour: The Lore and Culture of Crisis and Mystery in Rural Greece* (New York, 1970).

4. Mental Life in the Homeric Epics

Note: An earlier version of Chapter 4 appeared as B. Simon and H. Weiner, "Models of Mind and Mental Illness in Ancient Greece: I. The Homeric Model of Mind," *J. Hist. Behavioral Sciences* 2 (1966):303–314, and J. Russo and B. Simon, "Homeric Psychology and the Oral Epic Tradition, *J. Hist. Ideas* 29 (1968): 485–98.

1. For the nonspecialist, the most complete single reference work on Homer is A. J. B. Wace and F. H. Stubbings, eds., *A Companion to Homer* (London, 1962). Good general introductions are C. R. Beye, *The Iliad, the Odyssey, and the Epic Tradition* (New York, 1966), and A. Lesky, *A History of Greek Literature,* trans. J. Willis and C. de Heer (London, 1966), pp. 14–90. The translations used, unless otherwise indicated, are from R. Lattimore, *The Iliad of Homer,* 2d ed. (Chicago: University of Chicago Press, 1962. Copyright 1951, ©1962 by the University of Chicago) and *The Odyssey of Homer* (New York: Harper & Row, 1968).

2. For the problems of disentangling fact from history, see M. I. Finley, "Lost: The Trojan War," in his *Aspects of Antiquity* (New York, 1968), pp. 24–37.

3. See C. M. Bowra, "The Meaning of a Heroic Age," in *Language and Background of Homer,* ed. G. S. Kirk (Cambridge, 1964), pp. 22–47.

4. See esp. B. Snell, *The Discovery of the Mind,* trans. T. G. Rosenmeyer (Cambridge, Mass., 1953), and Russo and Simon, "Homeric Psychology."

5. D. Claus, "Psyche: A Study in the Language of the Self before Plato" (Ph.D. dissertation, Yale, 1969). I thank Professor Claus for several conversations and for access to an unpublished manuscript.

6. Although many scholars consider all or parts of Book 11 to be a later interpolation, the account of psyche is generally compatible with the rest of the *Odyssey* and the *Iliad.*

7. Translation mine.

8. But cf. *Odyssey,* 10.555, where psyche seems equivalent to "a breath of fresh air."

9. Homer's description of cremation and archaeological evidence on inhumation imply that the psyche survives after death, but not necessarily at the site of burial. See, for example, G. E. Mylonas, "Burial Practices," in Wace and Stubbings, *Companion to Homer,* pp. 478–88, and E. T. Vermeule, *Greece in the Bronze Age* (Chicago, 1964), pp. 297–304.

10. E. Rohde, *Psyche,* trans. N. B. Hillis from 8th German ed. (London, 1925), pp. 4–8.

11. See O. Rank, *The Double,* ed. and trans. H. Tucker (Chapel Hill, N.C., 1971), and also some relevant material in *Beyond Psychology* (privately published, 1941). I thank Dr. W. Meissner for these and other references that appear in his unpublished manuscript "The Double." See also J. P. Vernant, "La categorie psychologique du double," in *Mythe et pensée chez les Grecs* (Paris, 1971), vol. 2, pp. 65–78.

12. See H. Kohut, *The Analysis of the Self* (New York, 1971), Index, s.v. "Mirror transference"; C. Feigelson, "Mirror Dream," *Psa. Study Child* 30 (1975):341–55; and

the work of J. Lacan, best explicated in J. Laplanche and J. B. Pontalis, *The Language of Psycho-Analysis,* trans. D. Nicholson-Smith (New York, 1973), s.v. "Mirror phase."

13. This and other clinical examples are drawn from my clinical experience, with modification to ensure confidentiality. The technical term for the mirror phenomenon is autoscopic hallucination.

14. Note the anxiety dream cited in the *Iliad,* 22.199–200, used as a simile in the scene where Achilles chases Hector around the walls of Troy.

15. A useful brief survey of dreams in Homer may be found in A. Brelich, "The Place of Dreams in the Religious World Concept of the Greeks," in *The Dream and Human Societies,* ed. G. E. von Grunebaum and R. Callois (Berkeley, 1966), pp. 293–301). See also E. R. Dodds, *The Greeks and the Irrational* (Berkeley, 1951), pp. 104–107. S. Reid, "The *Iliad:* Agamemnon's Dream," *Am. Im.* 30 (1973):33–56, presents a psychoanalytic discussion of the dream in Book 2 of the *Iliad.* The entire scene has been a puzzlement to scholars, for Agamemnon's behavior in telling the troops to go home seems inconsistent with the manifest instructions in the dream, though it is consistent with Zeus's intent to deceive him. Reid's analysis is most instructive, especially his comments on l. 114 of Book 2 (repeated at l. 21 of Book 9), "Now he [Zeus] has devised a vile deception." See also G. Devereux, *Dreams in Greek Tragedy* (Berkeley, 1976), pp. ix–xxix and passim. Compare young children's theories of dreams in J. Piaget, *Play, Dreams, and Imitation in Childhood* (New York, 1962).

16. The exception is Penelope's dream in the *Odyssey,* 19.536–53. See G. Devereux, "Penelope's Character," *Psa. Q.* 26 (1957):378–86.

17. See Snell, *Discovery of the Mind,* pp. 12–17; Russo and Simon, "Homeric Psychology"; K. von Fritz, "*Noos* and *Noein* in the Homeric Poems," *CP* 38 (1943):79–93.

18. Snell, *Discovery of the Mind,* pp. 1–5.

19. Claus, "Psyche," and C. Watkins, "Indo-European and the Indo-Europeans," in *AHD,* pp. 1496–1502.

20. An instructive example is the verb *apelein,* to threaten, discussed in A. W. H. Adkins, *From the Many to the One* (Ithaca, N.Y., 1970), pp. 37–44.

21. Snell, *Discovery of the Mind,* pp. 5–8.

22. Ibid., p. 3.

23. Translation from Russo and Simon, "Homeric Psychology."

24. J. Joyce, *Ulysses,* Modern Library ed. (New York, 1934), p. 724.

25. See Dodds, *Greeks and the Irrational,* pp. 1–27.

26. See H. Fränkel, *Dichtung und Philosophie des frühen Griechentums,* 2d ed. (Munich, 1962), p. 85.

27. I am indebted to Dr. Norman Reider for the term in quotation marks.

28. See Freud, *Group Psychology and the Analysis of the Ego* (1921), SE 18:67–143, esp. p. 116.

29. Fränkel, *Dichtung und Philosophie,* esp. pp. 80–94.

30. The classic work that demonstrates the similarities among the thinking of children, preliterate peoples, and schizophrenics is H. Werner, *Comparative Psychology of Mental Development,* rev. ed. (New York, 1957). See also A. Storch, *The Primitive Archaic Forms of Inner Experience and Thought in Schizophrenia,* trans. C. Willard (New York, 1924). I know of only one work that systematically discusses the differences: H. Werner and S. Kaplan, *Symbol Formation* (New York, 1963). C. Lévi-Strauss, *The Savage Mind* (Chicago, 1966), gives a more recent view emphasizing the logic of the so-called savage mind.

31. See D. Stewart, *The Disguised Guest* (Ames, Iowa, 1976).

32. See C. Voigt, *Überlegung und Entscheidung: Studien zur Selbstauffassung des Menschen bei Homer* (Berlin, 1933). Note too the word *bussodomeuō,* brood, only in the *Odyssey* (e.g., Book 17, l. 66), which seems to be a more "inward" mental term (D.

Clay, personal communication). Even this word, however, is rather concrete ("building deep") and always takes a direct object, such as *kaka*, evil things.

33. See B. Simon, "The Hero as an Only Child: An Unconscious Fantasy Structuring Homer's *Odyssey*," *Int. J. Psa.* 55 (1974):555–62.

34. See C. H. Taylor, Jr., "The Obstacles to Odysseus' Return," in *Essays on the Odyssey: Selected Modern Criticism* (Bloomington, Ind., 1963), pp. 87–99.

35. This allusion to the myth of Heracles' delayed birth is thematically appropriate for it counterpoints the sense of sibling rivalry for pride of place which has marked the relationship between Achilles and Agamemnon.

36. For one thing, *atē* can serve to relieve private guilt as well as to mitigate public shame. Similarly, shame can be internalized as well as guilt, so that the distinction between guilt and shame on the basis of degree of internalization is not valid. I believe it more useful to consider shame and guilt as having developed independently, rather than to consider shame the more primitive affect.

37. Examples are most conveniently found in L. Sechan, *Etudes sur la tragédie grecque dans ses rapports avec la céramique* (Paris, 1926), and A. D. Trendall and T. B. L. Webster, *Illustrations of Greek Drama* (London, 1971); see "Lyssa" in index. A particularly beautiful illusration of Lyssa is found on a red-figured krater in the Museum of Fine Arts in Boston. Mania is shown in a scene of Heracles' madness on a krater in Madrid. See pp. 132 and 133 above.

38. Dr. F. Kudlien (personal communication). Similarly, berserk means wearing a bear shirt, i.e., raging like a bear (*OED*) (pointed out by Dr. T. Gutheil, personal communication).

39. Note, however, that this passage in Book 6 makes no reference to Book 5, the "Diomedeia."

40. For illustrations of Lykourgos in drama, see Sechan, *Etudes*, pp. 63–79, and above, p. 132.

41. Dr. George Devereux has suggested this as an instance of the cultural patterning of psychotic behavior. Not every culture considers being alone to be part of the stereotype of madness (personal communication).

42. Translation mine. This passage is the motto of Samuel Butler's *Way of All Flesh*.

43. In psychodynamic terms, Achilles' shame and guilt over his role in Patroklos' death prevent the resolution of his grief. Ambivalence toward the deceased (with the hatred unconscious) frequently underlies pathological grief.

44. The gods had at first urged that Hector's corpse be stolen and returned to Priam. Such a ploy, of course, would have been dramatically weak, short-circuiting the account of the human process of working through grief and rage.

45. Thetis, as a loving mother, grieves with her son, but urges him to take comfort from the pleasures of eating and sex (*Iliad*, 24.129–31). By the time Priam appears in his tent, Achilles has resumed eating but has not gone to bed with his concubine, Briseis. The reference to sexual intercourse was deemed improper by Alexandrian scholars, who therefore wished to reject this passage as an interpolation. See K. J. Dover, *Greek Popular Morality* (Oxford, 1974), p. 206.

46. We must note too that the gods serve as an external superego, by whose command Achilles is relieved of guilt and shame arising from unconscious hostility to Patroklos.

5. Epic as Therapy

1. *Hesiod*, trans. H. G. Evelyn-White, LCL (Cambridge, Mass., 1950), p. 85.

2. For discussion of the role of dance and song in relation to other cultural institutions, see A. Lomax, *Folksong, Style, and Culture* (Washington, D.C., 1968). See also G. Bateson and M. Mead, *Childhood in Bali* (New York, 1942). Some fascinating

material on how the rhythms of speech begin to pattern body movements in early infancy may be found in W. S. Condon and L. W. Sander "Neonate Movement Is Synchronized with Adult Speech: Interactional Participation and Language Regulation," *Science* 183 (1974):99–101.

3. See B. Simon and H. Weiner, "Models of Mind and Mental Illness in Ancient Greece: I. The Homeric Model of Mind," *J. Hist. Behavioral Sciences* 2 (1966):303–314, and J. Russo and B. Simon, "Homeric Psychology and the Oral Epic Tradition," *J. Hist. Ideas* 29 (1968):485–98.

4. Compare our colloquial use of the term "an open mind," which connotes the mind's being open to *new* influences.

5. See C. M. Bowra, "The Meaning of a Heroic Age," in *Language and Background of Homer*, ed. G. S. Kirk (Cambridge, 1964), pp. 22–47.

6. M. Parry, *The Making of Homeric Verse*, ed. A. Parry (Oxford, 1971), esp. Editor's Introduction; A. Lord, *The Singer of Tales* (Cambridge, Mass., 1960).

7. See Parry, *Making of Homeric Verse*, Editor's Introduction.

8. See J. Russo's review of A. Hoekstra, *Homeric Modification of Formulaic Prototype* (Amsterdam, 1965), in *AJP* 88 (1967):340–46. Also W. Whallon, *Formula, Character, and Context: Studies in Homeric, Old English, and Old Testament Poetry* (Cambridge, Mass., 1969); G. S. Kirk, *The Songs of Homer* (Cambridge, 1962); D. Young, "Never Blotted a Line? Formula and Premeditation in Homer and Hesiod," *Arion* 6 (1967): 279–324; R. Finnegan, "What Is Oral Literature Anyway?" in *Oral Literature and the Formula*, ed. B. A. Stoltz (Ann Arbor, 1976), pp. 127–76, and "Literacy versus Non-Literacy: The Great Divide?" in *Modes of Thought: Essays on Thinking in Western and Non-Western Societies* (London, 1973), pp. 112–44. The role of oral tradition in American black culture is discussed in A. Murray, *The Hero and the Blues* (Columbia, Mo., 1973). See also E. A. Havelock, *Prologue to Greek Literacy* (Norman, Okla., 1971).

9. See Whallon, *Formula, Character, and Context*, e.g., pp. 1–32.

10. Summaries of this material may be found in E. A. Havelock, *Preface to Plato* (Cambridge, Mass., 1963), and *Prologue to Greek Literacy*.

11. See the introduction to A. Medjedovic, *The Wedding of Smailagic Meho*, ed. and trans. A. B. Lord and D. E. Bynum, 2 vols. (Cambridge, Mass., 1974), and review by J. Foley, *Slavic and East European Journal* 20 (1976):195–99.

12. Lord, *Singer of Tales*, esp. chap. 5, discusses the way the performer may vary the contents of his story according to his audience.

13. E.g., Demodocus' song, *Odyssey*, 8.266–366.

14. *Odyssey*, 8.580.

15. Havelock, *Preface to Plato*, e.g., pp. 145–64.

16. See Simon and Weiner, "Models of Mind," and Russo and Simon, "Homeric Psychology."

17. The psychoanalytic literature contains a number of important discussions about fantasies surrounding the experience of inspiration, e.g., E. Kris, *Psychoanalytic Explorations in Art* (New York, 1952), pp. 291–320, and P. Greenacre, *Emotional Growth* (New York, 1971), vol. 1, pp. 225–48.

18. This statement is qualified in Finnegan, "What Is Oral Literature Anyway?"

19. Translation modified from Plato, *The Dialogues*, trans. B. Jowett, 3d ed. (1892; reprint Oxford, 1924). In ll. 533E–534A poetic inspirations are compared to Bacchic and Korybantic madness. Madness and inspiration are discussed in Chapter 7.

20. The gender of the Muses indicates that Greek culture saw the sources of poetry and song in the early mother-child relationship. The bard, in order to learn and be inspired, must be in touch with a certain mode of passive receptivity, which ordinarily we associate with the young child.

21. See H. Kohut, *The Analysis of the Self* (New York, 1971), for theoretical and clinical discussions of the concept of the grandiose self in relation to narcissism. Dr. C.

Ducey has suggested that *Ion,* 533D (quoted earlier) is an account of a fantasy of narcissistic enlargement of the self (personal communication).

22. E. R. Dodds, *The Greeks and the Irrational* (Berkeley, 1951), pp. 1–18.

23. This formulation is implicit in Dodds's comments in ibid., p. 14.

24. From this perspective, many primitive healing rituals (shamanistic rites) demand an extreme measure of loss of self on the part of the healer. He may fall into a trance as his soul departs to search for the soul of the sick person. Group ecstatic experience (see Chapter 13) also involves a form of loss of boundaries of the self. Modern theories that emphasize interpersonal aspects of psychological processes are discussed in Chapter 14.

25. Chapter 13 discusses the social and psychological implications of the medical theory of hysteria.

6. Mental Life in Greek Tragedy

1. From *Roman Drama,* translated by Frank O. Copley and Moses Hadas, copyright © 1965 by the Bobbs-Merrill Co., Inc.

2. See D. Clay's introduction to his translation of *Oedipus Rex* (Oxford, forthcoming).

3. W. Burkert, "Greek Tragedy and Sacrificial Ritual," *GRBS* 7 (1966):87–122, discusses the three possible ways of understanding "goat song."

4. I am referring principally to Jane Harrison, Francis Cornford, and Gilbert Murray. A succinct review and bibliography may be found in G. F. Else, *The Origin and Early Forms of Greek Tragedy* (New York, 1972), esp. chap. 1. Else is distinctly critical of these writers' emphasis on the primitive.

5. *Poetics,* 1453a17–22.

6. A review of psychoanalytic interpretations of the *Oresteia* may be found in R. S. Caldwell, "Selected Bibliography on Psychoanalysis and Classical Studies," *Arethusa* 7 (1974):115–34, esp. pp. 121–22. See also G. Devereux, *Dreams in Greek Tragedy* (Berkeley, 1976), chaps. 3, 4, 6; and D. Kouretas, *Anōmaloi karaktēres eis to archaion drama* [Abnormal characters in the ancient drama] (Athens, 1951), reviewed by G. Lyketsos in *Psa. Q.* 22 (1953):110–12. See also P. Hartcollis's review in *Int. J. Psa.* 57 (1976):365–67.

7. *On the Sublime,* sec. 16, para. 4, OCT, ed. D. A. Russell (Oxford, 1968), p. 26, alluding to Euripides' *Bacchae,* l. 317.

8. *Poetics,* 1449b24, 1449b36–50a15.

9. In fact, throughout the play Sophocles exploits the linguistic similarity between the verbs "to know" and "to see," which share an Indo-European root.

10. Dreams are also an exception, often represented as sent by an external agency, though not so conspicuously as in the Homeric epics (Devereux, *Dreams in Greek Tragedy*, p. 30n).

11. Unless otherwise indicated, all translations in Chapter 6 are from D. Grene and R. Lattimore, eds., *The Complete Greek Tragedies,* 4 vols. (Chicago: University of Chicago Press, 1959). *Oresteia* and *Eumenides* © 1953 by the University of Chicago; *Antigone* © 1954 by the University of Chicago; *The Bacchae* © 1958 by the University of Chicago.

12. Discussions of this speech typically pair it with Phaedra's speech (*Hippolytus,* ll. 373–430). These speeches are discussed in B. Knox, "Second Thoughts in Greek Tragedy," *GRBS* 7 (1966):213–32. Phaedra's speech is discussed in T. Irwin, "Euripides and Socrates," in *Essays on Attic Tragedy,* ed. R. L. Gordon (Cambridge, forthcoming). Claus, in "Phaedra," argues for the more archaic quality of Phaedra's

speech, disagreeing with the idea that the speech represents a unique internalization of mental and moral functions. I believe he overstates his case.

13. Modified from Grene and Lattimore: "courage" for "spirit" (*kardia*).

14. Euripides, *The Medea,* trans. Rex Warner (London, 1944). Used by permission of the publisher, John Lane, The Bodley Head Ltd.

15. Knox, "Second Thoughts."

16. See, however, Aeschylus, *Choephoroi,* ll. 390–92, for a concrete sense of *thumos.*

17. B. Snell, *The Discovery of the Mind,* trans. T. G. Rosenmeyer (Cambridge, Mass., 1953), and H. Fränkel, *Dichtung und Philosophie des frühen Griechentums,* 2d ed. (Munich, 1962), explain the differences between Homeric epic and tragedy in the portrayal of mental life as a historical development. Others (best represented by J. Russo, "The Inner Man in Archilochus and the *Odyssey,*" *GRBS* 15 [1974]:139–52, and his review of G. Kirkwood, *Early Greek Monody: The History of a Poetic Type* [Ithaca, N.Y., 1974], in *Arion* n.s. 1 [1974]:707–730) attribute the differences to genre. D. Bynum has pointed out (in unpublished lectures) that when narrative folktale is transformed into drama in other cultures, the portrayal of inner mental life becomes more prominent. I believe that both explanations are necessary.

18. The significance of the shift here from iambic trimeter, the usual meter of dialogue, is pointed out by L. H. G. Greenwood, *Aspects of Euripidean Tragedy* (Cambridge, 1953).

19. Ibid.

20. Translation from S. Barlow, *The Imagery of Euripides* (London, 1971), p. 38. See also ll. 1089–95.

21. Translation mine.

22. J. de Romilly, *La crainte et l'angoisse dans le théâtre d'Eschyle* (Paris, 1958), and Else, *Origin and Early Form,* pp. 97–98.

23. *Poetics,* 1449b27, 1451b38, and passim.

24. B. Snell, *Poetry and Society* (Bloomington, Ind., 1961).

25. I thank Dr. C. Ducey for this point. He also reminded me of the connection between the perception of human movement in the Rorschach test and the capacity for fantasy. J. L. Singer, *Daydreaming* (New York, 1966), elaborates this connection.

26. G. F. Else, *Aristotle's Poetics: The Argument* (Cambridge, Mass., 1967), e.g., pp. 383–85 and "Recognition" in index.

27. SE 4 and 5:262.

28. See G. Devereux's valuable discussion, "The Structure of Tragedy and the Structure of the Psyche in Aristotle's *Poetics,*" in *Psychoanalysis and Philosophy,* ed. C. Hanly and M. Lazerowitz (New York, 1970), pp. 46–75.

29. A detailed analysis of this dream may be found in Devereux, *Dreams in Greek Tragedy,* chap. 8. Translation mine, based on Devereux's translation and commentary, esp. pp. 262–64.

30. See O. Rank, *The Myth of the Birth of the Hero,* trans. F. Robbins and S. E. Jelliffe, ed. P. Freund (New York, 1932) (first published 1914 in *J. Nerv. and Mental Diseases*).

31. J. Mattes, *Der Wahnsinn in griechischen Mythos und in der Dichtung bis zum Drama des fünften Jahrhunderts* (Heidelberg, 1970), discusses madness in the lost plays.

32. *On the Sublime,* 15.3.

33. J. W. Gregory, "Madness in the *Heracles, Orestes,* and *Bacchae:* A Study in Euripidean Drama" (Ph.D. dissertation, Harvard, 1974), shows how madness is clearly integrated into the literary and artistic needs of the play.

34. Caldwell, "Selected Bibliography," critically reviews the psychoanalytically oriented literature on these plays.

35. The connection between tragedy and sacrifice is discussed in Burkert, "Greek Tragedy," and in F. I. Zeitlin, "The Motif of the Corrupted Sacrifice in Aeschylus'

Oresteia," TAPA 96 (1965):464–508, and "Postscript to Sacrificial Imagery in the *Oresteia," TAPA* 97 (1966):645–53.

36. SE 13:155–56.

37. Overtones of sacrifice may be detected in ll. 218–20.

38. Such an assumption informs P. E. Slater, *The Glory of Hera* (Boston, 1968), but it must be used judiciously.

39. Devereux, *Dreams in Greek Tragedy,* chap. 8, contains a detailed discussion.

40. Fancies=*doxai,* appearances. In later Greek medicine this word becomes a technical term for hallucination (see LSJ). It is an important term in Plato, where it indicates an inferior form of thinking.

41. With the exception of ll. 155–61, which are from Grene and Lattimore, eds., *Complete Greek Tragedies,* this and the other passages from the *Eumenides* are from Aeschylus, *Eumenides,* ed. H. Lloyd-Jones (Englewood Cliffs, N.J.: Prentice-Hall, 1970. Reprinted by permission of Prentice-Hall, Inc.)

42. This conflict contrasts with that of Lyssa, the figure of madness in the *Heracles,* who is torn by the question whether it is right to drive Heracles mad for no reason other than to obey the will of Hera.

43. The Greek notion of melancholia and its relation to modern psychodynamic concepts are discussed in Chapter 11.

44. Freud, "Mourning and Melancholia," SE 14:237–58; K. Abraham, *Selected Papers on Psycho-Analysis* (London, 1965), pp. 137–56. See also M. Klein, "Some Reflections on the *Oresteia,*" with emphasis on oral envy, in her *Our Adult World* (London, 1963), chap. 2, and the review by A. Green, *Rev. Fr. Psa.* 28 (1964):816–19. The studies reviewed in Caldwell, "Selected Bibliography," pp. 125–26, emphasize incest and oedipal configurations rather than this oral-incorporative material. For the most profound psychoanalytic views, however, see Slater, *Glory of Hera;* A. Green, *Un oeil en trop* (Paris, 1969); and forthcoming articles by R. Caldwell.

45. I am indebted to J. W. Gregory, "Madness in *Heracles,*" for her careful and psychologically perceptive studies of madness in Euripidean drama. I have also found A. P. Burnett, *Catastrophe Survived* (Oxford, 1971), especially useful. On the history of the word "paranoia," see A. Lewis, "Paranoia and Paranoid: A Historical Perspective," *Psychol. Med.* 1 (1970):2–12.

46. The Hypothesis of Aristophanes the Grammarian (in Euripides, *Fabulae,* 3 vols., ed. G. Murray, 2d ed. [OCT, 1913], vol. 3, pp. 21–22): "Except for Pylades, all the characters are scum."

47. On the subject of *philia* in Euripides, I am indebted to T. Haggerty for his unpublished manuscript "The Awakening to Philia," in which he points out that the theme of false and true *philia* is pervasive in Euripides' works.

48. L. 279; a slight change in pronunciation changes "calm" (after the storm) to "weasel."

49. Translation mine.

50. Orestes' taunting of the Phrygian slave for his effeminacy is projection, betraying Orestes' anxiety about his own inadequacy as a male.

51. Translation mine.

52. In an early, lost play of Euripides, the *Telephos,* the infant Orestes was held hostage by Telephos (with the collusion of Clytemnestra?) until the Greeks yielded to his demands. In taking Hermione hostage, Orestes is repeating with her what was done to him. The Telephos-Orestes-Clytemnestra scene is represented on numerous vase paintings and is parodied in Aristophanes' *Acharnians.*

53. *Anō katō,* upside down, occurs four times, more frequently than in any other Euripidean play. Barlow, *Imagery of Euripides,* esp. pp. 62–67, discusses shifts in spatial perspective that are almost parallel to cinematic techniques of moving from close-up to telescopic views and shooting the same scene from different angles.

54. M. Sendak, *Where the Wild Things Are* (New York, 1963).

55. Translation mine.

56. M. Arthur, "The Choral Odes of the *Bacchae* of Euripides," *YCS* 22 (1972):145–80, contains an excellent discussion of the political tensions in the *Bacchae*.

57. See now G. Devereux, "Le fragment d'Eschyle 62 Nauck². Ce qu'y signifie *chlounēs*," *REG* 86 (1972–73):278–84.

58. Greek homosexual males ridiculed effeminacy and strenuously suppressed male fantasies of being a woman (see Chapter 13).

59. W. Sale, "The Psychoanalysis of Pentheus in the *Bacchae*," *YCS* 22 (1972):63–82, presents a similar discussion of regression in the behavior of Pentheus.

60. In *Iphigenia in Tauris*, the crumbling of a house and its pillars in Iphigenia's dream symbolizes castration and destruction of the royal line.

61. Translation mine. Sale, "Psychoanalysis of Pentheus," and S. Halpern, "Free Association in 432 B.C.: Socrates in 'The Clouds,' " *Psa. R.* 50 (1963):419–36, contain fine discussions of dramatic dialogue as analogue to a psychoanalytic session.

62. The Greek stereotype of madness always emphasized visual distortion, rarely auditory distortion. In fact, while I have found instances of auditory hallucinations of sounds (usually flute music), I have found no hallucinated voices. See Chapter 2, n. 6.

63. B. D. Lewin has dealt at length with the relationship between oral wishes and the representation of fantasies of parental intercourse. He has pointed out that the nursing mother and child may be used regressively to represent parental intercourse. Pentheus regresses from desire to watch copulation to desire to be nursed. These points are scattered throughout Lewin's writings, but are presented with special cogency in *The Psychoanalysis of Elation* (New York, 1950) and *The Image and the Past* (New York, 1968). Primal scene themes are prominent in the *Bacchae*. In myth and fantasy special dangers await the person who views parental intercourse, including blindness and madness. If the viewer survives, he may then have acquired special magical powers (Tiresias exemplifies both the danger and the special powers). See Chapter 8 and notes.

64. Slater, *Glory of Hera*, discusses the interplay of orality, merging, and aggression in Greek myth, esp. in chaps. 7–8.

65. E.g., Aristophanes' *Ecclesiazusae*.

66. See *Hippolytus*, l. 120, and the last scene of the play, where human love comes to the fore after the goddess has left her favorite, Hippolytus. See too *Heracles*, ll. 1341–46. See Haggerty, "Awakening to Philia."

7. *Tragedy and Therapy*

1. I thank Douglas Stewart for access to his notes on madness in *The Wasps*.

2. "The Wasps," trans. D. Parker, in *Three Comedies by Aristophanes*, ed. W. Arrowsmith (Ann Arbor, 1969), p. 15. See too his Introduction.

3. J. Starobinski, "L'épée d'Ajax," in *Trois Fureurs* (Paris, 1974), pp. 12–71, contains an approach and conclusions very similar to mine. See also M. Faber, "Suicide and the 'Ajax' of Sophocles," *Psa. R.* 54 (1967):441–52, and R. Seidenberg and E. Papathomopoulos, "Sophocles' *Ajax:* A Morality for Madness," *Psa. Q.* 30 (1961):404–412.

4. See Aristotle, *Problemata*, 30. Note the tradition that the son of Asclepius who treated internal diseases diagnosed Ajax's depression (*barunomenon noēma*).

5. Unless otherwise indicated, all translations in Chapter 7 are from D. Grene and R. Lattimore, eds., *The Complete Greek Tragedies*, 4 vols. (Chicago: University of Chicago Press, 1959). *Ajax* © 1957 by the University of Chicago; *Heracles* © 1956 by the University of Chicago.

6. Translation mine.

7. These formulations derive ultimately from the writings of Freud on psychosis and the extensive clinical work of Harry Stack Sullivan. The work of Elvin Semrad in particular has pinpointed the sequence of onset and resolution. See E. V. Semrad et al., *Teaching Psychotherapy of Psychotic Patients* (New York, 1969).

8. B. Knox, "The *Ajax* of Sophocles," *HSCP* 65 (1961):1–37.

9. B. Knox, *The Heroic Temper: Studies in Sophoclean Tragedy* (Berkeley, 1964), pp. 32–34.

10. B. Simon, "The Hero as an Only Child: An Unconscious Fantasy Structuring Homer's *Odyssey*," *Int. J. Psa.* 55 (1974): 555–62.

11. *Heracles*, probably 418–417 B.C.; *Orestes*, 408; *Bacchae*, ca. 406.

12. U. von Wilamowitz-Müllendorff, *Euripides Herakles*, 2d ed. (Berlin, 1895), notes the later tradition that the stone was called the *sōphronestēr*, sanity stone. A. C. Vaughn, *Madness in Greek Thought and Custom* (Baltimore, 1919), also discusses the stoning of madmen. It is possible that stoning was conceived of both as a cure and as a means of keeping madmen at a distance.

13. In his introduction to his translation of the *Heracles* in Grene and Lattimore, eds., *Complete Greek Tragedies*, vol. 3, pp. 266–81.

14. Note the imagery of spatial dislocation in the play; e.g., ll. 735, 765, 1307.

15. See Hesiod, *Theogony*, l. 27, where the Muses tell *pseudea*, fictions—the term used by Homer to describe Odysseus' tales (*Odyssey*, 19.203). The Sirens (e.g., *Odyssey*, 12.39), while not explicitly lying, use their tales to enchant. Chapter 8 discusses Plato's attacks on myths told to children while he invents his own *pseudea*.

16. Compare Heracles' situation to that of Job, who similarly cannot accept the idea of an unjust god. Also see Xenophanes' fragments 11 and 12 in *Die Fragmente der Vorsokratiker*, ed. H. Diels with additions by W. Kranz, 5th–7th eds. (Berlin, 1934–54), on the maligning of the gods by the poets.

17. S. Becroft, "Personal Relationships in the *Heracles* of Euripides" (Ph.D. dissertation, Yale, 1971), properly argues that Theseus must offer material help (e.g., land) to Heracles if Heracles is to continue living. He is wrong, however, to minimize the importance of the emotional support and love that Theseus provides.

18. Modified from Grene and Lattimore, eds., *Complete Greek Tragedies*.

19. Some sixty passages in the *Heracles* contain *phil-*, compared with thirty in the *Ajax*. Only Euripides' *Alcestis* contains as many *phil-* words.

20. *JHS* 90 (1970):35–48.

21. Ibid. I disagree with Devereux's conclusion that Euripides has definitely portrayed Heracles as the victim of an epileptic seizure. It is true that Euripides needed to portray an attack of madness caused by an external agent; the evidence that Euripides intended to portray an epileptic seizure, however, is not conclusive.

22. Compare the reference to Sisyphus in the *Ajax* (l. 189), where the emphasis is on his trickery rather than his suffering. Ixion, mythology's first criminal, killed his father-in-law. Like Heracles, "he mixed for mortals kindred blood" (Pindar, *Pythian*, 2.32, trans. M. R. Lefkowitz, *The Victory Ode* [Park Ridge, N.J., 1976]). After being purified by Zeus, he attempted adultery with Hera and was punished by being tied to a rotating wheel.

23. For a discussion of *tlemosunē*, endurance, throughout Sophocles' plays, see C. H. Whitman, *Sophocles: A Study of Heroic Humanism* (Cambridge, Mass., 1951), *Tlemosyne* in index.

24. See Wilamowitz's commentary on l. 1234 in *Euripides Herakles*, p. 251.

25. Compare the end of the *Oedipus at Colonus*.

26. The reason Heracles must take Cerberus to Argos is discussed in Wilamowitz, *Euripides Herakles*, p. 276.

27. The figure of Socrates is important here. He is compared, on a number of

occasions, to one or another of the epic heroes, especially Achilles. See D. Clay, "Socrates' Mulishness and Heroism," *Phronesis* 27 (1972):53–60.

28. P. Laín Entralgo, *The Therapy of the Word in Classical Antiquity*, trans. L. J. Rather and J. M. Sharp (New Haven, 1970), pp. 186–87. His review of this mass of opinion and his own formulations of catharsis are invaluable.

29. J. Bernays, *Zwei Abhandlungen über die Aristotelische Theorie des Drama* (Berlin, 1880), p. 16, translated in Laín Engralgo, *Therapy of the Word*, p. 187. A. Momigliano, *Jacob Bernays* (Amsterdam, 1969), is a fine study of the scholarly life of Bernays.

30. H. F. Ellenberger, *The Discovery of the Unconscious* (New York, 1970), pp. 484 and 561. See also S. Gifford, "Theory of Abreaction and Catharsis before 1897," *International Encyclopedia of Neurology, Psychiatry, Psychoanalysis, and Psychology*, ed. B. Wolman (New York, 1977).

31. See "Purgation through Pity and Terror," *Int. J. Psa.* 54 (1973):499–504. See also D. Kouretas, "La catharsis d'après Hippocrate, Aristote, et Breuer-Freud," *Annales médicales* 1 (1962):627–61.

32. I am impressed by the commentary in G. F. Else, *Aristotle's Poetics: The Argument* (Cambridge, Mass., 1967). Else argues that critics have given disproportional weight to catharsis and underemphasized all the rest of Aristotle's discussion of the intricate balance of reason and emotion that goes into creating and responding to a great tragedy. I am less convinced, however, by his suggestion that catharsis applies to the characters in the play and not to the audience (at 1453b37–54a9). I have found particularly trenchant the views of L. Golden, as found in L. Golden and O. B. Hardison, Jr., *Aristotle's Poetics* (Englewood Cliffs, N.J., 1968); "Mimesis and Katharsis," *CP* 64 (1969):145–53; "*Katharsis* as Clarification: An Objection Answered," *CQ* 23 (1973):45–46; "The Purgation Theory of Catharsis," *J. Aesthetics and Art Criticism* 31 (1973):474–79. The constructions in Laín Entralgo, *Therapy of the Word*, are also consonant with the views expressed here.

33. *Psychoanalytic Explorations in Art* (New York, 1952), esp. pp. 62–64. See too G. Devereux, "The Structure of Tragedy and the Structure of the Psyche in Aristotle's *Poetics*," in *Psychoanalysis and Philosophy*, ed. C. Hanly and M. Lazerowitz (New York, 1970), pp. 46–75.

34. See R. Schafer, "The Psychoanalytic Vision of Reality," *Int. J. Psa.* 51 (1970):279–97, and H. Loewald, "Psychoanalysis as an Art and the Fantasy Character of the Psychoanalytic Situation," *J. Am. Psa. A.* 23 (1975):277–99.

35. *Glory of Hera* (Boston, 1968) and "The Greek Family in History and Myth," *Arethusa* 7 (1974):9–44.

36. E.g., the story of Phoenix, *Iliad*, 9.447–57.

37. An illuminating discussion of *Hamlet* as a play about plays, may be found in M. Rose, "Hamlet and the Shape of Revenge," *English Literary Renaissance* 1 (1971):132–43.

38. In the commentary to his edition of the *Bacchae*, 2d ed. (Oxford, 1960), p. 151. While Dodds has not really mustered the evidence to support this suggestion, he has hit on something important about the god.

39. Translation Dodds's; see his commentary in ibid.

40. Aristotle, *Poetics*, 1455a22–34. See also Else's commentary in *Aristotle's Poetics*, esp. pp. 496–502.

41. Gorgias, B23, in *Fragmente der Vorsokratiker*, ed. Diels. For useful comments on rhetoric as therapy, see Laín Entralgo, *Therapy of the Word*. See also C. P. Segal, "Gorgias and the Psychology of the Logos," *HSCP* 66 (1962):99–155.

42. D. W. Winnicott, "Transitional Objects and Transitional Phenomena," in *Collected Papers* (New York, 1958), pp. 229–42.

43. N. Cameron, *Personality Development and Psychopathology* (Boston, 1963), pp. 470–513. For daydreaming studies, see J. L. Singer, *Daydreaming* (New York, 1966), esp. pp. 195–98.

44. The implications of this formulation in relation to theater other than the Greek are worth considering. *Hamlet,* for instance, can be fruitfully reexamined, especially in light of the work of K. Eissler, *Discourse on Hamlet and "Hamlet": A Psychoanalytic Inquiry* (New York, 1971), and Rose, "Hamlet and the Shape of Revenge." The modern playwright who most conspicuously plays with the connections among madness, illusion, and theater is Luigi Pirandello, especially in *Henry IV.* The main character has become mad while playing a role in a pageant, and the plot revolves around an attempt to cure him by the staging of a new drama. Interestingly, the doctor who devised this strategem is named Dionysio. See, too, J. W. Krutch, "Pirandello and the Dissolution of the Ego"; D. Vittorini, "Being and Seeming: *Henry IV*"; and an excerpt from Pirandello's *Umorismo,* all in *Modern Drama: Annotated Texts,* ed. A. Caputi (New York, 1966), pp. 471–92. I thank Judith Kates for helpful discussion and useful references for madness and theater.

45. See M. Arthur, "The Choral Odes of the *Bacchae* of Euripides," *YCS* 22 (1972):145–80, for an analysis of the interplay of the instinctual and the political around the word *sophia.*

46. Cambridge, 1948.

47. This process is examined in detail in J. Croissant, *Aristote et les mystères* (Liège, 1932).

48. See E. R. Dodds, *The Greeks and the Irrational* (Berkeley, 1951), pp. 64–82, and I. M. Linforth, "The Corybantic Rites in Plato" and "Telestic Madness in Plato, *Phaedrus* 244DE," *University of California Publications in Classical Philology* 13 (1946):121–72.

49. See Croissant, *Aristote et les mystères,* and R. Klibansky, E. Panofsky, and F. Saxl, *Saturn and Melancholy* (New York, 1964), esp. chap. 1. This passage is discussed at greater length in Chapter 12 of this book.

50. Else, *Aristotle's Poetics.* The following discussion draws heavily on Else's commentary on this passage. The modern psychological literature on creativity is voluminous and often inconclusive. Two short and useful pieces, however, are: L. Edel, "The Madness of Art," *Am. J. Psychiat.* 32 (1975):1005–1012, and W. Niederland, "Psychoanalytic Approaches to Creativity," *Psa. Q.* 45 (1976):185–211, with bibliography.

51. Translation mine. See Else's commentary in *Aristotle's Poetics,* p. 460.

52. See, for example, Gorgias, *Encomium to Helen,* B11 and B11a, in *Fragmente der Vorsokratiker,* ed. Diels.

53. A. Vaughn, *Madness in Greek Thought and Custom* (Baltimore, 1919).

54. A. P. Burnett, *Catastrophe Survived: Euripides' Plays of Mixed Reversal* (Oxford, 1971), presents an elegant discussion of the complex sequences in Euripides.

55. G. Devereux, personal communication.

8. Plato's Concept of Mind and Its Disorders

Note: Chapters 8 and 9 are revisions and expansions of my articles on Plato: "Models of Mind and Mental Illness in Ancient Greece: II. The Platonic Model," *J. Hist. Behavioral Sciences* 8 (1972):389–404 and 9 (1973):3–17.

1. J. H. Randall, Jr., *Plato: Dramatist of the Life of Reason* (New York, 1970), and D. Clay, "The Tragic and Comic Poet of the *Symposium,*" *Arion* n.s. 2/2 (1975): 238–61, with references, esp. D. Tarrant, "Plato as Dramatist," *JHS* 75 (1955):82–89.

2. E. A. Havelock, "The Socratic Self as It Is Parodied in Aristophanes' *Clouds,*" *YCS* 22 (1972):1–18, gives a succinct review and bibliography of the relationship between Socratic and Platonic teachings. G. Vlastos's review of W. K. C. Guthrie, *A History of Greek Philosophy,* vol. 4, *Plato, the Man and His Dialogues: Earlier Period* (Cambridge, 1974), in *TLS* 12 (December 1975):1475–76, provides a brief overview of the current state of Platonic scholarship.

3. D. Clay's review of G. Vlastos, *Platonic Studies* (Princeton, 1973), in *Arion* n.s. 2/1 (1975):116–32, discusses the problems of deducing information about Plato himself from the Platonic dialogues. Plato is such a rich, imaginative thinker that it is difficult to equate any one of his imaginative creations with his own personality or conflicts. Yet certain themes and images run so constantly through the dialogues that they must represent his personal stamp. The most extensive study of the relationship between Plato's personal psychology and the vicissitudes of his philosophy is Y. Brès, *La psychologie de Platon* (Paris, 1968). An imaginative work, it is bedeviled by methodological insufficiencies from both a classical and a psychoanalytic perspective. It is reviewed in L. Brisson, "Platon psychanalysé," *REG* 86 (1973):224–31.

4. This highly condensed discussion of the pre-Socratics is based principally on H. Cherniss, *Aristotle's Criticism of Plato and the Academy*, vol. 1 (Baltimore, 1944); B. Snell, *The Discovery of the Mind*, trans. T. G. Rosenmeyer (Cambridge, Mass., 1953); and E. A. Havelock, *Preface to Plato* (Cambridge, Mass., 1963). J. Burnet, *Early Greek Philosophy*, 4th ed. (London, 1958), presents a contrasting view. Havelock's views about the pre-Socratics and Plato are controversial. His *Preface to Plato* is reviewed, sometimes quite critically, in F. Solmson, *AJP* 87 (1966):99–105; R. G. Hoerber, *CP* 59 (1964):70–74; N. Gulley, *CR* (1964):31–33 (the most sympathetic); and H. Myerhoff, *Gnomon* 36 (1964):422–24. I believe that none of the major objections raised by these reviewers is lethal to Havelock's main thesis, though they do require detailed rebuttal.

5. See references in LSJ, s.v. *Phusiologeō*. Aristotle calls the pre-Socratics *phusiologoi* (e.g., *Poetics*, 1447b19). These terms do not appear in the extant fragments of the pre-Socratics.

6. Translation modified from G. S. Kirk and J. E. Raven, *The Presocratic Philosophers* (Cambridge, 1962), pp. 372–73. I render *apeiron* "without boundary" instead of "infinite," which is more abstract than is appropriate here.

7. K. von Fritz, "*Noos, Noein,* and Their Derivatives in Pre-Socratic Philosophy," pt. 1, *CP* 40 (1975):223–42; pt. 2, *CP* 41 (1946):12–34.

8. H. Diels, ed., *Die Fragmente der Vorsokratiker*, with additions by W. Kranz, 5th–7th eds. (Berlin, 1934–54), Heraclitus, B45.

9. Ibid., Heraclitus, B119. D. Clay has pointed out to me the connection between this fragment and the Homeric *daimonie* (personal communication).

10. This is a minority opinion, argued in J. Burnet, "The Socratic Doctrine of the Soul," *Proc. Brit. Acad.* 7 (1916):235–59; Havelock, *Preface to Plato;* and D. Claus, "Psyche: A Study in the Language of the Self before Plato" (Ph.D. dissertation, Yale, 1969). The majority view sees a gradual evolution of psyche, not a Socratic "revolution."

11. See Havelock, "Socratic Self." The English word "self" derives from a root that also comes to designate words meaning "the group." Thus the original distinction between "self" and "other" seems to be based on the distinction between "our tribe" and "the others" (*AHD*).

12. Translation from T. M. Robinson, *Plato's Psychology* (Toronto, 1970), p. 11.

13. Ibid, p. 8. *Alcibiades I*, 130C: "*hē psuchē estin anthrōpos.*"

14. Claus, "Psyche," pp. 221–30 (Democritus) and 240–46 (the medical writers).

15. The idea of motion is often associated with psyche. Especially in the *Timaeus*, the psyche *is* a motion. As G. Vlastos points out, mental events in Plato (especially in the *Timaeus*) are described as motions: "The Disorderly Motion in the *Timaeus*" (1939) and "Creation in the *Timaeus*: Is It a Fiction?" (1964), in *Studies in Plato's Metaphysics*, ed. R. E. Allen (London, 1942), pp. 379–420. The significance of orderly versus disorderly motion is discussed later in this chapter.

16. E.g., *horos, Topics,* 101b39; *horismos, Poetics,* 91a1. On Aristotle's *Metaphysics*, 1078b, see R. Robinson, *Plato's Earlier Dialectic*, 2d ed. (Oxford, 1953), pp. 46–60.

Robinson agrees that Socrates and Plato did not have an abstract term for definition. T. Irwin argues (personal communication) that Robinson's examples in fact are contrary to his conclusion.

17. See T. Irwin, "Euripides and Socrates," in *Essays on Attic Tragedy,* ed. R. L. Gordon (Cambridge, in press).

18. See W. I. Grossman and B. Simon, "Anthropomorphism: Motive, Meaning, and Causality in Psychoanalytic Theory," *Psa. Study Child* 24 (1969):78–111.

19. Paraphrased from *Republic,* 588B–589A.

20. The sexual imagery in Plato brings up complex issues. Briefly, homosexual physical love is the first step on the road to love of the true, the good, the beautiful. Heterosexual love (or sexuality) is not so described. In the *Republic,* the *Symposium,* and the *Phaedrus,* the imagery of coming to see or know the highest good is heavily colored with the language of mystical fusion and transcendence. It includes the imagery of sexual union and reproduction, but the imagery tends to be typical of pregenital sexual fantasy. Nowhere in the Platonic dialogues, to my knowledge, do we find heterosexual lust praised (and it is only occasionally even described). The heterosexual aspect of Plato's vision of fusion with the good emphasizes yearning rather than lusting. The issue of Plato's personal homosexuality and its relation to his philosophy is enormously important, but it is explored here only indirectly.

21. Plato has chosen a term, *doxa,* that also has connotations of madness. For *doxai* as hallucinations, see Aeschylus, *Choephoroi,* l. 1052; also *mainomenē doxa* in the *Bacchae,* l. 887 (Chorus).

22. Best spelled out in A. W. H. Adkins, *Merit and Responsibility* (London, 1960).

23. Contrast the *Symposium,* where the sexual imagery emphasizes pregnancy, with the *Phaedrus,* where the imagery emphasizes (homosexual) excitement, erection, penetration, and mutilation.

24. F. M. Cornford incorrectly asserts that for Plato, *eros* comes from above and is then degraded ("The Doctrine of Eros in Plato's Symposium," in *The Unwritten Philosophy* [Cambridge, 1950]).

25. See Xenophon, *Memorabilia,* 1.1.15–18, where "What is *sōphrosunē?*" and "What is *mania?*" are listed as topics of Socratic inquiry. Note that the first *elenchus* (argument) in the *Republic* involves the example of whether or not it is just to return a dangerous weapon to a madman who has lent it to you (331C–D). See the discussion and bibliographical notes in W. Leibbrand and A. Wettley, *Der Wahnsinn* (Freiburg, 1961), pp. 59–66. See also Brès, *Psychologie de Platon,* pp. 287–319.

26. Plato did not originate the metaphor "sickness of the psyche," but he used it extensively (F. Kudlien, "Krankheitsmetaphorik in Laurentiushymnus des Prudentius," *Hermes* 90 [1962]:104–115; F. Wehrlis, "Ethik und Medizin: zur Vorgeschichte der aristotelischen Mesonlehre," *Mus. Helvet.* 8 [1951]:36–62, and "Der Artzvergleich bei Plato," ibid., pp. 177–84.

27. See J. Neu, "Plato's Analogy of State and Individual: The *Republic* and the Organic Theory of the State," *Philosophy* 46 (1971):236–54.

28. Translation from P. Shorey, *Plato: The Republic,* LCL (Cambridge, Mass., 1946).

29. First suggested to me by T. Irwin and borne out by my own preliminary investigations of political metaphors in the medical writings. See also G. Vlastos, "Slavery in Plato's Thought" and "*Isonomia Politikē,*" in his *Platonic Studies,* pp. 147–203.

30. Translation from R. G. Bury, *Plato,* vol. 8, LCL (London, 1920).

31. Translation mine. See also Plato, *Republic,* 571D; *Laws,* 689A.

32. Translation of this and following passages from Shorey, *Plato: The Republic.*

33. See Freud, *Interpretation of Dreams,* SE 4:67; 5:620.

34. "So it thinks" is my version of *hos oietai,* instead of Shorey's bowdlerized "in fancy."

35. Translation from Plato, *The Dialogues,* trans. B. Jowett, 3d ed. (1892; reprint Oxford, 1924).

36. *Statesman,* 268E–274E, esp. 271A; *Republic,* 414B–15D.

37. For the best review and critical evaluation, see A. Esman, "The Primal Scene: A Review and Reconsideration," *Psa. Study Child* 28 (1973):49–82.

38. M. Bonaparte, "Notes on the Analytic Discovery of a Primal Scene," *Psa. Study Child* 1 (1945):119–25.

39. Esp. Freud's analysis of the "wolf man" and of his dream, SE 17:29–47.

40. See P. Greenacre, "The Primal Scene and the Sense of Reality," *Psa. Q.* 42 (1973):10–41, and W. A. Meyers, "Split Self-Representation and the Primal Scene," *Psa. Q.* 42 (1973):525–38. See also N. Simon, "Primal Scene, Primary Objects, and *Nature Morte:* A Psychoanalytic Study of Mark Gertler," *Int. Rev. Psa.* 4 (1977):61–70.

41. Pointed out in Esman, "Primal Scene," 73, and in G. Devereux, "Primal Scene and Juvenile Heterosexuality in Mohave Society," in *Psychoanalysis and Culture,* ed. G. B. Wilbur and W. Muensterberger (New York, 1951), pp. 90–117.

42. William Faulkner, *Light in August* (New York, 1950), pp. 104–107, contains a brilliant description of such a sequence.

43. Plato's objections to theater would certainly be a corollary of this construction. That is, for him the prospect of *viewing* a presentation is invaded by a primal scene fantasy. The primal scene, in a sense, is bad theater, for it represents an excessive breakdown of boundaries, poorly modulated affect, and unsublimated fantasy. See H. Edelheit, "Mythopoiesis and the Primal Scene," *Psa. Study Soc.* 5 (1971):212–33 (which must be taken *cum grano salis*), and D. Dervin, "The Primal Scene and the Technology of Perception in Theater and Film," *Psa. R.* 62 (1975):269–304.

44. H. Kelsen, "Platonic Love," *Am. Im.* 3 (1949):1–70, presents the most extended discussion of Plato's homosexuality. G. Vlastos, "The Individual as Object of Love in Plato," in his *Platonic Studies,* pp. 3–42, gives a basically correct assessment of the relationship between Plato's homosexuality and his sense of love (the discussion is somewhat confused, however, and would benefit from more precise psychodynamic formulation). Clay's otherwise thoughtful review (cited in n. 3) unfortunately does not help dispel the confusion.

45. "Primal Scene Experience in Human Evolution and Its Phantasy Derivatives," *Psa. Study Soc.* 4 (1967):34–79.

46. Translation from Plato, *Dialogues,* trans. Jowett.

47. Ibid.

48. See *OCD*², s.v. Bendis.

49. See list in Shorey, *Plato: The Republic,* vol. 2, p. 143, n. 9.

50. Translation mine. Note also *mainomenōn,* insane, at 329D.

51. Herodotus (*Histories,* bk. 1, secs. 8–13) presented another version of the myth, in which the king insisted that Gyges hide in the bedroom to see the queen naked. For an elegant analysis of the Platonic version, see C. Hanly, "An Unconscious Irony in Plato's *Republic,*" *Psa. Q.* 46 (1977):116–47.

52. See too *Republic,* 560B. D. Clay has pointed out to me that *hupo skotou* is regularly a term for illegitimate birth (see J. Adam, *The Republic of Plato,* 2d ed. [Cambridge, 1963]). I believe, however, that in this passage the phrase is both literal and metaphorical.

53. D. E. Hahm, "Plato's 'Noble Lie' and Political Brotherhood," *Classica et Mediaevalia* 30 (1975):211–27, presents a thoughtful discussion of the theme of brotherhood in the *Republic.* Hahm's emphasis is on the adaptive aspect of Plato's scheme, while mine is on the unconscious conflict. The other dialogue with Plato's brothers (and his younger half brother and stepbrother) is the *Parmenides,* which deals with the categories, subdivisions, and "families" to which objects and their forms belong, and about complex interrelationships. See also *Republic,* 328B.

54. Translation from Shorey, *Plato: The Republic,* vol. 2, pp. 118–19, note a. Italics mine. My construction is, to my knowledge, the first of the Freudian "fantastic interpretations" to which Shorey alludes in his commentary on 514A, though I doubt it will be the last.

55. See G. F. Else, "The Structure and Date of Book 10 of Plato's *Republic,*" *Abhandlungen der Heidelberger Akademie der Wissenschaften* (Heidelberg, 1972) pp. 28–29, 39, and n. 57.

56. In Euripides' *Bacchae,* l. 1301, the same word is used for Agave's madness. At l. 1264 Cadmus urges her to look at the sun (sky?) to clear her head.

57. Translation mine. See *Republic,* 506E–507A, for the image of the "offspring of the good."

58. Translation from Shorey, *Plato: The Republic,* vol. 2, p. 143. See also Shorey's footnotes g and h on p. 143.

59. Other passages linking illicit sexual activity with bad government are 557B (a garment of many colors as equivalent to *polupragmosunē*), 558B, 560B.

9. The Philosopher as Therapist

1. Cambridge, Mass., 1963.

2. H. Diels, ed., *Die Fragmente der Vorsokratiker,* with additions by W. Kranz, 5th–7th eds. (Berlin, 1934–54), Xenophanes B1.

3. Book 3 focuses on the training of the guardians, Book 10 on the philosophers. Apparently the philosophers' renunciation of poetry must be far more stringent than the guardians'.

4. See P. Laín Entralgo, *The Therapy of the Word in Classical Antiquity,* trans. L. J. Rather and J. M. Sharp (New Haven, 1970), pp. 108–138.

5. G. F. Else, "Structure and Date of Book 10 of Plato's *Republic,*" *Abhandlungen der Heidelberger Akademie der Wissenschaften* (Heidelberg, 1972), p. 47.

6. Translation mine, based on A. Bloom, *The Republic of Plato* (New York, 1968).

7. H. Doolittle, *Tribute to Freud* (New York, 1956), discusses the role of images and shadows of ancient scenes in her brief analysis with Freud. Her "calcomanias" have primal scene connotations, but are also the images of her poetic creativity.

8. I thank Dr. Stanley Palombo for helpful discussion on these points.

9. Translation from Plato, *The Dialogues,* trans. B. Jowett, 3d ed. (1892; reprint Oxford, 1924).

10. See R. Robinson, *Plato's Earlier Dialectic* (Oxford, 1953); G. Ryle, *Plato's Progress* (Cambridge, 1966), esp. chaps. 4 and 6; A. J. P. Kenny, "Mental Health in Plato's *Republic,*" *Proc. Brit. Acad.* 55 (1969):229–53; and J. Stannard, "Socratic Eros and Platonic Dialectic," *Phronesis* 4 (1959):126–34; H. L. Sinaiko, *Love, Knowledge, and Discourse in Plato* (Chicago, 1965).

11. E.g., *Meno,* 75C–D.

12. E. R. Dodds, *The Greeks and the Irrational* (Berkeley, 1951), p. 64.

13. Stannard, "Socratic Eros."

14. Dodds, *Greeks and the Irrational,* pp. 207–224.

15. *Republic,* 620C. Odysseus chooses the psyche of the *apragmōn idiotēs,* the private, simple man, not caught up in *polupragmosunē.* See the discussion in V. Ehrenburg, "*Polupragmosunē*: A Study in Greek in Greek Politics," *JHS* 67 (1947):46–67.

16. A. E. Taylor, *Plato: The Man and His Work* (Cleveland, 1952), p. 351, argues that Plato does not agree that his theory of forms is fatally flawed, but rather that the dialogue is "an elaborate *jeu d'esprit.*" G. Vlastos has argued most cogently for the view that the dialogue is a "record of honest perplexity," and that Plato is willing to submit his own theory to an unusually searching critique. He also believes that, in fact, the arguments of the dialogue are a valid contradiction of Plato's theory. See

Vlastos, "The Third Man Argument in the *Parmenides*," in *Studies in Plato's Metaphysics*, ed. R. E. Allen (London, 1965), pp. 231–63, esp. 254–55, and 259–61. See also the other essays on the *Parmenides* in that volume, by G. Ryle, W. G. Runciman, P. T. Geach, and G. Vlastos.

17. Plato, *Dialogues*, trans. Jowett. Aristophanes' *Clouds* contains a caricature that anticipates (by seventy-five years) Plato's proposed *phrontistērion*, the think tank. Perhaps Plato's choice of name was intended as a rebuttal to Aristophanes.

18. See P. Rieff, *The Triumph of the Therapeutic* (New York, 1966), pp. 67–69.

19. There is much scholarly controversy about the nature of the activities and teachings of the Academy, particularly during Plato's lifetime. We do not know for certain which doctrines were taught, if any, or even whether dialectic was taught during Plato's lifetime. See H. Cherniss, *The Riddle of the Early Academy* (New York, 1962), and Ryle, *Plato's Progress*. For brief accounts, see Taylor, *Plato*, pp. 5–6, and H. I. Marrou, *A History of Education in Antiquity*, trans. G. Lamb (New York, 1956), pp. 102–105.

20. See E. A. Havelock, *Preface to Plato* (Cambridge, Mass., 1963), "Pre-Literacy and the Pre-Socratics," *Bull. Instit. Class. Stud.* 13 (1966):44–45, *Prologue to Greek Literacy* (Norman, Okla., 1971), and *A History of the Greek Mind*, vol. 2 (in preparation); M. McLuhan, *The Gutenberg Galaxy* (Toronto, 1962); W. J. Ong, *The Presence of the Word* (New Haven, 1967); R. Finnegan, "What Is Oral Literature Anyway?" in *Oral Literature and the Formula*, ed. B. A. Stoltz (Ann Arbor, 1976), pp. 127–76. See also I. Watt and J. Goodie, "Consequences of Literacy," *Comparative Studies in Society and History* 5 (1963):305–345. Some important remarks on the relationship between oral and literate culture and the "therapy of the word" may be found in W. J. Ong's foreword to Laín Entralgo, *Therapy of the Word*, pp. ix–xvi. Ong makes excellent use of Havelock's ideas and confirms the gist of my own arguments. See also A. G. Woodhead, *The Study of Greek Inscriptions* (Cambridge, 1967), pp. 6 and 15–16, and *OCD*², s.v. Alphabet, Greek.

21. Evidence from fifth-century vase paintings indicates that reading and writing were taught in adolescence, not at age six or seven.

22. This possibility adds another dimension to the intense conflicts around vision in the play: a reflection of conflict between fathers and sons over knowing how to read.

23. Havelock, "Prologue to Greek Literacy."

24. Plato himself says nothing about the introduction or spread of literacy in his day or the decades before him. In the *Phaedrus* (274C–279C) the attack on the use of writing is highly specific to the setting of that dialogue and does not have global application. H. Sinaiko, *Love, Knowledge, and Discourse in Plato*, argues cogently (p. 15) that Plato wishes to combine the best of both the spoken word and the written word. For references to writing and literacy in Plato, see the index to Plato, *Dialogues*, trans. Jowett, s.v. Letter, Syllable, and Writing.

25. Havelock, *Preface to Plato*, p. 200.

26. See R. S. Bluck's commentary in *Plato's Meno* (Cambridge, 1961), p. 344. See too S. Reid, "The *Apology* of Socrates," *Psa. R.* 62 (1975): 97–106.

27. See, however, Robinson, *Plato's Earlier Dialectic*, pp. 146–47, "A Conflict between Plato's Epistemology and His Methodology."

28. Suggested in Shorey and Bloom, *Republic of Plato*, p. 345.

29. Recall the tradition that Aristotle was known as the *nous* (mind) of the Academy, cited in J. H. Randall, Jr., *Aristotle* (New York, 1962), p. 13.

30. *OCD*², s.v. Education. The best single work on Greek education is still Marrou, *History of Education in Antiquity*.

31. See pp. 249 and 320, n. 29, for fuller discussion and references.

32. See E. A. Havelock, "Why Was Socrates Tried?" in *Studies in Honor of Gilbert*

Norwood, ed. M. E. White (Toronto, 1952), pp. 95–109, which forms the basis of the present discussion.

33. D. Clay, "Socrates' Mulishness and Heroism," *Phronesis* 27 (1972):53–60, demonstrates that Socrates *is* eros.

34. George Orwell's phrase from *1984*.

35. K. J. Dover prefers "superior discourse" and "inferior discourse" in his edition of the *Clouds* (Oxford, 1970), p. xxiii.

36. Dodds, *Greeks and the Irrational,* p. 61, n. 104; see also *Republic,* 562E, and P. Shorey, *Plato: The Republic,* LCL (Cambridge, 1946), vol. 2, p. 307, note g.

37. *Aristophanes: Three Comedies,* ed. W. Arrowsmith (Ann Arbor, 1969).

38. Ibid.

39. E.g., ll. 650–54, 924, 1371.

40. S. Halpern, "Free Association in 432 B.C.," *Psa. R.* 50 (1963):419–36, cleverly analyzes this interchange as a caricature of psychotherapy.

41. Dodds, *Greeks and the Irrational,* esp. chap. 2; G. Glotz, *La solidarité de la famille dans le droit criminel en Grèce* (Paris, 1904; reprint New York, 1973). Two important but neglected pieces are Z. Barbu, "The Emergence of Personality in the Greek World," in *Problems of Historical Psychology* (New York, 1960), pp. 69–144, and R. de Saussure, "Le miracle grec," *Rev. Fr. Psa.* 10 (1938):87–148, 323–77, 471–536.

42. Dodds, *Greeks and the Irrational,* chap. 7.

43. See R. Ekstein and R. L. Motto, *From Learning for Love to Love of Learning: Essays on Psychoanalysis and Education* (New York, 1969).

44. See Socrates' claim for such rewards from the city (*Apology,* 36).

10. Plato and Freud

Note: Chapter 10 is a revision and expansion of my article "Plato and Freud: The Mind in Conflict and the Mind in Dialogue," *Psa. Q.* 42 (1973):91–122.

1. SE 7:134.

2. E. R. Dodds, "Plato and the Irrational," *JHS* 65 (1945):16–100.

3. *The Ego and the Id,* SE 19:25.

4. *Three Essays on the Theory of Sexuality,* SE 7:134. The article Freud cites is M. Nachmanson, "Freuds Libido Theorie verglichen mit der Eroslehre Platos," *Int. J. Psa.* 3 (1915):65–83.

5. See index to SE 24 s.v. Plato.

6. Simon, "Plato and Freud." See in particular P. Laín Entralgo, *The Therapy of the Word in Classical Antiquity,* trans. L. J. Rather and J. M. Sharp (New Haven, 1970); E. Amado Levy-Valensi, "Verité et language du dialog platonicien au dialogue psychanalytique," *La Psychanalyse* 1 (1956):257–74; W. Leibbrand and A. Wettley, *Der Wahnsinn* (Freiburg, 1961). The most extensive recent work is Y. Brès, *La psychologie de Platon* (Paris, 1968) (see Chapter 8, n. 3). Useful articles written from a psychoanalytic perspective (but not primarily concerned with comparisons between Plato and Freud) are H. Kelsen, "Platonic Love," *Am. Im.* 3 (1942):1–110, and P. Plass, "Philosophic Anonymity and Irony in the Platonic Dialogues," *AJP* 85 (1964):254–78 and "Eros, Play, and Death in Plato," *Am. Im.* 26 (1969):37–55. A major contribution is C. Hanly, "An Unconscious Irony in Plato's *Republic,*" *Psa. Q.* 46 (1977):116–47.

7. Freud once said that his knowledge of Plato was fragmentary. As a young man he had translated some essays of J. S. Mill into German, including "Grote's Plato" (*Edinburgh Review,* April 1866). Freud was impressed by Plato's idea of *anamnesis,* recollection, which Mill treated sympathetically. See E. Jones, *The Life and Work of Sigmund Freud,* vol. 1, *1856–1900* (New York, 1953), pp. 55–56. Mill's essay is available in B. Gross, ed., *Great Thinkers on Plato* (New York, 1969), pp. 135–93.

8. Hence, in my view, Plato's tripartite model does not successfully solve the issues raised by the psyche-soma model.

9. For a succinct account of the history of changes in Freud's theories, see C. Brenner, *An Elementary Textbook of Psychoanalysis,* rev. ed. (New York, 1973). My view of this fundamental dichotomy running through all of Freud's changing formulations runs counter to much of the emphasis in current psychoanalytic thinking on the uniqueness and novelty of the structural theory. I believe the power of the structural theory lies in its clinical formulations rather than in its radicalness as a theoretical formulation. See W. I. Grossman and B. Simon, "Anthropomorphism: Motive, Meaning, and Causality in Psychoanalytic Theory," *Psa. Study Child* 24 (1969):78–111.

10. See W. I. Grossman, "Reflections on the Relationships of Introspection and Psycho-Analysis," *Int. J. Psa.* 48 (1967):16–31, and Grossman and Simon, "Anthropomorphism."

11. See G. Vlastos, "Slavery in Plato's Thought," in his *Platonic Studies* (Princeton, 1973).

12. "The Resistances to Psycho-Analysis," SE 19:218.

13. See S. H. Fraiberg, *The Magic Years* (New York, 1959), pp. 23–27 for an example in childhood. Modern ego psychology emphasizes that curiosity has roots independent of the scopophilic instinct, but that the two are closely intertwined. See H. Hartmann, E. Kris, R. Loewenstein, *Papers on Psychoanalytic Psychology,* monograph 14, *Psychological Issues* 4 (1964).

14. Roy Schafer, *A New Language for Psychoanalysis* (New Haven, 1976), represents a partially successful attempt to reformulate psychoanalytic propositions without the language of energy.

15. SE 1:283–397. The following discussion owes much to conversations with Dr. W. Grossman; see also W. Stewart, *Psychoanalysis: The First Ten Years, 1888–1898* (New York and London, 1967).

16. See in particular "Instincts and Their Vicissitudes" and the Editor's Note, SE 14:105–140, esp. 111–13. Freud speaks of instincts in two ways, as (1) "a concept on the frontier between the mental and the somatic . . . a psychical representative of the stimuli originating from within the organism and reaching the mind," and (2) a concept that differentiates between the instinct, which is more somatic, and the "instinctual representation," or psychic representation of an instinct. That is, Freud is not entirely clear on the allocation of somatic and psychic aspects of instinct.

17. This distinction was pointed out to me by T. Irwin. A major difference between Plato and Freud, of course, is that Freud has an elaborate notion of the emergence of instinctual drives in a great variety of derivative, symbolized, and disguised forms.

18. E.g., "Recommendations to Physicians Practicing Psycho-analysis," SE 12:109–120 (1920); "Analysis Terminable and Interminable," SE 23:209–253 (1937).

19. SE 22:79

20. SE 21:59–148; see pp. 123–45 for the very unplatonic notion of unconscious guilt.

21. See "On Psychotherapy" and "Psychical (or Mental) Treatment," SE 7:257–68 and 283–302.

22. I cannot locate the source of this quotation.

23. SE 12:108.

24. A. Gouldner, *Enter Plato* (New York, 1965), p. 148 and passim.

25. Dr. A. Tyson (personal communication).

26. J. Piaget, *Structuralism,* ed. and trans. C. Maschler (New York, 1970), pp. 106–119, contains an excellent discussion of the relationship between structures and the mind that does the structuring. See also Simon, "Plato and Freud," and Grossman and Simon, "Anthropomorphism."

27. M. Schur, *Freud: Living and Dying* (New York, 1972), esp. pp. 19–22 and 127–31 (where Schur speculates on the significance of Freud's probable repeated exposure to the primal scene before age four).

28. We have little autobiographical information on Plato, with the exception of the *Seventh Letter*, which most scholars believe to be genuine. (My own examination of the imagery of the letter leads me to conclude that it bears the same marks of a primal scene fantasy as parts of the *Republic*.) Surmises about the psychoanalytic formulations must come from the dialogues, and I have already noted the problems of using them as a source of statements about Plato himself (Chapter 8, n. 3). Be that as it may, I list here the points I feel must be considered in any psychoanalytic treatment of Plato, his character, and the relationship between his character and his work: (1) the known facts of his family life, including the death of his father and the remarriage of his mother; (2) suggestions of a characterological Hamlet-like hesitancy in politics (*Seventh Letter*); when he did leap, he botched it; (3) a depressive cast; (4) his proposal to eliminate the family in the *Republic*, a dialogue in which his brothers appear; (5) his idealization of and intense attachment to Socrates, accompanied by hints of some ambivalence (e.g., he was not present at Socrates' death); (6) the possibility that the trial and death of Socrates revived unresolved oedipal feelings around the death of his father and the remarriage of his mother; (7) the prominence of parricidal themes throughout the dialogues; (8) evidence of a homosexual orientation (e.g., his relationship to Dion, his lack of interest in or disdain of female sexuality and a lack of evidence of any heterosexual life, together with hints of ambivalence toward homosexuality (e.g., *Phaedrus*, 250E); (9) the prominence of primal scene imagery in the dialogues; (10) his emphasis on renunciation and control of instinctual drives and his disdain for the sensory and the sensual, pointing toward a severe superego; (11) the contents of his philosophical ideas and the sequence of their change and development, especially the scheme of degrees of reality, in which the forms are the most real; (12) his teaching methods, and the problem of promulgation and propagation of his teachings; (13) his ability to transform his individual malaise into a diagnosis and method of treatment of the malaise of society at large. See now C. Hanly, "Unconscious Irony in Plato's Republic."

29. *Moses and Monotheism*, SE 23:58, 66–72, and passim. See R. Robinson, *Plato's Earlier Dialectic* (Oxford, 1953), pp. 202–223. M. Black, *Models and Metaphors* (Ithaca, N.Y., 1962), contains a useful discussion (esp. chaps. 3 and 13) of the assets and debits of analogies and model making.

30. SE 2:305.

31. See P. Ricoeur, *Freud and Philosophy: An Essay on Interpretation*, trans. D. Savage (New Haven, 1970). The relationships between Freud and Kant, Hegel, and even Spinoza are just beginning to be explored by Ricoeur and others. C. Hanly, "Unconscious Irony in Plato's *Republic*," pp. 138–39, criticizes my comparison of Plato and Freud on the basis (*inter alia*) of the vast difference between modern and ancient philosophy (the Renaissance is the turning point). I believe Hanly is correct to emphasize this difference, but he misreads the main thrust of my discussion of the similarities in Plato and Freud and the differences between them.

11. The Hippocratic Corpus

1. The quotation originated with the neurophysiologist Dr. Ralph Gerard.

2. See M. Siegler and H. Osmond, *Models of Madness, Models of Medicine* (New York, 1974) esp. chaps. 4 and 5.

3. P. Laín Entralgo, *The Therapy of the Word in Classical Antiquity*, trans. L. J. Rather and J. M. Sharp (New Haven, 1970), p. 141 and references cited there.

4. A recent study is D. Goltz, *Studien zür altorientalischen und griechischen Heilkunde* (Wiesbaden, 1974). I have not been able to consult this work, but according to F.

Kudlien "it is . . . justifiedly skeptical with regard to the exact amount of 'contributions' or 'influences' from the Orient" (personal communication). See also F. Kudlien, *Der Beginn des medizinischen Denkens bei den Griechen von Homer bis Hippokrates* (Zurich, 1967), p. 13. The influence of Egyptian medicine is discussed in J. B. de C. M. Saunders, *The Transitions from Ancient Egyptian to Greek Medicine* (Lawrence, Kans., 1963).

5. E.g., Machaon, *Iliad,* 2.732 and passim. "For a doctor is worth many men" (ibid., 11.514).

6. E.g., O. Temkin and C. L. Temkin, eds., *Ancient Medicine: Selected Papers of Ludwig Edelstein,* trans. C. L. Temkin (Baltimore, 1967). Also Edelstein's "Nachträge" on Hippocrates in *RE,* supp. 6, pp. 1290–1345. E. B. Levine, *Hippocrates* (New York, 1971), offers a good survey, esp. his annotated bibliography, pp. 155–68, as does L. Bourgey, "Greek Medicine from the Beginning to the End of the Classical Period," in *Ancient and Medieval Science,* ed. R. Taton, trans. A. J. Pomeroy (New York, 1963). References to Hippocrates, unless otherwise indicated, are from E. Littré, ed., *Hippocrate: Oeuvres complètes,* 10 vols. (Paris, 1849).

7. See Kudlien, *Beginn des medizinischen Denkens,* "Einleitung," and his "Early Greek Primitive Medicine," *Clio Medica* 3 (1968):305–336. R. Joly, *Le niveau de la science hippocratique* (Paris, 1966), emphasizes (somewhat unduly) the irrational and fantasy elements in Hippocrates. I fully agree, however, with Joly's assessment of the works on sex and reproduction. L. Bourgey, *Observation et expérience chez les médecins de la collection hippocratique* (Paris, 1953), emphasizes the empirical element.

8. To the extent that one can distinguish Coan from Cnidian material (and this is problematic), I cannot find differences vis-à-vis mental activity or mental illness.

9. W. Leibbrand and A. Wettley, *Der Wahnsinn* (Freiburg, 1961), pp. 24–57, discusses and collates sources. Littré, *Hippocrate,* vol. 6, pp. 111–12, gives examples of the theory of the primacy of blood in relation to mental life. *Psuchē* is not an especially common or important term of mental life in Hippocrates and appears most frequently in *On Diet* (ibid., p. 466), which has been ascribed to the fourth century. Ibid., vol. 10, p. 479, lists passages containing *psuchē.* See also D. Claus, "Psyche: A Study in the Language of the Self before Plato" (Ph.D. dissertation, Yale, 1969), pp. 240–46.

10. *On Internal Diseases,* Greek text in Littré, *Hippocrate,* vol. 7, pp. 284–89. Translation mine, drawing heavily on Littré. *Kluzein* here means "purge," not "wash." (See LSJ and references there, esp. to Sophocles fragments.) Beet juice was considered a good purgative for excess bile (J. Stannard, "Hippocratic Pharmacology," *Bull. Hist. Med.* 36 [1961]:497–518), and the quantities suggest a purgative rather than fluid to wash in (hemicotyl=402 cc).

11. The Hippocratic corpus is particularly rich in terms for delirium. The ones I have collected are: *parapheromai, paraphroneō, paranoō, parakrouō* (*Epidemics,* books 1 and 3); *parakopē, ekmainomai, mainomai, mania; lēros* and *paralēros, paralērō; paralelao; paraplesia; phluareō* (*katanoeō*=to come out of a delirium). Not all of these terms are specific for delirium; they may also connote being "out of one's head." See W. H. S. Jones, trans., *Hippocrates,* 4 vols., LCL (London, 1923), vol. 1, p. lix.

12. Works on this treatise are O. Temkin, "The Doctrine of Epilepsy in the Hippocratic Writings," *Bull. Hist. Med.* 1 (1933):277–322, and *The Falling Sickness,* 2d ed. (Baltimore, 1971). Texts, commentaries, and translations are H. Grenseman, *Die Hippokratische Schrift, "Über die heilige Krankheit"* (Berlin, 1968), and Jones, *Hippocrates,* vol. 2. See also Levine, *Hippocrates,* pp. 107–110.

13. The description of the vascular anatomy is grossly inaccurate and indicates that the author of the treatise had no experience in dissection and was writing for an audience that also had no such experience. C. R. S. Harris, *The Heart and the Vascular System in Ancient Greek Medicine from Alcmaeon to Galen* (Oxford, 1973), contains a definitive discussion of Greek knowledge of the blood and heart. See also L. Edelstein,

"The History of Dissection in Antiquity," in *Ancient Medicine,* ed. Temkin and Temkin; F. Solmson, "Greek Philosophy and the Discovery of the Nerves," *Mus. Helvet.* 18 (1961):150–97.

14. Translation from Jones, *Hippocrates,* vol. 2, p. 175.

15. The sections referred to here and elsewhere are those in Jones, *Hippocrates,* vol. 2, the most accessible translation of this treatise. In modern medicine, idiopathic epilepsy is a disease characterized by seizures (of several possible varieties: grand mal, petit mal, psychomotor), with no associated (detectable) brain lesion, such as tumor, blood clot, infectious focus. Needless to say, the notion of a "lesion" changes as techniques for locating the epileptic focus become increasingly refined.

16. Falling, however, is not listed among the symptoms in this treatise.

17. Aristotle, *Problemata,* 30. See Chapter 7, n. 21. Temkin, in *Falling Sickness,* doubts that Euripides linked Heracles with epilepsy. He has revised his view on the word *hieros,* sacred, which he now argues does not have the ambivalent connotation of the Latin *sacer* (i.e., both holy and cursed).

18. A ten-year-old boy was afflicted with Sydenham's chorea, a neurological sequela of rheumatic fever and streptococcal infection producing involuntary jerky motions of the limbs. When asked what caused this condition, he explained that the doctors told him it was the result of a toxin from a bacteria producing an allergic reaction in his nervous system, affecting the parts of the brain that control movement. But *he* thought it had to do with what his teacher had always said—that he was a bad boy because he never sat still in school. The boy held both a physiological and a mythological view of his condition.

19. This impression is based on my limited reading in Galen, on a search of the index to the principal Greek edition, C. G. Kuhn, ed., *Claudii Galenii: Opera Omnia* (Leipzig, 1821–1823), i–xx, and on P. De Lacy, "Galen and the Greek Poets," *GRBS* 7 (1966):259–66. See Galen's passages on Medea in *De Placitis Hippocratis et Platonis,* ed. I. Müller (Leipzig, 1874), pp. 283–84, where he mentions that Euripides calls her *megalosplanchnos,* large-spleened, thereby illustrating the connection between anger and the spleen (though Medea was not generally considered insane). See also the injunction not to quote the poets in medical lectures, *Precepts,* sec. 12, ll. 1–8, in Jones, *Hippocrates,* vol. 1, pp. 326–27.

20. See H. Diels, *Die Fragmente der Vorsokratiker,* with additions by W. Kranz, 5th–7th eds. (Berlin, 1934–1954), s.v. Alcmaeon and Diogenes; also, s.v. Philolaus, B13; see commentary in G. S. Kirk and J. E. Raven, *The Presocratic Philosophers* (Cambridge, 1957), and Grenseman, *Hippokratische Schrift,* pp. 27–31, who cites an otherwise obscure physician, Abas, who also held to the primacy of the brain. Alcmaeon's political metaphors *isonomia* (equal rule) and *monarchia* are relevant to the discussion in Chapter 8 on the dominant role of brain and physician (see Chapter 8, n. 29); see also Solmson, "Greek Philosophy."

21. *On Wounds in the Head,* sec. 13 and 19, in *Hippocrates,* LCL, vol. 3, trans. E. T. Withington, pp. 33 and 44. In popular thought, the connection between head (or brain) injury and raving is taken for granted, as in Aristophanes' *Clouds,* ll. 1271–76 (*egkephalon seseisthai*).

22. See E. Clarke, "Aristotelean Concepts of the Form and Function of the Brain," *Bull. Hist. Med.* 37 (1963):1–14; D. H. M. Woollam, "Concepts of the Brain and Its Functions in Classical Antiquity," in *The History and Philosophy of Knowledge of the Brain and Its Functions,* ed. F. N. L. Poynter (Springfield, Ill., 1958).

23. R. Onians, *The Origins of European Thought* (Cambridge, 1951), esp. pp. 93–122, 186, 199, and 227–28.

24. See *Timaeus,* 69E–72D. The parts above and below the diaphragm, respectively, are compared to the men's and women's quarters, with the implicit comparison of women to the baser parts of the psyche.

25. Cf. the historian Christopher Hill's thesis about William Harvey and his views on the primacy of the heart, discussed in O. Temkin, "The Historiography of Ideas in Medicine," in *Modern Methods in the History of Medicine*, ed. E. Clarke (London, 1971), pp. 1–21.

26. Another parallel between the brain and the doctor is the function of diagnosis. See *On the Sacred Disease*, sec. XIX, for *diagnōsis* (discrimination) for the brain and sec. XX for *diaginōskein* (to discriminate) for the physician (Jones, *Hippocrates*, vol. 2, pp. 178–81).

27. In reference to the traditional statement that Hippocrates separated medicine from philosophy, see Kudlien, *Beginn des medizinischen Denkens*, p. 7. See too Edelstein, "The Role of Eryximachus in Plato's *Symposium*" and "The Relation of Ancient Philosophy to Medicine," in *Ancient Medicine*, ed. Temkin and Temkin; G. E. R. Lloyd, "Who Is Attacked in *On Ancient Medicine?*" *Phronesis* 8 (1963):108–126.

28. Translation from Plato, *The Dialogues*, trans. B. Jowett, 3d ed. (1892; reprint Oxford, 1924). For the numerous references to medicine in Plato, see Jowett's index s.v. Medicine. See also W. Jaeger, *Paideia*, trans. G. Highet (New York, 1944), vol. 3, pp. 3–45, and F. Wehrli, "Der Artzvergleich bei Platon," *Mus. Helvet.* 8 (1951):177–83. The most perplexing passage about medicine in Plato is *Phaedrus*, 270B, where Plato purports to describe the Hippocratic method of reasoning about the body. See R. Joly, "La question hippocratique et le temoignage du *Phèdre*," *REG* 74 (1961):69–92.

29. For examples of their use, see *On Internal Diseases* (Littré, *Hippocrate*, vol. 7, p. 274).

30. Laín Entralgo, *Therapy of the Word*, pp. 139–70, provides a good discussion of the communication between doctor and patient, emphasizing the connections between rhetoric and medical communication. The field of medicine was very much immersed in the oral modes of teaching and learning, and still is. The connections between medicine and the rise of literacy deserve exploration.

31. See *Regimen*, in *Hippocrates*, trans. Jones, vol. 4, pp. 420–47, the classic Hippocratic discussion of dreams. S. Silverman, a psychoanalyst, argues that in his clinical work he has found instances of physical illness revealed in dreams (*Psychological Cues in Forecasting Physical Illness* [New York, 1970]).

32. I. Veith, *Hysteria: The History of a Disease* (Chicago, 1965), p. 36. But see Apuleius, *Golden Ass*, bk. 10, sec. 2, ll. 4–8 (e.g., in the translation by J. Lindsay [Bloomington, Ind., 1962], p. 213) for the charge that doctors are inept at recognizing lovesickness.

33. E.g., as found in Caelius Aurelianus, *On Acute Diseases and on Chronic Diseases*, trans. I. E. Drabkin (Chicago, 1950).

34. See E. Glover, "The Therapeutic Effect of Inexact Interpretation," *Int. J. Psa.* 12 (1931):397–411. Glover hypothesizes that the use of cathartics and emetics in the treatment of psychological disturbances allows the patient the unconscious fantasy of purging all his bad *psychological* stuff.

12. Aristotle on Melancholy

1. The major works on the history of melancholy are H. Flashar, *Melancholie und Melancholiker in den medizinischen Theorien der Antike* (Berlin, 1966); R. Klibansky, E. Panofsky, and F. Saxl, *Saturn and Melancholy* (New York, 1964); F. Kudlien, *Der Beginn des medizinischen Denkens bei den Griechen von Homer bis Hippokrates* (Zurich, 1967) and "Schwärzliche Organe im frühgriechischen Denken," *Medizin historisches Journal* 8 (1973):53–58; A. Lewis, "Melancholia: A Historical Review," in his *The State of Psychiatry* (London, 1967), pp. 71–110 (with copious bibliography); W. Leibbrand and A. Wettley, *Der Wahnsinn* (Freiburg, 1961), pp. 43–89; and W. Müri,

"Melancholie und schwarze Galle," *Mus. Helvet.* 10 (1953):21–38; J. Starobinski, "Geschichte der Melancholiebehandlung von den Anfängen bis 1900" (*Documenta Geigy*), *Acta Psychosomatica* 4 (1960).

2. E.g., *Epidemics* bk.6, sec. 8, para. 31, in E. Littré, *Hippocrate: Oeuvres complètes,* 10 vols. (Paris, 1849), vol. 5, pp. 354–56.

3. Ibid., p. 272.

4. *On Diseases,* bk. 2, para. 72, in ibid., vol. 7, pp. 108–111. Translation mine, based on Littré. In modern terms, this is probably an agitated depression.

5. See R. Klibansky, E. Panofsky, and F. Saxl, *Saturn and Melancholy* (New York, 1964); Flashar, *Melancholie und Melancholiker.*

6. Klibansky et al., *Saturn and Melancholy,* and review by B. Simon, *Psa. Q.* 37 (1968):145–49.

7. Translation from Klibansky et al., *Saturn and Melancholy,* pp. 18–19.

8. For Aristotle on inspiration and madness, see Chapter 7 and nn. 49–50.

9. F. Brommer, *Vasenlisten zür griechischen Heldensage,* 2d ed. (Marburg, 1960), discusses depictions of Ajax in vase paintings.

10. Text in *Hesiod, The Homeric Hymns, Homerica,* trans. H. G. Evelyn-White, LCL (Cambridge, Mass., 1936), p. 524, frag. 5.

11. See W. Burkert, "*Goēs:* Zum griechischen 'Schamanismus,' " *Rh. M.* 105 (1962):36–55, esp. pp. 48–49, and the critical discussion of Empedocles as shaman in C. H. Kahn, "Religion and Natural Philosophy in Empedocles' Doctrine of the Soul," in *Essays in Ancient Greek Philosophy,* ed. J. Anton (Albany, 1971), pp. 3–38, esp. 30–38.

12. See H. Kelsen, "Platonic Love," *Am. Im.* 3 (1942):1–110.

13. Comic fragment cited in Diogenes Laertius, *Lives of the Philosophers,* bk. 3, sec. 27, in P. Friedlander, *Plato: An Introduction,* trans. H. Meyerhoff (New York, 1964), p. 99; see also p. 354, n. 23.

14. A. W. H. Adkins suggests the connection between melancholia and the kinds of intense competitive strivings he posits for Greek culture (*From the Many to the One* [Ithaca, N.Y., 1970], p. 206).

15. Paraphrased, based on the translation of W. S. Hett, *Aristotle: On the Soul,* LCL (Cambridge, 1964), pp. 16–17.

16. J. Croissant, *Aristote et les mystères* (Paris, 1932), chaps. 1 and 2.

17. For the original formulation of the catecholamine hypothesis, see J. J. Schild-kraut, "The Catecholamine Hypothesis of Affective Disorders," *Am. J. Psychiat.* 122 (1965):509.

18. Kudlien, *Beginn des medizinischen Denkens,* pp. 77–99, and "Schwärtzliche Organe."

19. W. H. S. Jones, *Hippocrates,* LCL (London, 1923), vol. 1, pp. 260–63. See W. Müri, "Melancholie und Schwarze Galle." Note the account in Theophrastus' *Characters,* 20, "Ill-breeding" (in *The Characters of Theophrastus,* trans. J. M. Edmonds, LCL [London, 1929], p. 91), of the ill-bred man who announces at dinner that the bean soup is as black as his stools were the last time he took hellebore. It is unlikely that his stools were black, but it is likely that he expected hellebore to purge black bile.

20. Plato (*Timaeus,* 71) introduces a kind of psychophysiological synthesis of depression. The *nous* (brain) can use the bile contained in the liver to threaten the lower parts of the psyche and punish them for disobedience. The Furies and their "hypochondriasis" are discussed in Chapter 6; discussion of Plato's analogous version of hysteria may be found in Chapter 13.

21. See H. Fabrega, "Problems Implicit in the Cultural and Social Study of Depression," *Psychosomatic Medicine* 36 (1975):377–98.

22. The relation between a *fantasy* explanation and a *theory* of mental phenomena is

discussed in G. Devereux, "Cultural Thought Models in Primitive and Modern Psychiatric Theories," *Psychiatry* 21 (1958):359–74, revised in his *Ethnopsychanalyse complementariste* (Paris, 1972), chap. 10. On the importance of analogy in Greek science and medicine, see G. E. R. Lloyd, *Polarity and Analogy: Two Types of Argumentation in Early Greek Thought* (New York, 1966). See also B. Farrington, *Greek Science* (Harmondsworth, 1961), esp. pp. 66–70 and 138–42. Important in this regard is Hippocrates' *Regimen* 1, secs. 11–24 (in *Hippocrates,* trans. W. H. S. Jones, LCL [Cambridge, 1967], vol. 4, pp. 251–63), for examples of the way a Greek physician made inferences about unobservable physiological processes, such as digestion, using as analogies observable processes in such crafts as cooking, dyeing, and metallurgy.

23. SE 14:237–58. That is, Freud takes fantasies about the body and mind and uses them as a beginning in the formulation of a theory.

24. A series of excellent articles reviewing and expanding our current knowledge may be found in E. J. Anthony and T. Benedek, eds., *Depression and Human Existence* (Boston, 1975); M. F. Basch's synthesizing attempt, chap. 21, is especially rewarding.

13. Hysteria and Social Issues

1. See I. Veith, *Hysteria: The History of a Disease* (Chicago, 1965), and H. F. Ellenberger, *The Discovery of the Unconscious* (New York, 1970), especially important for the eighteenth and nineteenth centuries.

2. E.g., S. Freud, *An Autobiographical Study,* SE 20:3–76, esp. 13–19.

3. See Chapter 2.

4. See B. E. Moore and B. D. Fine, eds., *A Glossary of Psychoanalytic Terms and Concepts* (New York, 1968), s.v. Hysteria. These various psychoanalytic formulations are discussed in J. Marmor, "Orality in the Hysterical Personality," *J. Am. Psa. A.* 1 (1953):657–58; B. R. Easser and S. R. Lesser, "Hysterical Personality: A Reevaluation," *Psa. Q.* 34 (1965):390–405; W. R. D. Fairbairn, *An Object-Relations Theory of the Personality* (New York, 1954); D. Shapiro, *Neurotic Styles* (New York, 1965); and E. Zetzel, "The So-Called Good Hysteric," in her *The Capacity for Emotional Growth* (London, 1970).

5. See in particular C. Smith-Rosenberg, "The Hysterical Woman: Sex Roles and Role Conflict in Nineteenth-Century America," *Social Research* 39 (1972):652–78, and C. Smith-Rosenberg and C. Rosenberg, "The Female Animal: Medical and Biological Views of Woman and her Role in Nineteenth-Century America," *J. Am. Hist.* 60 (1973):332–56. See also M. H. Hollender, "Conversion Hysteria," *Arch. Gen. Psychiat.* 26 (1972):311–14; S. Marcus, *The Other Victorians* (New York, 1966); and A. D. Wood, " 'The Fashionable Diseases': Women's Complaints and Their Treatment in Nineteenth-Century America," *Journal of Interdisciplinary History* 4 (1973):27–52.

6. Classification of hysteria may be found in J. C. Nemiah, "Hysterical Neurosis," *CTP²*, pp. 1208–31.

7. The delineation of Briquet's syndrome is important. See R. A. Woodruff, Jr., P. J. Clayton, and S. B. Guze, "Hysteria: Studies of Diagnosis, Outcome, and Prevalence," *J. Am. Med. A.* 215 (1971):425–28.

8. For *a* see O. Fenichel, *The Psychoanalytic Theory of Neurosis* (New York, 1945), p. 528; *b* is often called Münchhausen syndrome, defined in *Psychiatric Dictionary,* ed. L. E. Hinsey and R. J. Campbell, 4th ed. (New York, 1970); for *c,* the impostors, see P. Greenacre, *Emotional Growth* (New York, 1971), vol. 1, pp. 95–112.

9. The term "inner objects" (or "object representations") refers to the internal picture, or conception, of the important people in a person's life, past and present.

10. See J. Neu, "Fantasy and Memory: The Aetiological Role of Thoughts according to Freud," *Int. J. Psa.* 54 (1973):383–98, and "Thought, Theory, and Therapy," *Psa. and Contemp. Sci.* 4 (1975):103–143; Freud, "Hysterical Phantasies and Their

Relationship to Bisexuality," SE 9:155–66, and "Some General Remarks on Hysterical Attacks," SE 9:227–34.

11. My own clinical observation, which requires further confirmation.

12. See A. Kiev, *Transcultural Psychiatry* (New York, 1972), esp. pp. 52–56; S. Parker, "Eskimo Psychopathology in the Context of Eskimo Personality and Culture," *American Anthropologist* 64 (1962):76–96. Also J. T. Proctor, "Hysteria in Childhood," in *Childhood Psychopathology*, ed. S. I. Harrison and J. F. McDermott (New York, 1972), pp. 431–44.

13. I am not discussing cases that *we* might diagnose as hysterical conversions but were not so diagnosed by the Greeks. Thus I do not deal with some of the cases mentioned in the inscriptions at Epidaurus in the temple of Asclepius which might be psychogenic. See the selection of inscriptions in E. J. Edelstein and L. Edelstein, *Asclepius*, 2 vols. (Baltimore, 1945).

14. E. Littré, *Hippocrate: Oeuvres completès*, 10 vols. (Paris, 1849), vol. 8, p. 327. Translation mine.

15. Veith, *Hysteria*, p. 10. Fantasy in medical writings on reproduction is discussed in R. Joly, *Le niveau de la science hippocratique* (Paris, 1966).

16. W. Leibbrand and A. Wettley, *Der Wahnsinn* (Freiburg, 1961), pp. 54–59, discusses hysteria in the Hippocratic writings in detail.

17. Littré, *Hippocrate*, vol. 8, pp. 466–71.

18. A similar fantasy in reverse, in which men are seen as derivative of women, can be seen in M. H. Sherfey, "The Evolution and Nature of Female Sexuality in Relation to Psychoanalytic Theory," *J. Am. Psa. A.* 14 (1966):28–128.

19. The best treatment of sexuality in classical Greece is K. J. Dover, "Classical Greek Attitudes to Sexual Behaviour," *Arethusa* 6 (1973):59–73, and *Greek Popular Morality in the Time of Plato and Aristotle* (Oxford, 1974). The latter work comments on the problem of the relative puritanism in the classical period (p. 207). J. Marcadé, *Eros Kalos* (Geneva, 1962), contains material on sexuality in Greek art.

20. The position of women in Greek antiquity is discussed in S. B. Pomeroy, *Goddesses, Whores, Wives, and Slaves* (New York, 1975); W. K. Lacey, *The Family in Classical Greece* (Ithaca, N.Y., 1968); and H. Licht, *Sexual Life in Ancient Greece*, ed. L. H. Dawson, trans. J. H. Freese (London, 1932).

21. See the articles "Expositio" and "Infanticidium" by G. Glotz in *Dictionnaire des antiquités grecques et romaines*, ed. C. Daremberg and E. Saglio (Paris, 1892).

22. Dover, "Classical Greek Attitudes," p. 66. Dover also points out that, while homosexual scenes are common on vases, homosexual intercourse is rarely portrayed.

23. P. E. Slater, *The Glory of Hera* (Boston, 1968).

24. E.g., the myth of Tiresias, who claimed that women get 90 percent of the pleasure of intercourse and men 10 percent. See Dover, "Classical Greek Attitudes."

25. The splitting of the woman into mother and sexual object is discussed in Freud, "Contributions to the Psychology of Love," SE 11:163–208, and A. Parsons, "Is the Oedipus Complex Universal? The Jones-Malinowski Debate Revisited and a South Italian 'Nuclear Complex,' " *Psa. Study Soc.* 3 (1964):278–328.

26. M. R. Lefkowitz, "Classical Mythology and the Role of Women in Modern Literature," in *A Sampler of Women's Studies*, ed. D. G. McGuigan (Ann Arbor, 1973), pp. 77–84.

27. The role of females in the Academy is discussed in Diogenes Laertius, *Lives of the Philosophers*, bk. 3, sec. 46, and Mary Renault, *Mask of Apollo* (New York, 1966).

28. A similar point is made by E. Badian in his review of Pomeroy, *Goddesses, Whores, Wives, and Slaves*, in *New York Review of Books*, October 30, 1975, pp. 28–31.

29. H. I. Marrou, *A History of Education in Antiquity*, trans. G. Lamb (New York, 1956); Licht, *Sexual Life*; G. Devereux, "Greek Pseudo-Homosexuality and the 'Greek Miracle,' " *Symbolae Osloenses*, fasc. 42 (1967):69–92; Dover, "Classical Greek Attitudes" and *Greek Popular Morality*; Slater, *Glory of Hera*.

30. Dover, "Classical Greek Attitudes," emphasizes the economic aspects of Greek attitudes to sexuality. Sexuality that did not squander the resources of the extended family was condoned.

31. T. Vanggard, *Phallos* (New York, 1972), p. 62, citing a study by E. Bethe, "Die dorische Knabenliebe," *Rh. M.* n.s. 62 (1907):438–75.

32. Aristophanes' *Clouds* and homosexual modesty are discussed in Chapter 9.

33. The danger of death in childbirth also contributed to conflict for the Greek woman.

34. Freud tells of such a failure in "Fragment of an Analysis of a Case of Hysteria," SE 7:3–124, esp. 105–122.

35. See, in particular, A. Preuss, "Biomedical Techniques for Influencing Human Reproduction in the Fourth Century B.C.," *Arethusa* 8 (1975):237–63. Father-daughter relations in Greek tragedy are discussed in R. Seidenberg and E. Papathomopoulos, "Daughters Who Tend Their Fathers: A Literary Survey," *Psa. Study Soc.* 2 (1962):135–60.

36. I. M. Lewis, *Ecstatic Religion* (Baltimore, 1971); E. R. Dodds, *The Greeks and the Irrational* (Berkeley, 1951), pp. 270–82. Also G. Mora, "An Historical and Sociopsychiatric Appraisal of Tarantism," *Bull. Hist. Med.* 35 (1963):417–40.

37. Lewis, *Ecstatic Religion*, pp. 62–64.

38. G. Harris, "Possession 'Hysteria' in a Kenya Tribe," *American Anthropologist* 59 (1957):1047–66.

39. An impressive account of a contemporary ritual in which women are allowed to attack men may be found in K. E. Read, *The High Valley* (New York, 1965), pp. 171–77. In this New Guinea tribe, "male chauvinism" would be an inadequate description of the suppression of women by men. The women's rage is barely contained by the ritual that is supposed to permit its harmless expression. The men flee in genuine terror, not mock fright.

40. R. L. Fox, *Alexander the Great* (New York, 1973), pp. 44–45 and notes.

41. See I. M. Linforth, "Telestic Madness in Plato, *Phaedrus* 244D–E" and "The Corybantic Rites in Plato," *University of California Publications in Classical Philology* 13 (1946):121–72.

42. See D. M. Kolkey, "Dionysus and Woman's Emancipation," *Class. Bull.* 50 (1968):1–5.

43. See Aristophanes, *Frogs*, ll. 1305–1308. Euripides' Muse is a fellatrix and a whore. The exact rendering of these lines is not clear, though the derogatory tone is. See J. Henderson, *The Maculate Muse: Obscene Language in Attic Comedy* (New Haven, 1975), s.v. *lesbiazein*: "to perform fellatio," and R. Lattimore's translation and note in *Aristophanes: Four Comedies*, ed. W. Arrowsmith (Ann Arbor, 1969), pp. 79 and 99.

44. M. R. Lefkowitz (personal communication).

45. This rendering is based on the commentary of W. S. Barrett, ed., in Euripides, *Hippolytos* (Oxford, 1974).

46. The "sickness of virgins" is discussed in Chapter 11.

47. Except for ll. 181–82, which are mine, translations from Euripides' *Andromache* are by J. F. Nims in *The Complete Greek Tragedies*, ed. D. Greene and R. Lattimore (Chicago: University of Chicago Press, 1959). *Andromache* © 1956 by the University of Chicago.

48. Translation from Plato, *The Dialogues*, trans. B. Jowett (1894; reprint Oxford, 1953).

49. François Rabelais, "Pantagruel," in *The Portable Rabelais*, ed. and trans. S. Putnam (New York, 1946), pp. 477–78, cited in Veith, *Hysteria*, pp. 107–108.

50. Freud, SE 6:147.

51. V. Elwin, *The Muria and Their Ghotul* (Oxford, 1947).

52. See D. Wender, "Plato: Misogynist, Paedophile, and Feminist," *Aresthusa* 6 (1973):75–90.

53. K. Abraham, "Restrictions and Transformations of Scopophilia in Psycho-Neurotics," in his *Selected Papers on Psycho-Analysis* (London, 1965), pp. 169–234, contains an excellent discussion of the freedom to look in ancient Greece versus the inhibition in the biblical culture.

54. The most complete account of these theories is E. Lesky, "Die Zeugungs- und Vererbungslehren der Antike," in *Abhandlungen der Akademie der Wissenschaft und der Literatur* (Mainz, 1950), pp. 1227–1425. See also R. B. Onians, *The Origins of European Thought about the Body, the Mind, the Soul, the World, Time, and Fate* (Cambridge, 1951), and M. T. May, trans., *Galen on the Usefulness of the Parts of the Body [De usu partium]* (Ithaca, N.Y., 1968). I thank Joan Cadden for directing me to some useful bibliography.

55. Onians, *Origins of European Thought*, pt. 2, "The Immortal Soul and the Body," pp. 93–246.

56. See also Plato, *Laws*, 841A, and Slater, *Glory of Hera*, pp. 354–55.

57. F. J. Cole, *Early Theories of Sexual Generation* (Oxford, 1930), points out that the existence of the mammalian ovum was not proved until 1812.

58. Translation from Aeschylus, *Eumenides*, trans. H. Lloyd-Jones (Englewood Cliffs, N.J., 1970).

59. Lesky, "Zeugungs- und Vererbungslehren," pp. 1237–39. The Hippocratic treatises are: *On Generation, On the Sacred Disease*, and *Airs, Waters, Places*. Pangenesis is the theory that the reproductive cells (gametes) are formed by a contribution from each cell of the body; see *OED*. According to Lesky, the views of the atomists were more egalitarian; they believed that both male and female contributed to the embryo (e.g., Lucretius, bk. 4, ll. 1192–1287).

60. Littré, *Hippocrate*, vol. 7, p. 470.

61. E.g., *Aphorisms*, sec. 5, nos. 38, 48 (Littré, *Hippocrate*, vol. 4, pp. 544–45, 550).

62. See especially May, trans., *Galen.*

63. Veith, *Hysteria*, p. 39 (her translation from the Latin of *De locis affectis*, bk. 6, sec. 5, para. 519, in *Claudii Galeni: Opera Omnia*, ed. C. G. Kuhn, 20 vols. (Leipzig, 1821–1823), vol. 8, p. 420.

64. Compare this with May, trans., *Galen*, p. 643, and Marcus, *Other Victorians.*

65. See P. H. Blaney, "Implications of the Medical Model and Its Alternatives," *Am. J. Psychiat.* 132 (1975):911–14.

66. See L. Edelstein, "The Relation of Ancient Philosophy to Medicine," in *Ancient Medicine: Selected Papers of Ludwig Edelstein*, ed. O. Temkin and C. L. Temkin (Baltimore, 1967), and F. Kudlien, "Der Arzt des Körpers und der Arzt der Seele," *Clio Medica* 3 (1968):1–20.

67. F. Solmson, "Greek Philosophy and the Discovery of the Nerves," *Mus. Helvet.* 18 (1961):150–97. See too the important work of R. E. Siegel, *Galen: On Psychology, Psychopathology, and Function and Diseases of the Nervous System* (Basel, 1973). By Galen's time the position of the brain as the central controlling organ of the psyche was secure. Physicians resolved the question of the transmission of information along sensory and motor nerves by positing a *pneuma* that was carried by the cerebrospinal fluid from the ventricles of the brain to the muscles and organs through "pores" in the nerves.

68. See O. Temkin, *Galen and Galenism* (Ithaca, N.Y. 1973), esp. p. 91.

14. The Psychoanalytic and Social Psychiatric Models

1. See J. D. Frank, *Persuasion and Healing: A Comparative Study of Psychotherapy*, 2d rev. ed. (Baltimore, 1973).

2. Summaries of these viewpoints may be found in *CTP*², chaps. 8–10 and 30; J. Kovel, *A Complete Guide to Therapy* (New York, 1976), offers critical discussion.

3. His attack is also motivated by a fear of poetry and drama as excessively instinc-tual.

4. An important part of the Halloween ritual. M. McDonald, "Teaching the Be-ginner: Baptism by Fire," *Psa. Q.* 40 (1971):618–45, is study of teachers who were traumatized as students and go on to traumatize their own students.

5. S. R. Palombo, "The Dream and the Memory Cycle," *Int. Rev. Psa.* 3 (1976):65–83, contains formulations on the matching of past and present events in dreams.

6. SE 12:145–55 and "Working Through" in J. Laplanche and J. B. Pontalis, *The Language of Psycho-Analysis*, trans. D. Nicholson-Smith (New York, 1973).

7. See R. R. Greenson's invaluable discussions of transference, working-alliance, and the "real relationship" in *The Technique and Practice of Psychoanalysis* (New York, 1967) and Greenson and M. Wexler, "The Non-transference Relationship in the psy-choanalytic Situation," *Int. J. Psa.* 50 (1969):27–39.

8. See H. Weiner, "On the Psychology of Personal Freedom," *Perspectives in Biol-ogy and Medicine* 6 (1962–63):479–92.

9. New York, 1966. The following quotations are on pp. 32 and 36.

10. See Chapter 9, n. 40.

11. H. Diels, ed., *Die Fragmente der Vorsokratiker*, with additions by W. Kranz, 5th–7th eds. (Berlin, 1934–54), *Protagoras*, B4 and B1.

12. D. Clay, "Socrates' Mulishness and Heroism," *Phronesis* 27 (1972):53–60.

13. *Triumph of the Therapeutic*, pp. 66–70.

14. T. Rennie, "Social Psychiatry: A Definition," *Int. J. Soc. Psychiat.* 1 (1955):5–14. See also R. J. Arthur, "Social Psychiatry: An Overview," *Am. J. Psychiat.* 130 (1973):841–49.

15. New York, 1958.

16. See G. Rosen, "Some Origins of Social Psychiatry," in his *Madness and Society* (Chicago, 1968).

17. "Conceptions of Modern Psychiatry," in *The Collected Works of Harry Stack Sullivan*, 2 vols. (New York, n.d.), vol. 1, p. 10. My discussion of Sullivan owes much to the work of P. Mullahy, especially *The Contributions of Harry Stack Sullivan*, ed. P. Mullahy (New York, 1952).

18. See H. S. Sullivan, "The Study of Psychiatry," *Psychiatry* 10 (1947):355–71 for this and the previous quotation. G. Murphy and E. Cattell (in Mullahy, *Contributions*, p. 169) preface the second quotation, "And while one finds in Freud the Platonic conception of the magnificent isolation of the self—'Where Id was, there shall ego be'—one finds in Sullivan the following."

19. J. G. Kennedy, "Cultural Psychiatry," in *Handbook of Social and Cultural Anthro-pology*, ed. J. J. Honigmann (Chicago, 1973), pp. 1119–98, gives a succinct view. See too the collection of articles in A. Kiev, ed., *Magic, Faith, and Healing* (New York, 1964).

20. *The Drums of Affliction* (Oxford, 1968), a section of which is adapted in Kiev, ed., *Magic, Faith, and Healing.*

21. Ibid., in Kiev, ed., *Magic, Faith, and Healing,* p. 262.

22. Turner distinguishes between rituals of affliction (healing rituals) and life-pas-sage rituals, which are more fixed. J. Murphy, "Psychotherapeutic Aspects of Sha-manism on St. Lawrence Island Alaska," in Kiev, ed., *Magic, Faith, and Healing,* pp. 53–83, tells of the arrival of "Communist spirits." Kiev, ibid., p. 455, details the role of such rituals among Mexican-Americans.

23. See R. May, "Value, Myths, and Symbols," *Am. J. Psychiat.* 132 (1975):703–706, unfortunately marred by a silly statement about the absence of anxiety in classical

324   *Notes*

Greek literature. See also V. W. Turner, *Drama, Fields, and Metaphors: Symbolic Action in Human Society* (Ithaca, N.Y., 1974), esp. pp. 56–58.

24. See A. F. C. Wallace, "The Institutionalization of Cathartic and Control Strategies in Iroquois Religious Psychotherapy," in *Culture and Mental Health,* ed. M. R. Opler (New York, 1959), pp. 63–96.

25. R. Rabkin, *Inner and Outer Space: An Introduction to a Theory of Social Psychiatry* (New York, 1970), also compares the Homeric model with the social psychiatric model; we arrived at this formulation independently.

26. C. Ducey, "The Life History and Creative Psychopathology of the Shaman: Ethnopsychoanalytic Perspectives," *Psa. Study Soc.* 7 (1976):173–230, and "The Shaman's Dream Journey: Psychoanalytic and Structural Complementarity in Myth Interpretation," *Psa. Study Soc.* 8 (1977), in press. Ducey's work shows the close relationship between cultural pressures for merging and dissociation, the nature of shamanistic ritual, and the personality of the shaman. See also A. Kiev, "A Cross-Cultural Study of the Relationship between Child Training and Therapeutic Practices Related to Illness," *Psa. Study Soc.* 1 (1961):185–217.

27. C. Lévi-Strauss, "The Effectiveness of Symbols" and "The Sorcerer and His Magic," in his *Structural Anthropology* (New York, 1963). A necessary critique, however, is provided by J. Neu, "Lévi-Strauss on Shamanism," *Man* 10 (1975):285–92. See also D. Freeman, "Shaman and Incubus," *Psa. Study Soc.* 4 (1967):315–43.

28. V. W. Turner, *The Ritual Process: Structure and Anti-Structure* (Chicago, 1969) and *Dramas, Fields, and Metaphors.*

29. This discussion of ritual healing has glossed over the healing of intrapsychic conflict (see the works of Ducey cited in n. 26) and the physiological and psychological importance of altered states of consciousness. See, for example, C. T. Tart, *Altered States of Consciousness* (New York, 1972), and B. W. Lex, "Physiological Aspects of Ritual Trance," *Journal of Altered States of Consciousness* 2 (1975):109–122. Kennedy, "Cultural Psychiatry," presents evidence of the efficacy of such healing. G. Devereux, "The Psychotherapy Scene in Euripides' *Bacchae,*" *JHS* 93 (1970):36–49, doubts its long-term efficacy. N. E. Waxler, "Culture and Mental Illness: A Social-Labelling Perspective," *J. Nerv. and Mental Diseases* 159 (1974):379–95, suggests that ritual healing minimizes social disability and does not isolate the psychotic from the group as much as Western healing practices do.

30. Budd Hopkins, unpublished lecture.

31. M. McLuhan, *The Gutenberg Galaxy* (Toronto, 1962).

32. R. J. Lifton, *History and Human Survival* (New York, 1970), pp. 311–31. See too E. Erikson, *Dimensions of a New Identity* (New York, 1974), p. 104.

33. V. Ehrenburg, "*Polupragmosunē:* A Study in Greek Politics," *JHS* 67 (1947):46–67.

34. A. Wheelis, *The Quest for Identity* (New York, 1958) and N. D. Lazar, "Nature and Significance of Changes in Patients in a Psychoanalytic Clinic," *Psa. Q.* 44 (1975):127–38, propose that new clinical entities are arising in relation to changed social conditions. For discussion of narcissistic characters see H. Kohut, *The Analysis of the Self* (New York, 1971). See also L. Spiegel, "Youth, Culture, and Psychoanalysis," *Am. Im.* 31 (1974):206–231. For some comments on narcissistic character disorder in classical (esp. Roman) antiquity, see C. Ducey and B. Simon, "Ancient Greece and Rome," in *World History of Psychiatry,* ed. J. G. Howells (New York, 1974), pp. 1–38.

35. C. Lasch, "The Narcissist Society," *New York Review of Books,* September 30, 1976, pp. 5–13.

36. See G. Devereux, *Ethnopsychanalyse complementariste* (Paris, 1972).

37. H. Hartmann and R. M. Loewenstein, "Papers on Psychoanalytic Psychology," *Psychological Issues* 14, no. 2 (1964), and H. Hartmann, *Essays on Ego Psychology* (New

York, 1965); F. Weinstein and G. Platt, *Psychoanalytic Sociology* (Baltimore, 1973) and my review in *Psa. Q.* 43 (1974):668–74. For anthropological work, see G. Devereux, *Mohave Ethnopsychiatry and Suicide* (Washington, D.C., 1961); *Essais d'ethnopsychiatrie générale,* 2d ed. (Paris, 1973), and *Ethnopsychanalyse complementariste,* and the annual *Psa. Study Soc.* For surveys of psychohistory, see B. Mazlish, "Psychiatry and History," in *American Handbook of Psychiatry,* ed. S. Arieti, 2d ed. (New York, 1974), vol. 1, pp. 1034–45, and R. J. Lifton and E. Olson, eds., *Explorations in Psychohistory* (New York, 1974), with N. Birnbaum's introduction to a more Marxist approach (pp. 182–213). See also R. Jacoby, *Social Amnesia: A Critique of Conformist Psychology from Adler to Laing* (Boston, 1975), esp. on the work of the Frankfurt school (Adorno, Horkheimer, Marcuse, et al.). For information theory: E. Peterfreund, *Information, Systems, and Psychoanalysis* (New York, 1971), and Peterfreund and E. Franceschini, "On Information, Motivation, and Meaning" in *Psychoanalysis and Contemporary Science,* ed. B. B. Rubinstein (New York, 1973), vol. 2. For critique, see L. Friedman's review in *Int. J. Psa.* 53 (1972):547–54 and letters to the editor in ibid. 56 (1975):123–29. On general systems theory: L. Von Bertalanffy, *Organismic Psychology and Systems Theory* (New York, 1968), and J. G. Miller, "General Systems Theory," *CTP*[2], pp. 75–88. On object relations theory: W. R. D. Fairbairn, *Psychoanalytic Studies of the Personality* (London, 1966), and H. Guntrip, *Personality Structure and Human Interaction* (New York, 1964). On learning theory and psychoanalysis: L. Birk and A. W. Brinkley-Birk, "Psychoanalysis and Behavior Therapy," *Am. J. Psychiat.* 131 (1974):499–501; W. W. Meissner, "The Role of Imitative Social Learning in Identificatory Processes," *J. Am. Psa. A.* 22 (1974):512–36, with references to his other articles.

38. Translation mine, based on A. Bloom, trans., *The Republic of Plato* (New York, 1968), p. 303.

Index

Abreaction, 141–42. *See also* Catharsis.
Abstract thinking, 60–61, 159, 163, 165, 169
Academy (Plato's), 157, 188–89, 198–99, 311n19, 320n27
Acharnians (Aristophanes), 302n52
Achilles, 54–55, 62–67, 72–76, 86, 278, 283
Aeschylus, 89; *Agamemnon,* 91, 102; *Choephoroi,* 102–105, 146; *Eumenides,* 105–108, 264; *Oresteia,* 91, 102–108
Affects: in Plato, 170, 184–86, 192–93; in psychological theories, 200; in tragedy, 143–44
Agememnon, 62, 91, 244
Agamemnon (Aeschylus), 91, 102
Agave, 113–21, 148
Air, importance of, to brain, 220–23, 225
Airs, Waters, Places (Hippocrates), 264
Ajax, 62, 70, 97, 149, 152–53, 186, 229–31; suicide of, 126–30
Ajax (Sophocles), 92, 102, 124–30, 135–39, 146, 232
Alcestis (Euripides), 148
Alcibiades, 195
Alcibiades I (Plato), 161
Alcmaeon of Croton, 222
Alphabetic writing, 53–54
Amathia (ignorance), 167–68
Ambivalence: in Homer, 298n43; in Plato, 211–12; in tragedy, 89, 100–102, 135–39, 144
Amphitryon, 131–39
Anagnorisis (recognition), 93, 153, 261
Analogy: in Greek medicine, 318–19n22; in Plato and Freud, 210–11
Analytic attitude, 275–76
Anamnesis (recollection), 165
Anatomy, ancient study of, 223, 242, 265, 267–68, 315n13
Anaxagoras, 22, 158–60

Anaximander, 158
Anaximenes, 158
Androgyny, Plato's myth of, 175
Andromache (Euripides), 258
Anna O., case of, 142
Anoia (ignorance), 168–69
Anthropomorphism, 163, 200–204
Antigone (Sophocles), 92–93, 96, 144, 277
Aphrosunē (foolishness), 178, 310n56
Apology (Plato), 161, 191
Appetitive (part of psyche). *See Epithumetikon.*
Aretaeus, 43
Aristophanes, 153; *Acharnians,* 302n52; *Clouds,* 195–98, 321n32; *Ecclesiazusae,* 257; *Frogs,* 256; *Lysistrata,* 257; *Wasps,* 122–24, 140, 256; and women, 256–57
Aristotle, 163, 199, 223, 268, 277; *De Anima,* 233; on epic and tragedy, 54; *Generation of Animals,* 264; on human reproduction, 264; *Nicomachean Ethics,* 233; *Poetics,* 91–92, 97–100, 140–44, 147–48, 151, 153; on pre-Socratics, 158; *Problemata,* 229–34
Arrowsmith, Williams, 131–34
Asclepius, 123; sons of, 231; temple of, at Epidaurus, 320n13
Atē (infatuation), 67, 86, 298n36
Athena, 62, 66, 93, 146, 153
Audience: of epic poet, 78–79, 84–85, 191–92, 283; of philosopher, 188–99; of tragedian, 140, 143–46, 150, 153

Bacchae (Euripides), 113–21, 136–37, 146–50, 153–54, 252, 256
Bacchantes. *See* Maenads.
Barrie, James, 146
Bellerophon, 68–70, 229–32
Bendis, 176
Bernays, Jacob, 44, 141–42
Bernheim, Hippolyte, 24, 201